Healing Henan

Sonya Grypma

Healing Henan
Canadian Nurses at the North
China Mission, 1888-1947

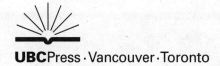

UBCPress · Vancouver · Toronto

16 15 14 13 12 11 10 09 08   5 4 3 2 1

Printed in Canada on ancient-forest-free paper (100% post-consumer recycled) that is processed chlorine- and acid-free, with vegetable-based inks.

Library and Archives Canada Cataloguing in Publication

Grypma, Sonya, 1965-
    Healing Henan : Canadian nurses at the North China Mission, 1888-1947 / Sonya Grypma.

Includes bibliographical references and index.
ISBN 978-0-7748-1399-0 (bound); 978-0-7748-1400-3 (pbk.)

1. Missions, Medical – China – Henan Sheng – History. 2. Nursing – China – Henan Sheng – History. 3. Missions, Canadian – China – Henan Sheng – History. 4. Protestant churches – Missions – China – Henan Sheng – History. 5. Nursing – Canada – History. I. Title.

R722.G79 2007   362.1'095118   C2007-905473-0

Canadä

UBC Press gratefully acknowledges the financial support for our publishing program of the Government of Canada through the Book Publishing Industry Development Program (BPIDP), and of the Canada Council for the Arts, and the British Columbia Arts Council.

This book has been published with the help of a grant from the Canadian Federation for the Humanities and Social Sciences, through the Aid to Scholarly Publications Programme, using funds provided by the Social Sciences and Humanities Research Council of Canada, and with the help of the K.D. Srivastava Fund.

Printed and bound in Canada by Friesens
Set in Stone by Artegraphica Design Co. Ltd.
Copy editor: Jillian Shoichet
Proofreader: Stacy Belden
Indexer: Patricia Buchanan

UBC Press
The University of British Columbia
2029 West Mall
Vancouver, BC V6T 1Z2
604-822-5959 / Fax: 604-822-6083
www.ubcpress.ca

For Martin, Janessa, and Mike

Contents

Appendices

Illustrations

Map

Table

Figures

Foreword

Janet C. Ross-Kerr

The letters published in the 1930s and 1940s in *Canadian Nurse* by a number of Canadian nurses commissioned by the Woman's Missionary Society of the United Church of Canada to work in Henan province, China, were seminal in the development of the intriguing program of research developed by Sonya Grypma. These letters from the North China Mission may have generated a great deal of interest at the time they were published and also encouraged other nurses to make a commitment to participate in the work in China under the banner of the United Church of Canada. But their serendipitous discovery by Dr. Grypma, who was looking for something else at the time she was perusing old issues of *Canadian Nurse*, led to questions such as who were these nurses, what was the nature of their work, how long did they serve in China, and what was the short- and long-term impact of their work?

Dr. Grypma has pursued these and other questions through painstaking searches for data in archival records in a number of repositories, contacts with descendants of the nurses, and searches for relevant documents and literature that might refer to, or shed light on, the nurses' mission and the situation in China that enveloped them and conditioned their work. She has left no stone unturned in her search for data and has made a number of visits to China to see where the original mission was established and to talk with nurses and health care personnel currently providing health services in the area. She clearly earned the trust of the descendants of the missionary nurses, including children of some of the missionaries. They have recounted their memories of their ancestors for her and shared documents in their possession that related to the professional work of the nurses. Some descendants have accompanied Dr. Grypma on each of her journeys to China to survey the site of the mission, search for information, and speak with local inhabitants.

The most fascinating element in terms of the reconstruction of the history of nursing and health care in the period of time that these Canadian missionary nurses lived and worked in China is that Dr. Grypma was able to share with the nurses and physicians who currently work in Henan province, and specifically in Weihui and Anyang, what was their own history. Since most records were destroyed with the advent of the revolution, there was virtually no knowledge among the local professionals of the health care and educational work that had been developed so many years ago. Early in her career, Dr. Grypma developed a nursing and medical exchange between Canada and Anyang, where one of the original hospitals was founded by Canadians. As a testament to the lasting contribution of this outstanding piece of work, Dr. Grypma was also invited to attend a ceremony held by the Weihui Hospital on the occasion of its 110th anniversary and concurrent establishment of a museum in the original hospital building. Her photographs and historical documents figure prominently in these museum displays. At this event, she was accompanied by eleven relatives of the Canadian missionaries who staffed the hospital over the sixty-odd years that they worked in China.

This powerful book, which records the contribution of Canadian nurses to the development of the health care system in the province of Henan, China, is unique because so little research has been undertaken on the work of nurses in the China missions. Physicians have figured prominently in research, but only two previous articles have focused upon nurses. Because of Sonya Grypma's work, the connection between North Henan province and Canada, which was so strong for so many years, has been re-established and strengthened.

I count it a privilege and an honour to have been involved in Dr. Grypma's journey to discover the nature and meaning of the work of the thirty Canadian missionary nurses who were associated with the North China Mission in Weihui, Anyang, and Huaiqing. As one of her former colleagues in the Faculty of Nursing at the University of Alberta, I was amazed by the precision, creativity, and passion with which Sonya Grypma pursued her questions. It is fitting that this book based on her work is now available for all to read.

Acknowledgments

When people ask how I came across such an interesting project, I must admit that I did not set out to study Canadian missionary nurses in China. A serendipitous discovery of missionary letters from China in archived issues of *Canadian Nurse* changed the direction of my research program and set the course for years of intriguing study. I could not have imagined that a fascination with these missionary nurses would take me across the country and halfway around the world. Gathering the history of these nurses into one cohesive whole has been a tremendous privilege. One of my greatest pleasures has been working with people and organizations whose enthusiasm and timely assistance made this project possible. I am indebted to a number of people who so freely gave of their time, energy, and knowledge. Many of these were from the University of Alberta. I would not have even considered undertaking this research were it not for the inspiration of Dr. Janet C. Ross-Kerr, whose dedication to nursing history is matched only by her keen interest in her students and her ability to guide novices through the complex world of professional scholarship. Dr. Pauline Paul has been a wonderful role model, leading me through the process of archival research and offering timely advice. I have also appreciated the support of Dr. Margaret Haughey. Dr. Shirley Stinson helped me to establish contact with a number of individuals and organizations whose input became central to the study, including the Canadian Association for the History of Nursing and the British Columbia History of Nursing Professional Practice Group.

To my knowledge, all the nurses named in *Healing Henan* are deceased. I am deeply indebted to the family and friends of missionary nurses who graciously shared their memories and private collections of letters and photographs. Thank you to all who contacted me after reading an advertisement in the *United Church Observer*. Some respondents (including Barb Putnam and Marilyn Harrison) helped me to identify key people for interviews; others became participants themselves. Those whom I invited to participate in this project were invariably gracious and generous with their time and resources.

Their participation helped bring the nurses to life. Muriel Gay and Irene Pooley were tireless in their collection of information about their aunt, Margaret Gay. Dr. Mary (Struthers) McKim was also an indefatigable resource. She and her cousin Isobel (Struthers) Staal provided documents and rare photographs of the North China Mission hospital work, which they had inherited from their fathers, Dr. E.B. Struthers and Dr. R. Gordon Struthers. Dr. McKim also gave excellent editorial advice. I must note that Dr. McKim, raised in China, never heard the term "mishkid" used in her childhood. I borrowed the term from Marion Menzies Hummels' *Memoirs of a Mishkid,* choosing it over the more cumbersome – yet more respectful, perhaps – "children of missionaries." Doug Skinner and Ward Skinner worked closely with their mother, Jean Skinner, to collect and copy private letters and photographs from their great-aunt Clara Preston. Betty Beatty and Judy Preston lent me their copies of Preston Robb's self-published book on his Aunt Clara; the late Dr. Preston Robb later gave me a rare copy of my own. Elizabeth Mittler, Bob and Beth Quesnel, Mike Hoyer, and Nancy Walkling helped me to locate copies of Henan missionary memoirs. Dr. Anne J. Davis gave me her rare copy of the 1926 history of the Nurses Association of China. Louise McLean offered insight into the life of her sister, Florence MacKenzie Liddell. Howard Parkinson and Rev. Doug Brydon gave insight into Janet Brydon. Yue Chi of Asian Adventure and Study Tours put me in contact with members of Coral Brodie's family; Arthur Kennedy, Dave Shepperd, Frances Fraser, and Karen James helped to round out my understanding of Coral Brodie. Retired missionaries Lillian Taylor, Peter Nelson, Doris Weller, Hazel Page, the late Helen Bergen, Daphne Rogers, and the late Dr. Wilf Cummings shared stories of their own missionary experiences in China, Taiwan, and Japan. Ms. Li Xiang Dong and Ms. Ren Jijuan provided valuable assistance from China, and Dr. Huihui Li and Ms. Jing Zhu assisted with translation. I must also thank the two anonymous reviewers for their invaluable suggestions.

I am especially indebted to Margaret (Gale) Wightman. Margaret shared a wealth of personal documents, photos, and a home movie from her parents, Dr. Godfrey and Elizabeth Thomson Gale. She also put me in touch with Elizabeth's sister Muriel. Most courageously, she allowed me – someone she had never met – to accompany her to China. It was Margaret's first trip back since leaving a Japanese internment camp in Shanghai in 1945.

Numerous archivists and assistants provided invaluable support in gathering data. I would especially like to thank Susanne Clark and Nancy Rosa from the United Church of Canada/Victoria University Archives; Dr. Glennis Zilm and Ethel Warbinek, who searched through the Vancouver General Hospital Archives; Anne Crossin from the Winnipeg General Hospital Alumnae Archives; Sister Rita McGuire from the Grey Sisters of Immaculate

Conception of Pembroke; Elysia DeLaurentis from the Wellington County Archives; Rose Carleton from the Overseas Mission Fellowship (formerly China Inland Missions); Greta Cumming, who searched Library and Archives Canada; and Dr. Mark Steinacher and Richard Jackson from McMaster Divinity College. I would also like to thank Asia historians Dr. David Wright of the University of Calgary and Dr. Luke Kwong of the University of Lethbridge for formally sharing their knowledge with me through independent guided studies. Thanks also to Jean Wilson of UBC Press for constant encouragement and to Alvyn Austin and Glennis Zilm for their outstanding advice. Finally, I wish to thank Dr. Janet Beaton, whose extensive knowledge about Canadian nurses at the West China Mission inspired and informed me.

A number of organizations provided funding for this project through various scholarships, grants, and awards. I am grateful to the Social Sciences and Humanities Research Council of Canada for a doctoral fellowship and the Izaak Walton Killam Memorial Trust for a doctoral scholarship. I am also grateful to the Canadian Association for the History of Nursing for their Margaret Allemang Scholarship, the American Association for the History of Nursing for their Student Researcher Award, the Alberta Association of Registered Nurses Educational Trust for their Helen Sabin Award, the Faculty of Nursing at the University of Alberta for their Dr. Shirley Stinson History of Nursing Award and Isobel Secord Award, and the Faculty of Graduate Studies at the University of Alberta for their Province of Alberta Graduate Fellowship and Walter H. Johns Graduate Fellowship. Travel grants for research and conferences were provided by the Mu Sigma chapter of Sigma Theta Tau, a University of Alberta J. Gordin Kaplan Award, and a Student Travel Grant from the Associated Medical Services/Hannah.

At the time that this book was going to press, I travelled to Henan with a group of nineteen Canadians whom I had invited to return with me on the request of the current presidents of the former North China Mission hospitals at Anyang and Weihui, Dr. Song Xianzhong and Dr. Zhang Xinzhong, respectively. Eight came as participants in a nursing/medical exchange in Anyang (now a twin city of Lethbridge, Alberta); eleven were relatives of Canadian missionaries described in these pages, including four "mishkids" returning to the place of their birth. We were all guests of honour at elaborate the 110th anniversary celebrations of the Weihui Hospital – the first Canadian-Chinese reunion of this scale in Henan since the North China Mission closed in 1947. The anniversary celebrations included the grand opening of the new museum of the First Affiliated Hospital of Xinxiang Medical University, housed in the building that had originally housed the Weihui hospital and training school for nurses. It was an unprecedented, profound, and moving experience – but, alas, another story for another time.

My family has provided encouragement and practical support throughout the years. To my parents, Henk and Cobi Visser, thank you for your intense interest in this project and for indulging me through innumerable after-dinner discussions. Thank you also for moving in to take care of things when I travelled. To my brother Mike Visser, thank you for your video expertise and excellent advice about visual images. To our children, Mike and Janessa, thank you for your constant reminder of the importance of play, for hugs, Boggle, and movie nights. Finally, to my husband, Dr. Martin Grypma, thank you for your constant encouragement, for taking time off work to take over household duties at particularly busy times, and for accompanying me to China twice, cameras in hand.

Spellings

Pinyin/Contemporary	Wade-Giles/Common
Anhui	Anhuei
Anyang/Zhangde	Changte
Aomen	Macao
Beijing	Peking/Peiping
Baoding	Paoting
Beidaihe	Peitaiho
Chengdu	Chengtu
Chongqing	Chungking
Chuwang	Chuwang
Daokou	Taokow
Fuzhou	Foochow
Fujian	Fukien
Guangdong	Kuangtung
Guangzhou	Canton/Kwangchow
Guiyang	Kweiyang
Guizhou	Kweichou
Hebei	Hopei
Henan	Honan
Huaiqing	Hwaiking
Huilong	Hwailung
Hupei	Hupeh
Jiangmen	Kongmoon
Jiangsu	Kiangsu
Jiaozhou	Kiaochow
Jinan	Tsinan
Liaodong	Liaotung
Lugouqiao	Lukouchiao
Nanjing	Nanking
Qingdao	Tsintao

Qilu	Cheeloo
Rongxian	Junghsien
Sanqui	Kweiteh
Shaanxi	Shensi
Shandong	Shantung
Shenyang	Mukden
Sichuan	Szechwan
Sincheng	Hsin-chen
Taibei	Taipei
Taiwan	Formosa
Tianjin	Tientsin
Wanxian	Wanhsien
Weihai	Weihaiwei (Shandong)
Weihui	Weihwei (Henan)
Weixian	Weihsien
Wuhan/Hankou	Wuhan/Hankow
Xian	Sian
Xinxiang	Hsin Hsiang
Yan'an/Fu-Shih	Yenan
Yunnan	Yunnan
Zhengzhou	Chengchow
Zhejiang	Chekiang
Zhifu	Chefoo

Abbreviations

CCC	Church of Christ in China
CIM	China Inland Mission
CMMA	Chinese Medical Missionary Association (later Christian Medical Association of China)
FAU	Friends Ambulance Unit
FMB	Foreign Mission Board (originally Foreign Mission Committee)
GMA	Glenbow Museum and Archives
NCM	North China Mission (originally Honan Mission and/or North Honan Mission)
NAC	Nurses Association of China
PUMC	Peking Union Medical College
RN	Registered nurse
TGH	Toronto General Hospital
UCCVUA	United Church of Canada/Victoria University Archives
UNRRA	United Nations Relief and Rehabilitation Administration
VGH	Vancouver General Hospital
WCUU	West China Union University
WCM	West China Mission
WCMA	Wellington County Museum and Archives
WFMS	Women's Foreign Missionary Society (later WMS)
WGH/HSCA	Winnipeg General Hospital Health Sciences Centre Archives
WMS	Woman's Missionary Society (originally Women's Foreign Missionary Society)

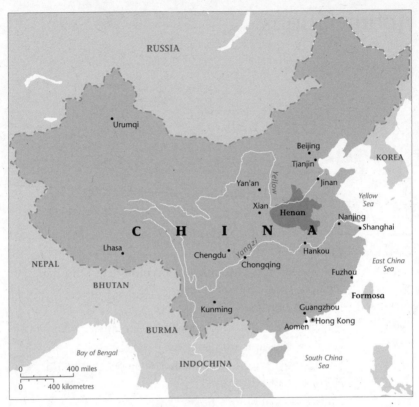

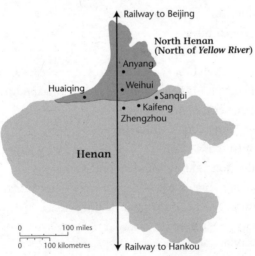

Map of China and Henan province
Cartographer: Eric Leinberger

Introduction

The founding of the nursing profession [in China] by Christians
was an even greater achievement than the introduction of modern
medicine; medical schools ... would have come sooner or later
anyway. But young [Chinese] women would not have taken up
nursing without the example set them by Christian women of
the West.

        – Unknown author, cited in Margaret Brown,
          History of the North China Mission

Bloor Street Church in Toronto was usually characterized by a solemn and
formal approach to worship – where, for example, ushers dressed in morning coats and striped trousers reportedly led worshipers down the aisles to
their numbered pews.[1] Yet on 17 June 1923, the excitement and curiosity
generated by a missionary designation service was palpable. On this Sunday, the sanctuary, which could seat 1,170, vibrated with emotion as the
congregation gathered to dedicate its latest group of missionaries, four of
whom were headed to the Presbyterian North China Mission in the province of Henan, China.[2] The North China Mission was one of the first overseas missions established by Canadians, in 1888.[3] By 1923, it had grown to
include three main mission compounds at Weihui, Anyang, and Huaiqing,
plus a number of smaller rural stations. Bloor Street Church had always
been mission-minded, forming its first Women's Foreign Missionary Society
auxiliary (a branch of the Presbyterian Women's Foreign Mission Society
[WFMS]) only two months after the congregation officially started, in January 1887. When the church sent Dr. James Menzies to Henan in 1895, it
became one of the earliest Presbyterian congregations in Canada to have its
own overseas missionary. The congregation dedicated $1,200.00 per month
to support Menzies in Huaiqing and then raised additional funds to build a
small hospital there.[4] Menzies' violent and untimely death in 1920 acted as

a catalyst in the decision to send four missionaries to Huaiqing: had the tragedy not occurred, it is possible that three of these missionaries – a physician and two nurses – would not have gone to China at all.

When Dr. James Menzies was killed by bandits at the Canadian mission compound at Huaiqing in 1920, his wife Davina was residing in Toronto, recovering from "sprue," a tropical disease she had contracted in China, and overseeing the education of the Menzies' daughters. Three years after her husband's death, the widowed Mrs. Davina (Robb) Menzies insisted upon returning to Henan as a missionary again in her own right (she had gone to Henan as a Woman's Missionary Society [WMS] missionary in 1896 before marrying James Menzies). Accompanying Mrs. Menzies would be Dr. Robert McClure, a young physician hired to replace her husband at the hospital at Huaiqing and oversee the construction of a new Menzies Memorial Hospital. "Bob" McClure, the China-born son of Dr. William McClure (one of the original Henan Seven), felt he had missed the "excitement" of the Great War and perceived the opportunity to take Dr. Menzies' place in China as a "chance for a great adventure."[5] Mrs. Menzies and Dr. McClure would be joined by the Menzies' eldest daughter Jean, who had recently graduated from the Toronto General Hospital Training School for Nurses (later Toronto General Hospital School of Nursing). Jean Menzies' decision to return to Henan as a missionary nurse was admirable and courageous. It was also unusual: Jean would not only be working in the shadow of her murdered father at a new hospital erected in his name, but would be doing so under the daily supervision of Miss Janet Brydon, the nurse her father had rescued from bandits the night he was shot. Still, Jean Menzies had plenty of support, from her mother and Bob McClure, whose family she boarded with at Weihui during grade school, as well as from Miss Coral May Brodie, her nursing school friend whose decision to go to China was encouraged – if not inspired – by Jean.[6]

The designation service in 1923 was a landmark event in Bloor Street history, remembered today as the date that the celebrated Dr. Bob McClure was designated. After a quarter-century of work in China, McClure went on to achieve legendary status within the United Church for his medical genius, dry wit, disregard for convention, and indefatigable pursuit of a new kind of Christian service. Although Jean Menzies and Coral Brodie (and other missionary nurses) are not even footnoted in most historical accounts of the United Church of Canada, their images are symbolically represented in the Narthex Windows of Bloor Street United Church. As Menzies and Brodie stood at the steps of the Bloor Street altar on 17 June 1923 to receive and recite vows related to their calling, nursing in Henan stood on the threshold of radical change. Jean Menzies and Coral Brodie arrived in China shortly after the opening of the first modern hospital and training school for nurses in Henan at Weihui, thus joining the group of Canadian nurses who collectively developed and nurtured an ideal of nursing practice that was adopted and adapted by the Chinese and continues in Henan today. Margaret Brown's suggestion that the work by missionary nurses was "a greater achievement than the introduction of modern medicine" echoes what many missionary nurses themselves believed: without modern nursing, China was somehow incomplete.

Canadian missionary nurses helped to transform the landscape of Chinese health care in Henan. Through the process, they found themselves transformed. Set against the backdrop of sociopolitical upheaval in China, this book examines the interplay of professional nursing with issues such as religion, gender, culture, health, and nation. Through periods of anti-foreign uprisings, national revolution, warlord rule, imprisonment under the Japanese, and civil war, nursing evolved out of existing tensions between personal, professional, and religious aims. Missionary nursing was characterized by an ongoing tension between evangelism and nursing service, an emphasis on cleanliness (the gospel of soap and water), a correlation between nursing development in China and Canada, and an adaptation of nurses to China and of China to nurses. The ability of nurses to respond to human suffering was mediated by sociopolitical forces within the North China Mission, the United Church, the National Association of Nurses, and the government of China. Over time, the mission became an unintentionally "cloistered" community where physically and socially constructed walls formed protected spaces in which Canadian and Chinese nurses developed a unique and progressive culture of medicine and health care.

Modern Nursing and China

In the following chapters, I will highlight ways in which the missionary nursing movement influenced the development of nursing in one region of China – but I wish to clarify one important point from the outset: Missionary nurses did not bring "nursing" to China. That is, if nursing is defined as a formalized system for attending to the physical needs of the ill, China had well-established nursing traditions long before missionaries came to China. According to Liu Chung-tung, nursing care in China ranged from care provided by female family members (following a strict system of hierarchy), to traditional healing practices provided by healers (including female *San gu liu po*), to paid care by male attendants (who had the status of servants).[7] What missionaries *did* bring to China was a particular and relatively new form of nursing practice rooted in Catholic and Protestant religious communities and adapted and popularized by Florence Nightingale after her success in caring for British soldiers in the Crimean War.[8] This system of professional nursing – variously called modern, Western, or scientific nursing – became the standard of nursing practice in Canada and around the world. In other words, missionary nurses brought "modern" nursing to China.

When Western missionary nurses began arriving in China in the 1880s, Nightingale's method of nurses' training was at its peak of popularity, and Canada was beginning to experiment with similar training methods at newly opened, hospital-based nursing schools. The Toronto General Hospital Training School for Nurses, for example, was opened in 1881, and by 1894 was the largest nursing school in Canada.[9] Nightingale introduced a system of care that emphasized a clean, airy, bright, quiet, and organized environment, believed to support patients' natural healing processes. In the days before antibiotics, cleanliness played a vital role in preventing infectious disease and promoting healing and, although Nightingale did not at first accept the germ theory, her meticulous attention to hygiene did much to prevent infection, and therefore morbidity and mortality. Under the Nightingale system that came to characterize nursing in the West from the late nineteenth century onward, nursing care was carried out with military efficiency; physicians' orders were to be obeyed, treatments were to be on time, and observations of patients were to be carefully recorded. Nurses' training took place in hospitals, where students progressed through various levels of apprenticeship over the course of training. Hospitals were staffed mainly by nursing students, who were paid a small wage. Although secular, Nightingale's system was influenced by the nursing care she observed in religious communities. In Canada as elsewhere, nursing students (all single women) lived together in residences and were expected to portray an image of purity, with well-groomed appearances, standardized uniforms, respectful demeanours, and morally upright behaviour that included chastity and abstinence from alcohol. Christian ideals and rituals were incorporated into training and practice, including regular prayers and bible study. Nursing became known as a respectable vocation for young women, with values that were congruent with those espoused by religious-minded women.[10]

For women interested in missionary work in the late nineteenth century, nurses' training provided practical skills deemed valuable in the mission field, where individual nurses could work as assistants to physicians and caregivers to ill missionaries and their families. Over time, as medical missionary care became more formalized and increasingly hospital-centred, so did missionary nursing care. And, as Canadian nursing became increasingly organized, with standardized education and professional criterion reflecting acceptable national and international nursing norms, so did missionary nursing practice. By the early twentieth century, the practice of nursing in Canada had become increasingly associated with hospitals; advances in medical science and technology brought the practice of modern medicine into hospitals designed to support medical diagnosis and treatment, and nurses became vital to the smooth functioning of these modern, physician-run hospitals. The hospital-based system became the model for modern nursing in China. Missionary nurses who graduated from Canadian training schools in the 1920s brought to China a desire to replicate the state-of-the-art nursing practice taught them in Canada. As Margaret Gay declared in her Vancouver General Hospital (VGH) 1926 graduating class yearbook, her aim was to "plant a bit of VGH in the Orient."[11]

Canadian missionary nurses who worked at the United Church of Canada North China Mission (originally the Presbyterian Church in Canada North "Honan" Mission) in the province of Henan between 1888 and 1947 were part of a broader missionary movement in China through which Christian nurses from Western nations collectively catalyzed the birth and incipient growth of professional nursing in China (see Appendix 1: Missionary nurses at the North China Mission). The earliest American missionaries were committed to Chinese nursing education. They established China's first training school for nurses in 1889, just five years after the first missionary nurse, Elizabeth McKechnie, arrived in Shanghai.[12] In contrast, it took thirty-four years from the time of Canadian nurse Harriet Sutherland's arrival in China in 1888 for the North China Mission to establish its first nursing school in Henan. In 1923, the Canadians opened the Weihui (Huimin) Hospital and Training School for Nurses, and the nursing profession in Henan enjoyed a period of growth. By the start of the Sino-Japanese War in 1937, Canadian-trained Chinese nurses had joined the Nurses Association of China and could be found in hospitals and public health programs in both rank-and-file and supervisory positions. When the Canadian nurses left Henan during the 1939 Anti-British Movement, their Chinese protégés took responsibility for nurses' training and services. Canadian nurses returned to Henan after the Sino-Japanese War ended in 1945 with visions of rehabilitating the war-damaged hospitals, but their dreams were short-lived; they found themselves in the centre of the Communist-Nationalist conflict. In 1947, Communist troops entered the mission compounds. Canadian and Chinese nurses fled; the Canadians did not return.

To Be a China Missionary: The North China Missionary Nurse in Perspective

The Presbyterian (later United) Church was not the first mission in Henan. Henan's first missionaries were Catholics from the Milan Missionary Society, who established their first bishopric at Weihui in the 1860s. Hudson Taylor's China Inland Mission began work in Henan in 1875, opening its first station there at Zhoukoushen in 1884. By 1940, an additional twelve missions were active in Henan, from the United States, Britain, Scandinavia, the Netherlands, Italy, and Canada.[13] At least seven of these missions developed dispensaries and/or hospitals in Henan. The early hospitals were small and relatively unsophisticated, "native-style" set-ups where patients stayed in shelters and their families cooked and cared for them.[14] Both Canadian Anglicans and Presbyterians developed modern hospitals with nursing schools; in 1926, Canadians operated three nursing schools in Henan recognized by the Nurses Association of China.[15] Although not the earliest mission in Henan, the Presbyterian Church in Canada North "Honan" Mission was the largest, covering the entire northern triangle of the province, north of the Yellow River.

The Canadian presence in China as a whole during the missionary era was most recognizable through six main missions: the Presbyterian Church in Canada mission in Taiwan (then Formosa, and at the time a province of the Chinese Empire, est. 1871), the Presbyterian mission in North Henan (est. 1888), the Methodist Church of Canada mission in Sichuan (est. 1891), the Presbyterian mission in Guangdong (est. 1902), the Catholic Scarboro Foreign Mission Society in Zhejiang (est. 1902), and the Anglican Church of Canada mission in Henan (south of the Yellow River, est. 1910).[16] The Presbyterian mission in Taiwan was the first overseas field of the Canadian Presbyterian Church, but the eccentricity of founder George Leslie MacKay, its remoteness from mainland China, and its continuance with the Presbyterian Church after "Union" kept Taiwan on the fringe of Canadian missions.[17] The union of all Methodists and most Presbyterians into one United Church of Canada in 1925 set the United Church apart as the largest Canadian mission in China, with sites in Henan (renamed the "North China Mission"), Sichuan ("West China Mission"), and Guangdong ("South China Mission"). Predictably, United Church missions figure dominantly in Canadian mission scholarship.

The United Church was the largest employer of Canadian missionary nurses (the North China Mission hired twenty-one WMS nurses, and the West China Mission hired twenty-four, compared with five Grey Sisters of Immaculate Conception associated with the Scarboro Foreign Mission Society.)[18] An estimated one hundred or more Canadian nurses worked in at least nine provinces of China during this period.[19] Other sponsoring agencies included the British-based inter-denominational China Inland Mission, the (Communist) Aid to China Council (which sent former Catholic missionary Jean Ewen to accompany Dr. Norman Bethune in 1938), and, after the Second World War, the United Nations Relief and Rehabilitation Agency. The majority of Canadian nurses worked in modern hospitals established by Presbyterian, Methodist, and Anglican missions in Sichuan, Guandong, Henan, and Taiwan. Smaller groups worked in Catholic dispensaries – such as the Grey Sisters of Immaculate Conception of Pembroke, Ontario, who provided medical services through the Scarboro Foreign Mission Society in Zhejiang between 1929 and 1952.[20] A further, inestimable number of Francophone and Anglophone nurses worked in French, American, and British hospitals scattered throughout China.[21]

Despite the ubiquitous nature of Canadian nursing in China, the work of nurses is eclipsed by studies of the work of physicians, evangelists, politicians, and mission boards. Most references to Canadian nurses are in association with protagonists of the missionary era. Some nurses were close colleagues of prominent Canadians such as Dr. Norman Bethune (Jean Ewen), Dr. Bob McClure (Coral Brodie, Jean Menzies), and Rev. Jonathan Goforth (Margaret Gay). Others were married to famous expatriates, such as 1924 Olympic gold medallist Eric Liddell (Florence MacKenzie). Still others were daughters of pioneering China missionaries, including Drs. Omar and Retta Kilborn (Cora Kilborn).[22] Alvyn Austin's use of the phrase "Florence Nightingales of the Orient" to describe female physicians rather than nurses in *Saving China: Canadian Missionaries in the Middle Kingdom, 1888-1959*, underscores this point: nursing has not received its due attention in historiography.[23] That said, Austin is one of only a handful of scholars to include Canadian missionary nurses in his work. In *Saving China*, Austin chronicles Canada's sixty-year missionary era, giving voice to a wide range of missions, from that of the well-known United Church of Canada to lesser-known Missions-Etrangères such as the Soeurs Antoniennes de Marie in Manchuria. Throughout, Austin emphasizes the experiences of individual Canadians, paying particular attention to how they responded to China's changing political and social life. He is one of the few authors to mention nurses by name, including West China Mission nurse Caroline Wellwood (Sichuan) and Grace Emblem (an inadvertent participant in the Communist Long March), and Anglican missionary Susie Kelsey (who interned under the Japanese in Shandong).[24] Published in 1987, *Saving China* set the standard for China-Canadian mission historiography. Emphasizing diversity and particularity, Austin's seminal work on Canadian missions underscores the complexity of the missionary era.[25]

In *The Golden Hope: Christians in China*, Peter Stursberg argues that the three main Canadian missions in China – Presbyterian, Methodist, and Anglican – were characterized by an emphasis on medical care.[26] Among the first Methodist and Presbyterian missionaries were physicians who were also ordained ministers. Missionaries believed that those who experienced physical healing would more easily receive the Gospel message: By healing bodies, medical missionaries could "open hearts to Christ."[27] Although Stursberg does not describe the role of Canadian nurses in missionary medicine, he does give a hint as to why modern nursing took so long to develop in Henan. He notes that, while the Methodist mission in Sichuan embraced medical missions early on, there was a lack of official support for modern hospital care in Henan. When two Montreal physicians arrived in 1906 to find Henan "totally lacking in nursing service," they rallied for attention to be paid to the need for modern facilities.[28] Initially, the Henan Presbytery agreed to raise funds to improve four hospitals, but after pressure from

pioneer missionary evangelist Jonathan Goforth, the proposal was turned
down as having "materialist" and "non-religious" purposes. Stursberg notes
that eventually Henan embraced medical services as legitimate expressions
of the Gospel rather than simply as a means to an evangelistic end. As will
be seen, the shift from evangelism to service had important implications
for missionary nursing. Although there had been at least one missionary
nurse at the North China Mission since its inception, the mission did not
expect her to make full use of her nursing skills. Only one physician in the
early years actively supported nursing care. Dr. James Frazer Smith lobbied
for the establishment of a position for a missionary nurse to assist him in
his work – to help soothe patients, change dressings, manage medical instruments, and sit with ill patients in their homes or in Chinese inns. After
an illness forced Dr. Frazer Smith to resign in 1894, there was little practical
support for nursing. The other physicians were not interested in having
nurses assist them in their work, and no efforts were made to develop organized nursing services. Margaret MacIntosh, the sole nurse at the North
China Mission between 1891 and 1914, turned to evangelistic work as her
main focus after Frazer Smith left. Although later missionary nurses criticized MacIntosh for her emphasis on evangelism, her relative disregard for
nursing practice seems inevitable. It was not until formal in-patient services
were developed that the North China Mission formally accepted organized
nursing services as essential to the aims of the mission.

   In contrast to Peter Stursberg, sociologist Yuet-wah Cheung is unimpressed
by the achievements of Canadian medical missionaries. In *Missionary Medicine in China,* Cheung examines missionary medicine at the United Church
West China Mission (Sichuan) and South China Mission (Guangdong) before 1937.[29] In a separate article with Peter Kong-Ming New, Cheung examines "North Honan" (Henan), but only up to 1900, when the mission was
evacuated during the Boxer Uprising.[30] For his study of the West China Mission and the South China Mission, Cheung takes a sociological approach to
determine whether medical missionaries were successful change agents. He
concludes that, while foreign missionaries were successful in introducing
modern medicine into China, their efforts were sporadic and localized and
did not improve Chinese health as a whole. Although American medical
missionaries had been in China since 1835, Cheung suggests that China did
not officially recognize Western medicine until after it proved itself during
the epidemic of pneumonic plague in Manchuria (1910-11). Afterward, China
became heavily dependent on foreigners to build the infrastructure of modern medicine. Hospitals and dispensaries run by the West China Mission
and the South China Mission became the major or sole source of modern
health care in their regions. Although the Nationalist government made
ambitious health plans to establish a national health care scheme after

1928, these remained largely unfulfilled, leaving existing medical facilities – however inadequate – as the backbone of modern health care in China.

Despite their success in introducing modern medicine to China, Cheung contends that medical missionaries ultimately failed because the extent of the change they achieved was disturbingly small. He identifies five reasons that Canadian missionaries did not make a larger impact on Chinese health. First, their instrumental goal of "winning souls" was at odds with public health work: Only curative medicine served evangelistic purposes. Second, the serious shortage of manpower and finances limited public health services and medical education. Third, missionary doctors preferred to work in hospitals because this is where they could influence patients to join the church. Fourth, there was little empathy and homophily (resemblance due to common ancestry) between missionaries and their Chinese patients. Finally, missions failed to mobilize financial support from the Chinese because their high standard of living and "flamboyant" facilities obscured any financial difficulties the missions may have experienced. Cheung despairs at the lack of public health emphasis in missionary care before 1937. To Cheung, the development of public health would have made a more lasting impact on China than the development of hospitals. Yet, unlike the establishment of hospitals, which could be locally developed and individually administered by groups of missionaries, the successful development of a nationwide public health program was dependent on governmental support. While Cheung suggests that the Nationalist health scheme was ineffectual, historian John Watt contends that, once the Ministry of Health made public health and nursing education a priority after 1928, both flourished.[31] At the North China Mission, nurses made impressive strides in the development of public health programs before 1937, but had to abandon their plans in the face of flooding and the Sino-Japanese War. In the destructive wake of natural disaster and war, the collective energy of physicians and nurses was spent caring for the wounded, the ill, and the dispossessed.

What is most intriguing about Cheung's and Stursberg's work is that they respond slightly differently to the question of whether missionaries were successful in their health care and evangelistic aims. Cheung found that Canadians' evangelistic aims interfered with their ability to effect significant health care change, whereas Stursberg found that Canadians were relatively successful in providing illness and injury care, but were failures at evangelism. Either way, in terms of volume (numbers of converts, hospitals, or public health programs), Canadians are presented as failures. Yet, if one considers longevity, it appears that the Canadian (and other) missionaries were actually successful. According to A. Donald MacLeod in 2001, Henan is one of the more Christianized of the thirty provinces that make up the

People's Republic of China.[32] Current members of the Anyang Christian Association agree, reporting to me in 2005 that the Christian church established by Canadians has flourished. Although the number they give is not verifiable (eighty thousand Christians in the Anyang area), a church built on the former mission site in 1995 seats three thousand, and four worship services are reportedly conducted each week. In the area of health care, former Canadian hospitals at Anyang and Weihui are currently providing state-of-the-art Western medicine and modern nursing services.[33] That Henan has chosen to preserve and commemorate its former relationship with Canadians sixty years after their departure indicates that Canadian missionaries were successful after all, albeit in unanticipated ways.

To Be a Missionary: Nurses as Missionary Women

The history of Canadian nurses at the North China Mission between 1888 and 1947 is a story about the evolution of a profession. It is also a story about the transformative experiences of women within that profession. Missionary nursing was a form of paid work, but it was more than a job: it was an identity. Missionaries in China were generally like-minded Christian men and women whose collective goal was to bring the "good news of Christ" to the people of China, through word and deed. Those with the designation "WMS missionary" were single women who had been successful in their formal applications to the Women's (later Woman's) Missionary Society and had been publicly commissioned by a local congregation.[34] Missionaries could anticipate spiritual and financial support from the church and, particularly in the early years, admiration from the Canadian public. Although the WMS hired only single women, both married and unmarried nurses contributed to the North China Mission and are included here. WMS nurses who married were required to resign – even if they married China missionaries, which many of them did. Missionary wives became affiliated with their husbands' mission boards. Despite no longer being officially recognized (or paid) as "missionary nurses," missionary wives offered nursing services when necessary – for example, during war-related medical crises.

What did it mean for a woman to be a missionary? Jane Hunter, Rosemary Gagan, Ruth Compton Brouwer, Myra Rutherdale, and Mary Ellen Kelm have each studied the lives of missionary women overseas and in Canada. With the exception of Jane Hunter (whose focus was on American missionary women in China), these scholars have included Canadian nurses in their studies. Because comparatively little has been written about Canadian nurses in China (only two article-length studies have been published to date),[35] current understanding of Canadian missionary nurses has been influenced by these seminal works on missionary women. Yet, as will be seen in the following chapters, experiences of Canadian nurses at the North China Mission differed in important ways from those described in broader studies of missionary women. For example, Canadian nurses in general were less cosmopolitan than Hunter's American missionary women, less evangelistic than Brouwer's Canadian Presbyterian women in India and China, less fearful than Gagan's Canadian Methodist women, and less effective colonizers than Rutherdale's and Kelm's women in First Nations communities. Some of these differences may be explained by differences in the periods under review. For example, the studies by Hunter, Gagan, and Brouwer focus on the turn of the twentieth century, whereas this book extends into the chaotic interwar and postwar years, when missionary nursing came into its own. Thus, while early missionary nurses at the North China Mission may display features similar to those of other Presbyterian women described by Ruth Compton Brouwer (1876-1914), later missionary nurses do not. Other differences may be attributable to differences in setting. For example, Rutherdale and Kelm included nurses in their studies of missions in Canada, but the evolution of missionary nursing in Canada differed from that of missionary nursing in China. In Canada, missionaries were part of an increasingly influential cultural majority, whereas, in China, missionaries remained part of a cultural minority whose colonial power diminished over time. In Canada, the dominant Anglo-European culture considered Aboriginal culture to be pagan and primitive, and Aboriginal persons were characterized as subhuman. In China, there was a discourse of difference, but it was mutual. If the Chinese were a mass of heathen millions, Canadians were long-nosed, large-footed barbarians and *yanggui* (foreign devils). Canadian missionary nurses may have perceived the Chinese "other" through what Myra Rutherdale calls the "imperialist gaze,"[36] but they were also keenly aware of their own tenuous position as cultural outsiders.

Overseas Missions: Socially Sanctioned Independence for Women

In *The Gospel of Gentility: American Women Missionaries in Turn-of-the-Century China,* Jane Hunter documents the surprisingly genteel lives of Protestant American women missionaries in China.[37] Missionary women had been encouraged to go to China because male contact with Chinese women was extremely limited due to Chinese social customs. By 1890, married and single women comprised 60 percent of the mission force in China. These American women found a unique opportunity to wield authority in China. Married women hired cooks for their American diets, nannies for their children, coolies for their heavy loads, and houseboys for the housework. Influenced by the British society in the internationalized treaty ports where they resided, some acquired upper-class standards of refinement, which included maintaining strict social separation from the Chinese. These women came to view the Chinese as particularly suited to menial work, seldom considering that institutionalizing racial hierarchies in their homes might compromise their missionary work. The lifestyle of relative ease for American missionaries in the cosmopolitan treaty ports contrasts sharply with the lives of early Canadian missionaries in China's harsh and isolated interior. If American missionary women in the treaty ports reinvented themselves as upper-class urban ladies, Canadian missionary women in Henan reinvented themselves as brave and adventurous rural pioneers who struggled through regular periods of violence and threats of disease.

Within the foreign missionary society hierarchy described by Hunter, single missionary women had low social standing. They were viewed as less feminine, unattractive, and unrefined. Yet single women had opportunities to fulfill vocational aspirations that were not available to married women, since husbands and mission boards chivalrously discouraged both the physical and mental strain of their wives. While the single Christian women described by Hunter were not self-consciously feminist, this was an unprecedented, socially sanctioned opportunity for them to preach, teach, and practice medicine without opposition from familiar patriarchal structures. Mission service could be a retreat from conventional marriage pressures and an opportunity to pursue a complex calling that was, in part, a commitment to self-determination. In contrast, for the Canadian nurses at Henan, missionary work was perceived as an opportunity to meet and marry like-minded men; of the twelve WMS nurses who resigned to be married, nine married China missionaries. One of Hunter's aims was to identify and expose inequitable power structures inherent in missionary women's life patterns, and she presents a well-supported argument that inequity existed between male and female missionaries, between single and married women, and between missionaries and the Chinese. In contrast, Canadian nurses after 1920 had surprisingly collaborative relationships with physicians – surprising since nurses in Canada were more typically subordinate to physicians during that period. Over time, Hunter contends, the goal of missionary work for women changed from the salvation of souls to the maintenance of the missionary presence – less in preparing God's kingdom than in managing a domestic empire that exploited it. Because of hierarchical social structures unique to China, American missionary women lost Christian and evangelistic purpose but gained power and self-determination. Canadian missionaries also shifted their aim away from evangelism over time, but their emphasis was on humanitarian service and outreach.

The early Canadian missionaries described by Ruth Compton Brouwer were less cosmopolitan than their American counterparts described by Hunter. In *New Women for God*, Brouwer examines Canadian Presbyterian women's involvement in missions between 1876 and 1914.[38] Although focused on India, Brouwer sheds light on the Western division of the WFMS, which also sent missionaries to China. According to Brouwer, a woman's decision to become a missionary was influenced by factors such as religious upbringing, exposure to popular evangelists, and participation in inter-denominational youth movements. "Missionary propaganda" emphasized women's particular obligation to spread the Gospel since women had the most to gain from Jesus' teachings on the equality of women, their "heathen sisters" had great spiritual and social needs, and converting women to Christianity would multiply into conversion of families and, eventually, the nation. Mission work was understood as an expression of personal religious faith and altruism. The belief that missionary work was God's will empowered women to leave security and familiarity for distant and hazardous lands. Prospective missionaries typically spoke of a longing to spread knowledge of Christianity and provide Christian service. But Brouwer points out that their religious motivation cannot be neatly separated from the allure of career opportunities or romantic adventures. For single women facing spinsterhood, missions offered possibilities not otherwise available, including positions of authority in their mission field and celebrity status in Canada. Still, Canada offered interesting opportunities for ambitious young nurses. For example, Elizabeth Thomson had a promising career as a nursing administrator in Toronto. Nurses like Thomson were attracted to the professional challenges inherent in cross-cultural work and found a sense of purpose and place of belonging in the community of missionaries, and nurses, in China. Just like the WFMS missionaries in Brouwer's study, Canadian nurses who left Canada with simple, arrogant beliefs about "the heathen" found that, over time, these beliefs emerged into more complex understandings as they came to know non-Christians and learn something of another culture. Their relationship with, admiration of, and respect for the Chinese nurses they trained and later worked alongside translated into a vision of professional nursing for the region – one that was neither fully Canadian nor Chinese, but reflected the changing values of each.

In her study of Methodist missionary women, Rosemary Gagan affirms Hunter's and Brouwer's findings that missionary women were religiously devout women whose experiences of missionary life contradicted their initial expectations. All expected evangelistic success, yet few achieved it. In *A Sensitive Independence,* Gagan focuses on more than three hundred single women hired through the WMS of the Canadian Methodist Church from its inception in 1881 until it was absorbed into the United Church of Canada WMS in 1925.[39] These missionaries included physicians, nurses, and teachers working in China, Japan, and remote parts of Canada. In trying to understand the motivation of women missionaries, Gagan mirrors Hunter's interest in demographic background, family structure and education, training, and life cycles, and Brouwer's interest in altruism and a deeply rooted sense of Christian vocation. Before the turn of the century, mission candidates were selected on the basis of their staunch Christian conviction. Later, missionaries were required to have a good education and professional experience. WMS missionaries emerged as an "elite well-educated middle-class company of pious single women drawn largely from the small towns and rural areas of Ontario and the Maritimes."[40] Like Presbyterian missionaries, Methodist missionaries were socialized in the church and influenced by youth organizations. Their most enduring incentive for missions, however, was a requisite call from God – exquisitely felt, earnestly received, and readily testified. Experiencing this call marked an entry into a select club of women who shared a common bond of assurance of salvation and purpose in life.

According to Gagan, once they arrived in their fields, the WMS missionaries became overwhelmed with fear. They became concerned for their safety, their work's success, and the spiritual and moral well-being of their constituents. They "reverted to an unwavering dependence and trust in Jesus and God as their own personal protectors," sometimes to the point of "abdicating any responsibility for, or control over, their own actions."[41] Work in West China was particularly difficult. The lives of WMS missionaries Amelia Brown and Jennie Ford illustrate why about 20 percent of WMS West China missionaries were "lost" to physical and mental breakdown – and death – between 1891 and 1925. Brown, a "woman with no medical qualifications," was grudgingly hired by the WMS because it was unable to find a female physician in 1891.[42] Within months of sailing to China, Brown became engaged to Canadian physician David Stevenson, effectively and disappointingly "defecting" from the WMS, although remaining at the West China Mission. Jennie Ford, the first Canadian nurse at the West China Mission, arrived in 1894 to assist the new WMS physician Retta (Gifford) Kilborn. In 1895, WMS missionaries faced a startling charge: the Chinese believed that "foreign barbarians" ate the flesh of human beings and kidnapped children, and they accused the women of eating babies and digging out their eyes for medicine. Accordingly, placards hung during a dragon boat festival warned the Chinese to watch their children, lest the missionaries kidnap and roast them. A threatening mob engulfed the missionaries, eventually destroying the mission compound. In the initial rioting, Amelia Brown Stevenson was beaten and her child was temporarily lost in the crowd. Although the missionaries were evacuated safely to Shanghai, Brown suffered a nervous breakdown along the way. She did not return to West China. In 1897, Jennie Ford died of meningitis. Missionary work in China was risky. According to Gagan, even a deep passion and high levels of education and experience could not shield women missionaries from missionary work's inherent dangers.

At the North China Mission, early missionary experiences with violence and death helped to shape the image of missionary work in China as dangerous. For example, stories about the attack on missionaries during the Boxer Uprising of 1900 and the deaths of missionaries and their children by disease[43] were told and retold, and new missionaries were praised for their courage as well as their piety. Still, only two of the thirty nurses associated with the North China Mission resigned due to illness (Jennie Graham, in .1891, and Coral Brodie, in 1940), and none died in China. In Gagan's study, WMS women dealt with the realities of Chinese society matter-of-factly, putting the best possible face on the situation for the Canadian public, often concealing the risks they took in the name of Christ. In contrast, North China missionaries emphasized the dangers they faced. Missionary nurses expected danger and hardship but also relied, consciously and unconsciously, on extant physical, political, and social barriers to shield them.

According to Gagan, WMS missionaries succeeded best when their expectations and abilities addressed "real needs." When medical missions were given increasing legitimacy in the early twentieth century, WMS missionaries in West China found a tangible place to invest their energies by participating in the development of a women's hospital and a training school for Chinese nurses. The hospital gave visible meaning to the missionaries' commitment. By 1925, WMS missionaries at the West China Mission had found a way to "turn their passion for Christian social activism into an instrument to advance their own personal independence, professional development, and social standing."[44] In a similar way, missionary nurses at the North China Mission turned their collective attention to modernizing and professionalizing nursing service after the first modern hospital was opened at Weihui in 1923.

Home Missions: Nurses as Colonizers

Seen through twenty-first-century eyes, Margaret Brown's suggestion that "young women would not have taken up nursing without the example set them by Christian women of the West" situates missionary nurses in China directly in the centre of current debates on the colonialist and imperialist nature of missionary medicine. Here I use the term "imperialism" to mean one nation extending power over another through political or economic control. It is an extreme form of nationalistic ethnocentrism based on an assumption of superiority and entitlement. I borrow from Mary Ellen Kelm's definition of "colonialism" as a process linked to imperialism that includes "the provision of low-level social services [and] the creation of ideological formulations around race and skin color, which positions the colonizers at a higher evolutionary level than the colonized."[45] Although their focus was not on nurses, in their respective studies of Canada's colonialist relationship with First Nations, both Mary Ellen Kelm and Myra Rutherdale present evidence that missionary nurses were collaborators in Euro-Christian hegemony. As missionaries, Canadian nurses in China are inevitably linked with the "imperial project," whereby Britain asserted power over other nations in an effort to subdue and subsume them into the expanding British Empire.[46] I argue that while Canadian nurses in China may have reflected and even embraced imperialist ideals, they were indifferent – and ineffective – colonizers.

In their respective studies, Kelm and Rutherdale successfully argue that missionary work supported both government and church agendas of directed cultural change. In her study of Aboriginal health and healing in British Columbia, Mary Ellen Kelm demonstrates the degree to which imperial efforts to dominate Aboriginal health in Canada were successful. Missionary nurses played a role in what Kelm has termed "colonizing bodies" through their support of assimilating First Nations into the dominant culture, noting that medical practitioners, including nurses, were among those intent on "expanding the frontiers of Anglo-European ascendancy" and were "imbued with the collective experience of empire-building" apparent in Asia and elsewhere.[47] In British Columbia, nurses and field matrons instructed Native women in the domestic arts (aiming to improve cleanliness and sanitary conditions of Native homes), helped with medical emergencies, made home visits to expectant and new mothers, and dispensed simple remedies "such as are found in average homes in white communities."[48] Some field matrons were without special training; those who were "trained" were often nurses. Together, nurses and field matrons served to build "Aboriginal confidence in the paternalism of the department [of Indian Affairs] and generate interracial goodwill."[49] Similarly, in her study of Anglican missionary women in British Columbia, Myra Rutherdale found that the Anglican Church of Canada acted "in tandem with the federal government in an attempt to assimilate Aboriginal peoples into Canadian society."[50] Thirty-four of the Anglican women missionaries working in northern Canada were trained nurses. These nurses assisted in the colonialist aim of assimilation through their work in residential schools, homes, and hospitals.

The link between colonialism and missionary nursing in Canada suggests a similar link between colonialism and nursing in China. After all, missionary nurses in China and Canada were often drawn from the same pool of candidates. That is, nurses hired by the United Church WMS could work at home (in WMS hospitals across Canada), or abroad, in countries such as China, Japan, Korea, and India.[51] In fact, China nurses Clara Preston and Janet Brydon worked at WMS hospitals in Canada when wartime conditions made China inaccessible – Preston at Hearst, Ontario, and Brydon at Smeaton, Saskatchewan. In both cases, the nurses found the Canadian settings lacking; Brydon described her working conditions at Smeaton as "very bad; primitive."[52] In comparison with work in China, with its large population, ancient culture, and mission community, work in remote areas of Canada could be isolating and depressing. Thus, while there was a link between missionary nursing in China and Canada, there was also much dissimilarity. In China, Canadian nurses benefited from being British subjects (for example, as recipients of extraterritoriality rights), and undoubtedly – if not unwittingly – came to China with ethnocentric ideals. But expressions or displays of cultural or national superiority tempered over time as nurses became more fluent in Chinese language and customs and identified more with Chinese colleagues and friends. Far from providing "low-level social services" associated with colonizers of First Nations, Canadian nurses in Henan were among those who envisioned and created Henan's first modern hospital and nurses' training school, which was, by all accounts, a state-of-the-art institution, comparable to hospitals in Canada.

The extent to which mission discourse has spilled over into nursing historiography can be seen in two seminal articles on nursing history in China, by Liu Chung-tung and Kaiyi Chen.[53] In both articles, the authors commend missionary nurses for their role in developing modern nursing, but express disapproval of the imperialist and colonialist impulses that characterized missionary work. To Chung-tung, missionaries were "the velvet glove of imperialism frequently backed up by the mailed fist, its effort in China [being] effective for a time in undermining Chinese self-determination."[54] To Chen, the missionary nurses' primary goal was to convert the Chinese to Christianity through "saving the soul."[55] In mission discourse, evangelism is closely tied to imperialism and colonialism, with "Christianizing" and "civilizing" heathen nations both being understood as ways to subvert self-determination. Because conversion to Christianity is understood as the first step toward assimilation of Anglo-European values, missionary work is necessarily seen as supporting imperialist aims. Chen and Chung-tung take up the view that (American) missionary nurses were primarily evangelistic and colonialist, but they do not provide evidence to support such claims.[56] While the lack of comprehensive studies makes it difficult to know whether and how American missionary nursing contrasted with Canadian nursing, emerging research on Canadian nursing challenges Chen's and Chung-tung's assumptions that missionary nurses in China had an imperialist agenda, damaged Chinese self-determination, and sought primarily to evangelize. That is, Janet Beaton's work on missionary nursing at the United Church West China Mission[57] and letters written by Canadian missionary nurses in China to *Canadian Nurse* between 1935 and 1947[58] portray nurses as aligning themselves more closely to internationalized, professional ideals than to nationalized, church ideals. As will·be seen, church and nation were important influences on missionary nursing at the North China Mission, but these constructs are only part of the story.

The relationship between evangelism and nursing practice at the North China Mission is best illustrated by the evolution of Margaret Gay's missionary career in China (1910-41). Gay, who went to China as an evangelistic missionary, came to perceive professional nursing as a better, more tangible expression of her faith and desire to serve the needs of the Chinese. While Margaret MacIntosh (1889-1927) focused on evangelism to the virtual exclusion of nursing service, and while post-1920 nurses focused on nursing practice to the virtual exclusion of evangelism, Gay saw a place for both. To Gay, evangelism was precisely what differentiated missionary nursing from other forms of nursing practice. Although other nurses did not generally integrate teaching the Christian Gospel to patients as part of their professional nursing service, missionary nursing came to be understood (and is still understood) as a form of evangelism.

Through their seminal studies, Hunter, Brouwer, Gagan, Rutherdale, and Kelm help to situate nursing in the broader movement of missionary women. These authors highlight the oft-overshadowed world of women's work for women, the influence of gender on missionary work, and the ways that women unexpectedly wielded power in male-dominated societies and organizations.[59] They also introduce the notion of women missionaries as inadvertent feminists and colonizers, themes reflected in the scant literature on nursing history in China. Their emphasis on the collective voice of women contrasts with mission records and scholarship that privilege the voices of men – particularly physicians, administrators, and evangelists who held dominant positions in the Presbyterian and the United Church. In both cases, the story of missionary nurses tends to be fragmented or hidden altogether in the extant literature. While gender bias partially explains the invisibility of nurses, the fact that greater attention is paid to female physicians than to nurses in China mission scholarship (despite an estimated MD:RN ratio of 1:4 at the West China Mission)[60] suggests that the invisibility of nurses must also be understood in the context of the historic power relationship between nurses and physicians. To accept the silence surrounding missionary nursing is to accept an image of nursing as an incidental, inconsequential, ancillary arm of medicine.

To Be a Nurse: Missionary Women as Trained Professionals
Missionary nurses at the North China Mission between 1888 and 1947 were "graduate nurses" (also called "trained nurses"). This meant that they had met the standards of qualification set by a recognized nurses' training school – normally a two- to three-year hospital-based apprenticeship program of study in Canada.[61] Some nurses went on to earn certificates in public health nursing at Canadian universities after the Red Cross Society began sponsoring one-year postgraduate certificate programs in five universities after 1919.[62] Graduate nurses wore distinctive uniforms, caps, and school pins, which helped to distinguish them from lesser-qualified lay nurses and subsidiary health workers. In Canada, nursing uniforms served an important function since different styles and colours indicated one's relative rank and position. This tradition was transferred to China, where nurses' training took place

in mission hospitals. For example, Chinese nursing students wore blue uniforms with white aprons, foreign and Chinese graduate nurses wore all white, and head nurses wore a black stripe on their white nursing caps. Because of the different uniform styles, patients could tell at a glance whether a nurse was a probationer (new student), senior student, graduate nurse, or nursing supervisor.

Prior to the construction of new, modern hospitals in Henan, Canadian nurses worked with physicians in patient homes, makeshift clinics, Chinese inns, mission dispensaries, and in what Clara Preston later referred to as "old-style" hospitals – one-story, Chinese-style structures with paper windows and rooms facing a central courtyard. The change from old-style to modern hospitals in the 1920s was catalyzed by four events. First, a new generation of missionary men and women began work in Henan after the First World War, including Dr. Bob McClure and Jean Menzies. Second, missionaries began to see a need for hospital services. For example, evangelistic worker Margaret Gay pursued nursing studies after feeling increasingly concerned by the prevalence of unmet medical needs. Third, professional nursing practice and education in Canada was becoming increasingly sophisticated, standardized, and organized: the *Canadian Nurse* journal started publishing in 1905, the Canadian National Association of Trained Nurses was formed in 1908, and the first baccalaureate program for nurses was established at the University of British Columbia in 1919. Finally, and perhaps most importantly, a widely distributed, comprehensive report of mission hospitals across China listed Henan hospitals as among the worst in the country in terms of facilities and staffing.[63] This may have shamed the Canadians into action or at least given weight to the appeals being made by some of the younger missionaries for modern medical care. After the first modern hospital and training school for nurses was built at Weihui, the community of nurses broadened to include Chinese women and men, and nurses became increasingly committed to the expansion of nursing services through education, professional networking, and standard setting. During the interwar years, nursing in Henan was developing at a pace similar to that of Canadian nursing at home.

According to former North China missionary Margaret Brown, Chinese women took up nursing because of the example set them by missionary nurses. This assertion is problematic. Although Brown's statement seems accurate in terms of missionary impact on nursing development in general, it is not clear that this was the situation in Henan. That is, while Brown suggests that Chinese women took up nursing out of admiration for missionary women, it seems equally plausible that, in Henan, Chinese women took up nursing out of admiration for Chinese nurses, or for other reasons altogether. By the time nurses' training started for Chinese nurses at Weihui, professional nursing was already established in the larger urban centres of

China, Western medicine had gained increased acceptance, and roles for women in China in general were changing. Because the earliest Chinese students at Henan were members of what would become the Church of Christ in China (a church initiated by, but separate from, the United Church and other denominations),[64] it is as likely that they were inspired by fellow Chinese Christians as by foreign nurses. Either way, we do not know what the perspective of Chinese nurses was, since the Chinese voice is typically left out of mission documents. Where Chinese nurses are described, it is always from the missionary perspective; data reveal more about the Canadian values and beliefs (for example, about the Chinese "other") than about the Chinese per se. While it is clear that the Chinese supported nursing and that nurses adopted structures and traditions of modern nursing, nursing practice in Henan differed from Western nursing in important ways (for example, its inclusion of male nurses, something virtually unheard of in Canada). It is difficult to say whether Chinese nursing in Henan was grounded in Christian ideals. Certainly Chinese nurses were well versed in Christian ideology, as members of the Chinese Church and even graduates of mission primary schools. But the degree to which they internalized Christian values is unclear from the record. What we do know is that Canadian nurses believed and expected their Chinese protégés to have similar values, and based their relationship with Chinese nurses on a belief that they had similar religious convictions.

Both Liu Chung-tung and Kaiyi Chen raise doubts about whether Chinese women adopted Western and Christian ideals related to nursing. To Chung-tung, nursing in China is best understood as a "transition within an extremely complex and ancient society" rather than an "extraneous implant" from the West.[65] Drawing attention to ancient traditions of healing and caring, Chung-tung identifies value conflicts experienced by the Chinese as they made the transition from ancient to modern practices. These included the Chinese expectation of gender segregation (for example, females could not take care of males), the low status of individuals who performed menial duties or touched the human body, and the general hatred and suspicion of foreigners. As the nursing profession came increasingly under Chinese leadership, the ideals of missionary nursing were reinterpreted in a specifically Chinese way. To Chung-tung, missionary nurses may have been catalysts for reform, but they were not reformers. Kaiyi Chen similarly suggests that missionary nurses' role in the development of professional nursing was commendable but transitory; Western values and beliefs were tolerated rather than embraced. To Chung-tung and Chen, the Chinese may have mimicked Western *structures* in their development of professional nursing, but Chinese nurses ultimately rejected both Western and Christian *ideology*.

Although missionary nurses played a key role in the introduction of modern nursing to China, it is impossible to conclude whether or not modern nursing would have developed in China without them. If, as Brown contends, modern medicine would have "come sooner or later anyway," so, too, would have modern nursing. Modern medicine, with its emphasis on hospital care, relied as much on nursing services as nurses relied on physicians; medicine was neither separate nor separable from nursing. Thus, while it is possible that physicians would have been able to provide care at dispensaries and small hospitals (where meals and personal care of patients were provided by family members), the modern model of organized in-patient care in Western-style hospitals demanded highly structured nursing care. Without nurses, modern hospital care was inconceivable. By the time the North China Mission was ready to modernize its medical care, missionary nurses were ready to rise to the challenge.

Methodological Notes: Gaps, Silences, and Opportunities

Since the earliest days of the profession, nurses have used history to celebrate individual achievement, acknowledge professional milestones, and socialize new nurses. With the replacement of nursing history by nursing theory as a professionalizing discourse, nurses have become disconnected with their historical roots.[66] Sioban Nelson recently lamented, "our education systems are producing nurses without a historical identity" who "equate nursing history with tales of Nightingale and old matrons."[67] But this is changing. Nurse historians have perceived a new path of historical possibilities, opened, in some measure, by feminist historians. As a response, Patricia D'Antonio and others have called for a "new historiography" in nursing.[68] In feminist biography, for example, historiography has moved from an "era of heroic biography to an era more interested in the archeology of humbler lives," making work on the ordinary daily lives of subjects increasingly possible and desirable.[69] The shift toward a new historiography in nursing allows attention to be given to what Kathleen Cruikshank calls the "lives of unknown or lesser known figures, exploring what their experience can offer to our understanding of an era, a movement, or a culture."[70] Canadian missionary nurses assist us to understand the Canadian role in the missionary era, the culture of missionary nursing, and the globalization of modern nursing.

In an effort to understand both the public and private spheres of Canadian nurses' lives, I sought out professional and personal, published and confidential, and official and unofficial sources. The public record (archives, published documents, newspapers) most readily spoke to the professional, communal aspects of missionary *nursing,* whereas private documents (family papers, letters, diaries) tended to reveal the personal, individual lives of *nurses.* Unfortunately, the Toronto General Hospital (TGH) nursing alumnae archives were not available during the period of this study; they were in temporary, private storage awaiting procurement of a permanent repository. Since most of the nurses were TGH graduates, information in this collection would undoubtedly assist in our understanding of the preparation of missionary nurses. Also missing is mission correspondence prior to 1912. According to a United Church of Canada/Victoria University Archives finding aid on the overseas mission board (Honan Mission), virtually all correspondence prior to 1912 "has been lost due to disturbances (e.g., the Boxer Uprising) or simply misplaced."[71] For this reason, I have depended upon memoirs of early missionaries and the unpublished history compiled by Margaret Brown for much of the chronology and early history of the mission. I recognize that each of these sources represents a particular agenda and a limited perspective on mission history.

By collecting and comparing a variety of independent perspectives on a specific event or experience, I have tried to substantiate (or contradict) the authenticity, origin, and originality of documents.[72] That is not to say that conflicting evidence or inconsistencies invalidate data, however. Like gaps and silences, conflicting data raised new questions, opening new possibilities for analysis. For example, in his study of missionary medicine at United Church missions in China before 1937, Yuet-wah Cheung suggested that conscious misrepresentation in missionary letters and reports could arise when success in the field was exaggerated in order to solicit greater support from the home church; unconscious misrepresentation might occur because of an error in memory or a passing mood.[73] While steps were taken to unravel inconsistencies in the data, I, like Cheung, strove for an "approximation rather than a completely accurate rendering of an historical event" through critical examination of the best available sources.[74]

Rather than limiting the study to the twenty-one WMS nurses, I chose to include others associated with the North China Mission, notably married nurses. Since married nurses were not officially part of the mission, they are rarely named in official mission documentation. Moreover, once married, even those who remained in Henan under the auspices of the United Church Foreign Mission Board were difficult to trace since their first names were no longer recorded. Tracing married nurses was an arduous but essential task: Maisie McNeely became, simply, "Mrs. Forbes," while Isabel Leslie became "Mrs. Fleming" (a matter further complicated by the fact that Leslie was actually the second Mrs. Fleming at Henan). Nurses were often left unnamed in mission records and photographs, and no comprehensive list of Canadian nurses existed. Because of this, I felt a thrill of discovery whenever I stumbled across the name or image of a Canadian nurse. For example, I first came across the name Margaret MacIntosh in an obscure record of the attack on a group of missionaries during the 1900 Boxer Uprising; Margaret Gay was in the preface of the 1935 edition of Jonathan Goforth's *Miracle Lives in China;* and Florence MacKenzie was in a documentary film on Scottish Olympian and China missionary Eric Liddell. Nurses who were well represented in the data inevitably became more dominant in the resultant text. That is, the relative lack of information on nurses who where missionaries for only a short period meant that these women (Harriet Sutherland, Jennie Graham, Eleanor Galbraith, and Margaret Straith) are mentioned only in passing, while nurses who lived in China for long periods (Margaret MacIntosh, Margaret Gay, Jeanette Ratcliffe, Janet Brydon, and Clara Preston) are covered extensively – as are nurses whose families I was fortunate to have as participants (for example, Elizabeth Thomson, Coral Brodie, and Helen Turner, among others). My greatest regret is the lack of information about Chinese nurses and students; the majority of these remain unidentified. One notable exception is the names of Chinese nurses at Weihui between 1937 and 1939, graciously provided to me recently by the administration of the First Affiliated Hospital of Xinxiang Medical University (formerly the North China Mission Weihui Hospital).

Throughout my analysis, I have tried to be mindful of subtle ways in which surviving documents privilege the worldview of missionaries. In an analysis of Chinese conversion stories from the North China Mission, Margo Gewurtz concluded that conversion narratives were shaped to serve the missionary purpose. I recognize, with Gewurtz, that the North China Mission narrative tends to ignore or reinvent the Chinese perspective.[75] Thus, while I am inclined to accept Gewurtz's assertion that "years of intimate contact [between the North China missionaries and the Chinese] changed both sides,"[76] my reliance on English-language sources necessitates an emphasis on the Canadian perspective of events.

Two final notes: First, I have chosen to translate the original place names into Pinyin for the benefit of contemporary readers, wherever possible (for example, "Henan" rather than the old spelling "Honan"). The Wade-Giles spelling is kept in rare cases where Pinyin spellings could not be ascertained. Although the Wade-Giles system was used by missionaries during the period under review, my aim is to allow readers to more easily relate the events to present-day settings. (See the list of Pinyin and Wade-Giles spellings earlier in the book.) Second, as careful as I was to corroborate sources, incorporate a wide range of perspectives, and invite feedback from those with firsthand experience in China missions, it is entirely possible that I have overlooked or missed some points, or interpreted some events differently from those who actually lived through them. Any errors are my own.

Overview of Chapters

Canadian missionary nursing was characterized by personal and professional struggle in an era and vocation where struggle was both expected and admired. Compared to life in Canada, missionary work in China was

dangerous, and narratives of disease, grief, threats, and violence predomin-
ate in mission correspondence, personal letters, and public reports. Events
such as the Boxer Uprising (1900), the murder of Dr. James Menzies (1920),
the Great Missionary Exodus (1927), the Anti-British Movement (1939), the
Sino-Japanese War (1939-45), and the Communist takeover of Henan (1947)
were constructed within an overarching narrative of survival, whereby nurses
are presented as strong, resilient, and committed. The emphasis on victory
and achievement in mission discourse is consistent with a Western image
of Christianity as a triumphant religion of glory and imperial power. Yet
missionaries also struggled with self-doubt, failure, and personal shame.
Although public displays of fear or doubt are rare in the mission record,
evidence of these common human emotions makes the story of missionary
nursing more poignant and familiar. For example, Clara Preston's angry
outburst directed at Chinese nurses who secretly fled the Weihui Hospital
compound the day before Communist troops attacked in 1947 seems as
significant as her heroic efforts to evacuate patients from the compound
under gunfire. Disappointment and failure, so pervasive in the human experience, are as necessary to the story of missionary nursing as accomplishment and triumph. Yet they are rare in surviving records.

According to WMS records, the story of the North China Mission "is the
story of repeated disturbances and wars, with repeated withdrawals and
returns of the missionaries."[77] To capture the narrative of danger and survival as well as the evolutionary nature of missionary nursing, I have organized the material into seven chronological chapters, using significant
sociopolitical crises as markers to define each time period. Each chapter
covers the period of time leading up to a particular crisis that had a significant impact on the North China Mission. The focus of this study is not on
the crises themselves, but rather on the work of Canadian nurses within the
context of these crises and the intervening years. In Chapter 1, I discuss the
nature of early missionary nursing and how its dependency on the broader
missionary agenda shaped its (lack of) progress from 1888 until the time of
the Boxer Uprising in 1900. In Chapter 2, I examine early attempts to modernize medical and nursing care, from 1901 until the 1920 Menzies murder.
Chapter 3 addresses the establishment and progression of modern nursing
and nurses' training, from 1921 until the Great Missionary Exodus of 1927.
In Chapter 4, I examine the period of unprecedented expansion and nursing innovation from 1928 until the 1937 Japanese invasion. In Chapter 5, I
discuss the period of upheaval during the Sino-Japanese War as North China
Mission nurses were scattered around China and Canada between 1938 and
1940. In Chapter 6, I consider the experiences of those who remained in
China under the Japanese after Pearl Harbor, between 1941 and 1945. Finally, in Chapter 7, I discuss the brief period of postwar rehabilitation until
the North China Mission was permanently closed in 1947.

1

The Gospel of Soap and Water, 1888-1900

> Some houses are saturated with deadly germs and need the gospel of soap and water, light and fresh air. Cleanliness, as well as godliness, is profitable for the life that now is, in Honan [Henan] as elsewhere.
>
> > – Murdoch MacKenzie, *Twenty-five Years in Honan*, 1913

Nurses were not part of the original plan for missionary work in Henan. When the General Assembly of the Presbyterian Church in Canada appointed the first two Canadian missionaries to Henan – Reverend Jonathan Goforth and Dr. James Frazer Smith – in June 1887, the option of sending single missionary women to China had not been considered.[1] It is ironic that Jonathan Goforth, who would later oppose the development of modern nursing in Henan, was indirectly responsible for the appointment of Harriet Sutherland, the first Canadian missionary nurse in China. Having learned from local missionaries upon arriving in China in 1888 that Chinese mores would not allow missionary men to have contact with Chinese women, Goforth wrote to the Foreign Mission Committee (later the Foreign Mission Board [FMB]), requesting "single lady missionaries" because "I am told that without the latter the women can scarcely be reached."[2] Dr. Frazer Smith, seeing an opportunity to procure assistance with his own medical work, pressed the FMB to appoint a nurse.[3] On 25 May 1888, the FMB appointed Harriet Sutherland. Her salary was paid by the Women's Foreign Missionary Society (later the Woman's Missionary Society [WMS]). During the next three years, while the expanding group of "North Honan" missionaries made unsuccessful attempts to procure property on Henan soil, Dr. Frazer Smith engaged the services of two additional nurses, Jennie Graham and Margaret MacIntosh, with the idea that they would assist him in his growing work of treating the illnesses of the rural Chinese. By 1891, Sutherland and Graham had resigned (due to marriage and illness, respectively), leaving Margaret MacIntosh as the sole nurse at the mission.

Under the aegis of Dr. Frazer Smith, MacIntosh brought to China her knowledge of nursing as learned at the Toronto General Hospital (TGH) Training School for Nurses. Started in 1881, the TGH nurses' training school was one of the largest and most progressive training schools in Canada. In 1894, it was the largest in Canada, having graduated 210 nurses, with room to accept only 53 of the 647 applications for admission.[4] In 1889, the year MacIntosh graduated from TGH, the terms "trained nurse" and "graduate nurse" had come to represent the best in nursing care. According to the inaugural address at the opening of the Johns Hopkins Training School for Nurses in 1889 by Miss Isabel A. Hampton (whose *Principles and Practice of Nursing* would become the first nursing textbook to be translated into Chinese),[5] of all the professions open to women, none met with more public favour than that of the trained nurse: "While all of the various types of nurses which existed before her time, still exist to a more or less degree, the trained nurse is acknowledged superior by both physician and patient, for the simple reason that the world at large readily recognizes the fact that in this work, as in all others, technical skill can only be acquired by a systematic course of practical and theoretical study under competent teachers."[6] Nurses were expected to "morally recognize the sacredness of the work they engage in," to be "fairly intellectual" and "strong and enduring physically."[7] State-of-the-art nursing practice in 1889 was considered an extension of physician care, where "the hands of a nurse are a physician's hands *lengthened out* to minister to the sick."[8] Nurses were to "yield implicit obedience and loyalty to the physician, faithfully carry out his directions, and in his absence watch over the welfare of his patient, and further his scientific study of disease by intelligently fulfilling his orders, in administering medicines, taking account of the range of pulse and temperature, regulating the sanitary condition of the sick room, noting every unusual symptom in the patient, and reporting the various changes in his condition, as the patient responds to treatment." As patients convalesced, trained nurses would provide companionship and entertainment, "not with gossip over the affairs of her last patient, or with accounts of her hospital life and experiences," but with her familiarity with current events, art, literature, and science.[9]

In addition to providing trained vigilance at the bedside, nineteenth-century nurses were trained in hygiene and sanitation. The "gospel of soap and water, light and fresh air" described by Henan missionary Murdoch MacKenzie *(Yin Cimu)* in 1913 was consistent with Florence Nightingale's theories of illness, health, and nursing care. To Nightingale, a clean, well-ventilated, bright, and quiet environment was essential to the healing process. Although Nightingale did not at first accept the germ theory, her meticulous attention to personal and environmental cleanliness helped to prevent the spread of communicable disease and other infections. The significance of careful attention to hygiene and sanitation in the era before antibiotics cannot be overstated; cleanliness was the best protection against the microorganisms that caused morbidity and mortality. Nurses who were trained in the late nineteenth century were expected to be skilled at ventilating rooms (including determination of air purity and moisture), determining water potability, disinfecting "clothing, rooms, and bodily discharges," and sanitizing "dwellings."[10] Surgical nurses were additionally expected to understand the "absolute importance of perfect asepsis" in all surgical operations. If the Gospel of Christ was central to the "missionary" aspect of missionary nursing, the gospel of soap and water was central to the "nursing" aspect of their work.

From the appointment of Harriet Sutherland in 1888 until the resignation of Dr. James Frazer Smith in 1894, the purpose of missionary nursing was to support the practice of missionary medicine – specifically, Frazer Smith's medical practice. Once Frazer Smith resigned, Margaret MacIntosh's interest in evangelistic work took precedence over her nursing work and, as will be seen, little progress was made in terms of organized nursing care between 1894 and the time of the Boxer Uprising in 1900. During these years, however, several sociopolitical forces helped to shape the foundation upon which subsequent nursing services were built, including the development of missionary medicine, the establishment of a Chinese Christian community, and incidents of violence that contributed to the emerging image of China as a vehemently anti-foreign and inherently dangerous country.

Harriet R. Sutherland and the Henan Seven

On 27 July 1888, a group of three Canadians from Ontario boarded a ship in Vancouver to commence their greatly anticipated voyage to China. Graduate nurse Miss Harriet R. Sutherland and the newly married Dr. and Mrs. James (Minnie) Frazer Smith considered themselves "adventurers going out in faith."[11] They were on their way to the treaty port of Zhifu in Shandong province, to meet up with fellow Canadians Rev. and Mrs. Jonathan (Rosalind) Goforth, who had arrived a few months earlier, in March. Bachelors Dr. William McClure (*Luo Weiling*) and Donald MacGillivray soon added to their number, bringing the total to seven. Dubbing themselves "the Honan [Henan] Seven" (after the famous "Cambridge Seven" group of British missionaries who had gone to China in 1886), this small band of Canadians was to take up the daunting task assigned to them by the Presbyterian Church in Canada – to establish a Christian mission in Henan, the "second most hostile province in the whole of China."[12] Unaware of the struggle that lay ahead, these first Canadian missionaries to China began to lay plans to settle in the triangular section of Henan north of the Yellow River.[13] It was not until six years later that Donald MacGillivray was finally able to secure property in Henan: in 1894, MacGillivray obtained a fifty-year lease on twelve *mu* (two acres) just outside the city wall of Anyang (also Zhangde), an important centre of local government in North Henan, thus officially establishing the first Canadian mission in Henan province.[14]

The province of Henan was the cradle of Chinese civilization; seven of China's nineteen historic capitals were located in this region. Although the word "Henan" means "the land south of the river," about 30 percent of the province lies north of the Yellow River.[15] This triangular region, referred to as North Henan, had three main *"fu"* or prefectural cities: Anyang, Weihui, and Huaiqing. After the Canadians secured sites at Weihui and Huaiqing in 1902, their mission became, and remained, the largest foreign mission in Henan. In 1904, a railway from Beijing to Hankou was completed, and passed through Weihui and Anyang, making these sites more accessible.[16] Although the mission established a number of smaller stations (for example, in Daokou in 1908), the mission stations at Anyang, Weihui, and Huaiqing became the largest and most developed. It was at these main mission stations that the first modern hospitals were built in the 1920s.

Harriet Sutherland never reached Henan. While in Zhifu in 1888, she nursed the ill wife of Rev. Dr. Hunter Corbett of the American Presbyterian Mission (North), and looked after his children after Mrs. Corbett passed away. In February 1889, Sutherland resigned from the WMS to be engaged to Corbett, only seven months after arriving in China.[17]

New Recruits Jennie Graham and Margaret MacIntosh

Sutherland's resignation was a blow to the WMS. Early missionaries signed seven-year contracts, which included a round-trip ticket to Canada, expenses related to travel and outfitting, and a one-year furlough.[18] Missionaries who resigned early were expected to pay for their own return costs to Canada. Considering that graduation from nursing school frequently coincided with the age of marriage eligibility, appointing single nurses to the mission field for seven years was a risky endeavour. Losing nurses through marriage was to become a familiar lament for the WMS: of the twenty Canadian nurses who succeeded Sutherland as WMS missionaries, nine resigned to marry China missionaries, mostly from other missions (see Appendix 2: WMS nurses who resigned to be married). For her part, Harriet Sutherland-Corbett remained in China under the auspices of the American Presbyterian Board in Shandong, giving "a life time of splendid service" there.[19] After her husband passed away, she remained in Zhifu until her own death sometime before 1937.[20] That most of the Canadian nurses remained in China after marriage provided little consolation to the WMS administrators, who were left to recruit their replacements.

Sutherland's engagement was doubly disappointing to the WMS. Not only had they lost their first missionary nurse, they had lost their first Henan missionary. It was also disappointing to Dr. Frazer Smith. He immediately appealed to the FMB for two more nurses for Henan, convinced as ever that there was "work to be done in China which must be done by *women* alone ... Through a lady with a partial knowledge of medicine, or a practical nurse, I could prescribe and treat numbers of women who would never come to the dispensary or a hospital."[21] To Frazer Smith, the role of a missionary nurse was to assist in medical work as well as to visit homes and teach women – something a male missionary would not be allowed to do in China. He recommended that the WMS appoint two nurses this time, for the following reasons: two nurses could help and encourage one another in studying the language; house rent would be the same for one as for two; and once the anticipated second mission was opened in Henan, each station could have a nurse.

Not everyone agreed with his plan. In a letter to the FMB, MacGillivray strongly protested the idea of assigning single women to the young mission. The policy of other missions, he chided, was to hold off the appointment of single women until missions were officially organized and an untarnished reputation among the Chinese was secured. MacGillivray was concerned that the Chinese would misconstrue the relationship between single women and male missionaries and presume that they were being "kept for immoral purposes." More to the point, MacGillivray feared that his own reputation as a celibate bachelor (and that of the other bachelor Dr. McClure) would be tainted by the close proximity of single women. For that reason, he insisted that, "if young ladies come out, they must work with [the married] Dr. Frazer Smith."[22] By the time the FMB received MacGillivray's letter of protest, it was too late: the two nurses were already appointed and ready to sail. It had taken less than three months to find replacements for Harriet Sutherland. As Sutherland prepared for her September wedding, Miss Janet (Jennie) Graham and Miss Margaret I. MacIntosh prepared for their voyage to China with Revs. MacVicar, MacDougall, and MacKenzie and their wives.[23] This group of "McAlls" arrived at their final destination in December.[24]

The new nursing recruits, Margaret MacIntosh and Jennie Graham, were born in Ontario and were graduates of the University of Toronto Training School for Nurses.[25] Like virtually all the Canadian nurses to follow her, MacIntosh finished her training shortly before leaving for China, in 1889. Yet MacIntosh had worked for a number of years before entering nurses' training and was already thirty-two when she sailed for China. Graham was thirty-one. Hiring such "old" women went against conventional mission wisdom. For example, in 1890, several articles written by Canadians and Americans from various Protestant denominations were published together in a book by B.F. Austin entitled *Woman: Her Character, Culture and Calling*. In a chapter dedicated to "Missionary Work in China," the author declared that single female recruits should be younger than twenty-five years, since it became more difficult after that age to acquire language skills.[26] By hiring two spinsters, the Presbyterian WMS may have hoped to avoid the problem of losing them to marriage, as happened with Sutherland.

MacIntosh and Graham were ideal mission candidates – experienced, educated, and evangelistic. Besides having trained as nurses, each had been familiar with all kinds of church work before coming to China. MacIntosh had been interested in the William and Elizabeth Street Missions in Toronto, and worked for more than ten years in city mission work before undertaking nurses' training to "fit herself better for foreign work."[27] She developed an interest in foreign missions through her pastor, Dr. Wardrobe. Both women were reportedly "devoted to winning women for Christ." Margaret MacIntosh (called *Ma Chiao Shih*) went on to serve in China for thirty-eight years in total, whereas Jennie Graham remained for less than a year.[28] Graham caught a cold en route to China and never regained her health. The cold was reportedly aggravated by bitter winter weather, a difficult journey inland, and unsanitary conditions in China's interior.[29] Graham resigned in January 1891 and returned to Canada.

Margaret MacIntosh: Sole Nurse for a Quarter-Century

Jennie Graham's untimely departure left MacIntosh as the sole WMS nurse in Henan for the next twenty-three years, until Maisie McNeely arrived in 1914. Initially, no appeal was made for a colleague for MacIntosh because of miscommunication between the Henan Presbytery (that is, the local mission governing body), the FMB, and the WMS. Although the WMS recruited, appointed, and sponsored female missionaries, in the hierarchical structure of the Presbyterian Church, the WMS was subordinate to the FMB. The FMB determined staffing needs and then made recommendations to the WMS. In 1891, the FMB decided that the work of single women missionaries was to be directed by the Henan Presbytery. The Presbytery assumed that the FMB was sending out another single woman, so did not make any requests. The FMB interpreted this silence as an indication of the Presbytery's "unfavorable attitude" toward single women, so no new missionaries were recruited.[30] Finally, a year later, in January 1892, the Presbytery forwarded a request for another single female worker. This time it specified a preference for "a fully qualified physician."[31] By August 1892, malaria and dysentery were sweeping through the mission, and the Presbytery's request for a doctor was upgraded to "urgent." Jennie Graham's sister, Dr. Lucinda Graham, arrived in 1892 to replace Jennie. That summer, the MacDougall family became ill, and Margaret MacIntosh accompanied them to the healthy air of the coast. The MacDougalls recovered, but the young sons of Dr. Frazer Smith and Rev. Goforth died.

Illness took a tremendous toll on early missionaries and their children. Cholera, dysentery, typhus, smallpox, and malaria were among the communicable diseases that plagued the Canadians. The death rate for children was the highest. In the first twenty-five years of the mission, nineteen children died; altogether, the Goforths buried five children in China.[32] MacIntosh's main nursing function was to attend to the physical needs of sick missionaries and their children, to provide companionship to missionaries during convalescence, to assist Dr. Frazer Smith with his medical treatment, and to sit with and observe Chinese postoperative patients operated on by Dr. James Frazer Smith, Dr. William McClure, Dr. William Malcolm, and, presumably, Dr. Lucinda Graham. In a letter dated 25 January 1893, MacIntosh outlined what she called "Encouraging Incidents" during her first three years as a North Henan missionary nurse. She provided one example of her nursing service: "There was work awaiting me here [in Sincheng], for almost immediately after our arrival I was called to sit up all night with a young girl upon whom the doctors had operated in the afternoon. The operation was of rather a serious nature, and a good deal depended on the care she received, especially at first."[33] It is interesting to note that despite the girl's need for "good nursing care," MacIntosh spent only one night caring for her. The following day, MacIntosh headed off to do evangelistic work, leaving the patient under her mother's sole charge. Even at this early date, it is clear that MacIntosh preferred evangelistic work over nursing, and she spent considerable time with other female evangelistic workers such as Rosalind Goforth, bringing the Christian Gospel message to Chinese women and children, at fairs, in Sunday school classes, and in their homes. Her main concern was not the state of health of these women and children, but the high rate of illiteracy among the women; it bothered MacIntosh that women were unable to read the tracts and printed hymns provided them.[34]

In 1894, Margaret MacIntosh's nursing skills were severely tested. MacIntosh was living with Dr. Lucinda Graham, the Frazer Smiths, and the MacVicars in their "rather restricted quarters" in Sincheng.[35] That summer, MacIntosh nursed Dr. William Malcolm's wife, Christina Malcolm, through a virulent case of smallpox. Mrs. Malcolm, a trained nurse from Guelph, was the only missionary wife during this period with nurses' training. She had always been considered to be of delicate health, and many criticized the FMB for having passed her as medically fit.[36] When Christina Malcolm was well enough to travel, MacIntosh accompanied the Malcolms to a resort in Japan to help restore Christina's health. They returned together to the treaty port of Tianjin in October 1894, only to find that Mrs. Malcolm was ill again – this time with cholera. Dr. Lucinda Graham was called to join MacIntosh and the Malcolms in Tianjin. Unlike Mrs. Malcolm, Dr. Graham was considered to be robust and strong. Her coworkers admired her jovial disposition and keen sense of humour.[37] While attending to Mrs. Malcolm, Graham contracted "a severe type of Asiatic cholera" and died after only eighteen hours of illness, on 13 October 1894. Mrs. Malcolm died eight days later.[38]

Margaret MacIntosh was stunned by the untimely death of her two friends. Compounding her sense of grief in 1894 was the unanticipated departure of Dr. Frazer Smith. While MacIntosh was nursing Mrs. Malcolm through smallpox during the summer, Dr. Frazer Smith became sick with typhus. Heavy medical and administrative duties combined with the "anti-foreign environment" of Sincheng had caused him strain, and he had been experiencing insomnia. He recovered from the typhus, only to be smitten by pneumonia. A thrombosis in his right thigh followed the pneumonia. By this time, Frazer Smith was critically ill and had to return to Canada. The journey home was no easy task in those days. Eight men carried Frazer Smith on a stretcher over the course of a mile to a river. He made the river journey to the treaty port of Tianjin by houseboat, and then took a steamer ship across to Canada – typically a four- to five-week trip. Travel from the port of Vancouver to Ontario was made by rail, on the newly completed Canadian Pacific Railway. Frazer Smith survived his ordeal but did not recover sufficiently to return to the harsh field of China. He was retired from the North Henan Mission in 1896. For her part, MacIntosh was "so shattered" by the deaths of Dr. Lucinda Graham and Mrs. Christina Malcolm that a furlough to Canada was advised.[39] She returned temporarily to Canada with the widowed Dr. William Malcolm.[40]

The tragic events related to illness in the summer of 1894 arguably changed the direction of missionary nursing in North Henan for the next three decades as nursing care became sporadic and informal, and attention shifted away from the care of Chinese patients to the care of missionaries themselves. It is ironic that firsthand experience with the virulent nature of communicable disease would stall, rather than jumpstart, the development of formal nursing services at the Canadian mission in Henan. By the same token, with the loss and departure of three trained physicians (Graham, Frazer Smith, and Malcolm) and two trained nurses (Mrs. Malcolm and Miss MacIntosh) that summer, perhaps it is more surprising that health care continued at all.

The lack of trained nurses at Henan meant that the task of attending to the sick had to be shared among the missionaries, particularly the physicians and missionary wives, who cared for ill children. Considering the prevalence of illness, it is little wonder that Maisie McNelly, the next WMS nurse appointed to the mission in 1914, was specifically directed to care for

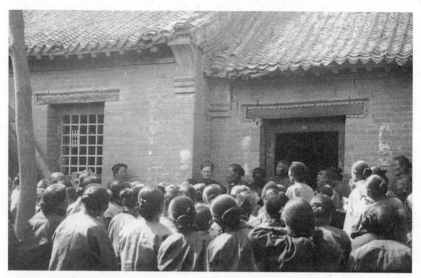

Figure 1 Margaret MacIntosh just before retirement, c. 1926.
UCCVUA 1999.001P/1737

missionaries and their families.[41] It was not until the 1920s that nursing attention turned once again to the care of the Chinese.

Although MacIntosh returned to China, and although she presumably helped to care for ill missionaries as necessary, there is no evidence that she ever took up formal nursing duties again. MacIntosh made the transition from nurse to evangelistic worker after 1894 with neither difficulty nor regret. In 1905, for example, MacIntosh spent 267 days holding classes in nine mission "out-centres" with Rosalind Goforth and Minnie Pyke.[42] Although she went on to work in Henan until age seventy (see Figure 1), MacIntosh's abandonment of nursing was considered by some as a shameful waste of talent. As Canadian missionary nurse Clara Preston (1922-47) later wrote, "How different the story [of the development of modern nursing before 1920] might have been if Miss Margaret MacIntosh, our first nurse, had used her gifts, with her courage and consecration in pioneering our nursing work instead of the evangelistic work."[43] Despite such criticism, MacIntosh's decision to pursue explicit evangelistic activity was not incongruent with the aims of the Presbyterian mission in Henan at the time. Nor was it inconsistent with the stated purpose of missionary medicine. Indeed, while nursing went through a period of dormancy in Henan, missionary medicine flourished and formed a foundation upon which professional nursing practice was eventually built. To understand the context from which missionary nursing emerged, we now turn to an examination of the nature of early missionary medicine.

Early Missionary Medicine: To Heal and to Preach

Take up the White Man's Burden
The savage wars of peace
Fill full the mouth of famine
And bid the sickness cease

– Rudyard Kipling, *The White Man's Burden,* 1899

From the outset, medical care was an integral part of the pioneer mission work of the Canadian Presbyterian mission in Henan. With two physicians and a nurse among them in 1888, the Henan Seven were, perhaps unintentionally, following in the footsteps of their missionary counterparts from other countries, many of whom were concentrating efforts on caring for the ill and injured in China. It had been more than fifty years since Dr. Peter Parker founded China's first hospital (1835) and medical training school in Guangzhou (1837). By 1890, thirty Protestant mission societies were involved in medical work; twenty-three had established mission hospitals.[44] Over the next thirty years, the number of mission hospitals in China would increase to 250, and within fifty years, at least seven different mission organizations would be operating hospitals in Henan alone (Canadian Anglican, Augustana Lutheran, Baptist, Catholic, China Inland Mission, Lutheran United Mission, and United Church of Canada).[45] Intentionally or not, the Presbyterian mission at Henan was part of a broader movement to establish Western medicine and nursing in China.

When they first arrived in China, it is possible that the Canadian Presbyterian missionaries hoped to eventually accomplish in China's harsh and remote interior what other foreigners were accomplishing in the internationalized treaty ports – namely, the development of dispensaries, hospitals, and training programs for physicians and nurses. But in 1888, their goal was not so much to bring a program of medical and nursing training to China as to provide direct medical treatment to individual Chinese. Through teaching and implementing Western theology and science, missionaries could root out physical, spiritual, and social disease: "Even a cursory examination of the four Gospels shows that healing and teaching or preaching were closely associated in the ministry of Jesus Christ ... the healing ministry of the missionary is parallel to the healing miracles in our Lord's public ministry ... and Christian workers in Mission fields earnestly desire to relieve bodily suffering, which is ever in evidence, as well as minister to the soul."[46]

Two of the earliest physicians in Henan had degrees in theology as well as medicine: Dr. James Frazer Smith (arrived 1888) and Dr. James R. Menzies *(Meng Yi Shi)* (arrived 1895). Yet it was the non-medical missionaries and mission boards, not the missionary physicians themselves, who tended to emphasize the value of medical practice as an evangelistic strategy, aimed at gaining the trust of prospective converts. Thus, while the earliest Henan missionaries considered medicine as an important component of mission work, there was disagreement over how much emphasis it should be given at the North Henan Mission. As long as medical practice supported the greater aim of the mission – that is, the establishment of a Christian community – it was welcomed and promoted. There was always the risk, however, that medicine's humanitarian purpose would overshadow its evangelistic purpose and that its concern with bodily suffering would take priority over concern with spiritual affliction. Thus, dissension arose whenever medical missionaries sought to expand their services. Jonathan Goforth, for one, perceived missionary medicine as simply a means to an evangelistic end. According to his wife Rosalind, Jonathan Goforth never veered from his evangelistic aims during his forty-eight years in China. As she later wrote, "[Goforth's aim was to put] aggressive evangelism *first* and in overwhelming proportion to all other phases of mission work. [He additionally urged] that any line of mission work, whether medical, education, or any other kind, could only be justified when made means to the one great end – the propagation of the Gospel of the grace of God in Jesus Christ."[47]

Goforth's convictions were consistent with those held by his contemporaries in other parts of China. According to what was being published in early Methodist and Christian Reformed missionary literature, for example, China "was opened to the Gospel at the point of a lancet [by Dr. Parker]," that "medicine has been the wedge used to open doors of hundreds of unfriendly homes," and that medical missionaries there were "[winning their] way to the hearts of the people and find[ing] opportunity multiplying upon [them], every day and hour, for preaching the Gospel in the most effective way."[48] Similarly, the Missionary Education Movement of the United States considered missionary medicine as an important means of "converting many to Christ."[49] Physicians were expected to be as effective at teaching the Christian message as they were at alleviating physical suffering. In Henan, Rev. Murdoch MacKenzie believed that "the doctor longs as ardently as the pastor to see [patients] become followers of Jesus Christ, and they often know him as a spiritual adviser before they receive his medical attention."[50] Henan missionary Margaret Brown also held this view, later writing that medical work in Henan served two purposes: "One, to bring people to the Chapel within sound of the Gospel and two, to show the love of Christ in deed."[51] Of these, the "first was the more important." Yet while non-physicians wrote about medical practice as an evangelistic strategy, physicians themselves focused their attention on treating physical ailments. The apparent demand for treatment of physical symptoms left little time for anything else. While memoirs by Rev. Goforth and Rev. MacKenzie emphasize the importance of preaching to patients, Dr. Frazer Smith's memoir focuses on specific

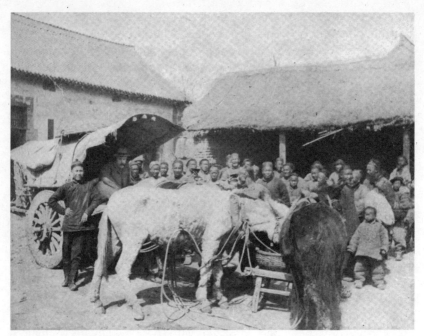

Figure 2   Dr. William McClure at a village inn, c. 1900.
Murdoch MacKenzie, *Twenty-five Years in Honan*

experiences with individual patients and on the tremendous need for medical care.

Shortly after arriving in China in 1888, Dr. James Frazer Smith and Dr. William McClure took some journeys through the countryside in mule-drawn carts, looking for potential patients and converts (see Figure 2). They attracted curious crowds of up to three hundred people, and estimated that seven out of every ten of those gathered were in need of medical treatment or surgical aid.[52] Common ailments included blood poisoning, dysentery, typhoid, smallpox, pneumonia, malarial fever, plague, boils, "felons," abscesses, toothaches, tumours, and blindness due to cataracts or trachoma. The need was overwhelming.

Memoirs written by Dr. Frazer Smith in 1937 provide a rare glimpse into the early days of missionary medicine in Henan. The medical kit for his journeys, Frazer Smith wrote, comprised "a pocket-case of instruments, a small assortment of medicines, and three pairs of forceps for extracting teeth."[53] News that one of the strange foreigners was a doctor would "spread rapidly," and soon large numbers of "sick-folk ... the maimed, and especially the blind," would crowd the courtyard of the inn where the missionaries spent the night. Frazer Smith helped many in the crowd on the spot but estimated that, for every one he treated, he turned six away. He dreamed of the day when the Canadians could build a hospital "where all who were sick and suffering could be treated."[54] When he became sick with typhus and pneumonia in 1894, Frazer Smith experienced feverish dreams. His recollection of these gives some insight into the prevailing view among medical missionaries that China's most urgent need was for medical facilities and "proper" hospital care: "When delirious, one source of great anxiety to me was the vast numbers of Chinese ... who seemed to be coming in an unending procession, a boundless sea of pained and troubled faces, hundreds and thousands, afflicted with all manner of diseases and putrid sores, all clamouring to be relieved of their pain and suffering ... Over and over again, as I tossed to and fro, my call sounded out, 'They're coming! They're coming! More room! More room! Make the hospital ready!'"[55]

Although mission narratives emphasized the need for, and practice of, evangelism, a tension existed between evangelistic expectations and the demand for medical treatment. For example, American author Harlan P. Beach noted in 1905 that physicians in China "are always tempted to leave to others the ministration to soul needs."[56] Similarly, Mrs. Howard Taylor of the China Inland Mission in Henan brought attention to the difficulty of integrating medicine and evangelism when she cited an article "written by Dr. Gibson" beseeching physicians to "save men and women, boys and girls, from spiritual death, which in horror, hatefulness and pathos far exceeds the mere corruption of flesh and blood. The command is plain, but it is appallingly easy to put time and brains and strength into the medico-scientific side of one's work to such an extent that the command is all but forgotten. This is, at any rate, the experience of the writer ... it is far easier to spend oneself in the operating room or in the office than in the quest for souls."[57]

At the Canadian Presbyterian mission at Henan, physicians did not necessarily ascribe to the mandate "to heal and to preach." For example, Dr. William McClure's son, Dr. Robert McClure, later insisted that his father "was strictly medicine [and] never did any preaching or anything like that." Then again, William McClure was also, according to his son, "a notorious liberal, and regarded as quite lost by many of his senior colleagues in the theological field."[58]

There is evidence that the dual practice of healing and preaching was exaggerated in mission reports at the Presbyterian mission. For example, in Murdoch MacKenzie's 1913 memoir published by the Presbyterian FMB, an early photo featuring Dr. James R. Menzies standing and reading before a small, Chinese audience is entitled "Preaching to Patients," but the caption of the original photo reads, "Dr. Menzies with his workmen at morning prayers" (see Figure 3).[59] There is a subtle but significant difference between the notion of patients receiving biblical instruction from a physician before receiving medical care, and employees participating in morning prayers.

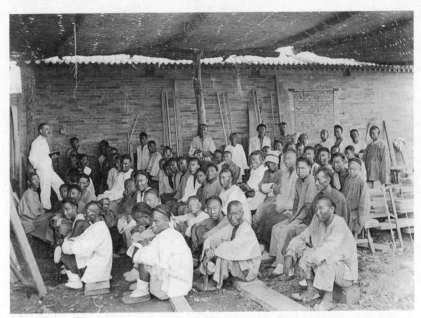

Figure 3   Original photograph later published as "Preaching to Patients," c. 1910.
UCCVUA 1999.001P/1712 N

Illness and injury makes patients particularly vulnerable to exploitation, making it possible that conversion to Christianity could be interpreted as the "cost" of treating ailments, or Christian rituals as magical cures. But to Canadian audiences at the time, a photo depicting a missionary physician preaching to patients would have affirmed that medical missionaries were doing what they were being paid to do.

The medical work of Dr. James Frazer Smith and Dr. James Menzies produced two early defining moments of the missionary work in North Henan that solidified support for medical missionaries within the Presbyterian community, and inadvertently contributed to the decision of at least one Chinese woman to enter nursing practice. Two of the earliest Henanese to embrace Christianity, Chou Lao-Chang and Li Chi Ching, were blind patients cared for by Frazer Smith and Menzies.[60] "Old Blind Chou" was the first Christian convert. Prior to his conversion, Chou was an opium addict and a low-status *yamen* runner (policeman) whose eyesight had begun to fail in his forties. After meeting Goforth and Menzies at a large fair in 1889, Old Chou had his cataracts removed by Dr. Frazer Smith a year later. He had been blind for seven years and now could see. In 1892, Chou and his son were baptized as the mission's first converts – an event heralded and chronicled in mission discourse as proof of the value of the mission. In an analysis of conversion stories, Margo Gewurtz suggests that descriptions of the conversion of Old Chou written by Frazer Smith in *Life's Waking Part* and the Goforths in *Miracle Lives of China* are actually "colonizing texts" insofar as they locate Old Chou within the corrupt imperial system, then narrate the story of blindness, cure, and conversion.[61] Pointing out inconsistencies between private and public accounts written by Frazer Smith, Gewurtz suggests that the Canadians ignored or distorted the facts (by, for example, leaving Chou's opium addiction out of the accounts and misrepresenting him as a scholar rather than a low-status *yamen*) and projected their own interpretation (and therefore agenda) onto the events. Still, this was the beginning of a Chinese Christian community in North Henan, which itself became central to the development of nursing there. Not only was Chou's granddaughter among the first group of Chinese students to enter nurses' training at the Weihui Hospital in 1923,[62] but the Church of Christ in China became the main pool from which Chinese nursing students were drawn.

Choosing Missions: Perspectives on Women's Work for Women
Jonathan Goforth's original appeal for single missionary women in 1888 was catalyzed by information from other missionaries that a strict gender separation existed in Chinese society. Missionaries with the China Inland Mission (CIM), for example, perceived that the "better class" of Chinese women was isolated from all men, whereas poorer women, who were "compelled by circumstances to be seen and move about freely," were not as isolated but were inaccessible to male strangers, including male missionaries.[63] Interestingly, in Murdoch MacKenzie's assessment of the issue, gender separation in Henan does not appear to have been as restrictive as that portrayed by the CIM. As MacKenzie described it, if Chinese women were found listening to men in public places, it would be a "violation of custom" if women were seen to be engaged in conversation with men in public places.[64] Although this would change, the prevailing view of missionaries at the time was that Chinese mores forbade interaction between Chinese women and male missionaries. Thus, only women could work with women. In *Woman: Her Character, Culture and Calling*, B.F. Austin of the CIM reported that openings for women's work in China in 1890 were "practically unlimited," and the need for additional workers was "very urgent."[65] Although almost half of the CIM missionaries in China at that time were single women, there were estimates that "the proportion of *three* or *four* lady workers to *one* male missionary would not be too large" because of the unique nature of women's work in China.[66] To the CIM, women's work was a particularly important Christian ministry because "when Jesus Christ came He found women systematically degraded, debased, imbruted by philosophy and pagan religion. He came, her truest friend, to give her a social resurrection, to formulate principles and illustrate them ... The tendency of Christianity is to lift woman up, to elevate her to a higher plane. It has given to woman a

larger sphere and has increased her intellectually."[67] If women's mission work in China was a virtuous calling, missionary nursing was an almost beatific vocation. In *Woman,* nurses Florence Nightingale and Clara Barton were praised as "moral queens ... nursing the world's ills and shedding the radiance which alone springs from Christian women over battle fields, hospital and home."[68] Accordingly, prospective missionary nurses to China could expect to become "missionary angels stooping to lift the whole world's girlhood and womanhood, its wifehood, motherhood and widowhood up to the realization of God's ideal of woman."[69] Such social elevation of women missionaries offered unmarried, educated, and religiously devout Canadian women an unprecedented and socially sanctioned opportunity to fulfill personal ambitions.

In a similar way, the Canadian Presbyterians believed that the "rightful destiny" of woman could not be reached apart from Christ, and that "nowhere outside of lands influenced by His Gospel has a woman been accorded her rightful sphere."[70] Christian women were to be treated with respect. This is not to say that women had authoritative equality, however. The WMS was subordinate to the FMB, and Presbyterian women in Canada and China could be neither elders nor voting members of the Presbytery in the Presbyterian Church.[71]

Canadian Presbyterian women interested in missionary work in China were not restricted to working with the Presbyterian WMS. Those who were interested in becoming missionaries had the option of joining the interdenominational CIM. But despite its attractive views on the eminent role of women, the CIM held other, less appealing views. First, unlike the salaried Canadian Presbyterians, CIM missionaries were expected to be entirely dependent on unsolicited contributions. Second, CIM missionaries were expected to adopt native dress and live among the Chinese themselves, whereas the Presbyterians lived together in small clusters – which later grew into large, walled, insulated (and insular) communities. Third, while the CIM insisted that their women workers be young (preferably less than twenty-five years in age), the Presbyterians came to prefer older women. Finally, the CIM did not value preconceived "methods and plans" as much as the Presbyterians did. To the CIM, the most important characteristic of a prospective missionary was "unreserved consecration and submission to the will of God, and that filling with the Holy Ghost without which the most earnest work will fail and be ineffectual. To be filled with the spirit is supremely important."[72]

Being "filled with the Holy Spirit" involved relying completely on God, trusting Him for daily requirements, direction, and, when necessary, miraculous intervention. Devotion and zeal were more valuable than particular skills or goals. God would lead. While Rev. Jonathan and Rosalind Goforth held a CIM-like view of missions as wholly reliant on an "outpouring of His

Holy Spirit" that would come only through regular prayer, scripture study, a surrender of one's will, and suppression of personal desires, the North Henan missionaries as a group were arguably more pragmatic and academic than the CIM. The Presbyterians valued educational preparation, institutions and governing bodies, and pre-determined goals. Prospective Presbyterian missionaries were required to have formally professed their Christian faith and commitment to evangelical ideals; they were also required to have specialized skills, of which nursing was one possibility.

Beliefs about Health and Illness

New missionaries in China invariably commented on perceived environmental differences between Canada and China. Early missionary physicians focused on the presence of unsanitary – and disease-causing – conditions, including offensive odours, sewage, dirt, and insects. To the Canadians, bringing the gospel of soap and water, light, and fresh air was an essential task – and one that was later taken up by nurses. As Dr. James Frazer Smith wrote,

> the reason why such a large proportion of the people are ill and suffering is the general lack of scientific knowledge and skill, and the woeful ignorance among all classes, of the fundamental principles of health and hygiene. Add to this the want of proper nourishment, of shelter and heat, the absence of all sanitary precaution, the myriads of germ-laden mosquitoes, the unhindered multiplication of fleas, flies, bedbugs, lice and all other disease carriers, the wonder is that there are so many people in China who are healthy and vigorous. The theory of "survival of the fittest" is fully exemplified, as the mortality in infancy and childhood is very high, and only the most robust children are able to survive.[73]

Perhaps what is most interesting about Frazer Smith's description is not the presence of unsanitary conditions, but that, despite these, *something* was contributing to health and vitality among the Chinese. Frazer Smith recognized the value of traditional Chinese medicine, crediting the Chinese for "their efforts in research work, as some native works on medicine go back to about twenty-five hundred years before the Christian Era."[74] Similarly, North Henan missionary Murdoch MacKenzie noted that some native methods of treatment were beneficial, and that "certain herbs are known to have marked value in the relief of certain forms of disease."[75] Despite any acknowledgment of the value of Chinese medicine, however, Henan was considered a land of Western medical opportunity. According to CIM missionary Mrs. Howard Taylor, Henan was dubbed "the open sore of the world."[76] Henan seemed to be teeming with communicable disease, dental abscesses, infections, and tumours – conditions that medical missionaries were generally equipped to effectively treat.

In light of Western science, the traditional Chinese theories of the cause and cure of disease seemed very crude to foreign missionaries. At best, Chinese medicine was seen as an outmoded approach to disease – valuable to a degree, but outpaced by advances in Western scientific knowledge. Chinese practitioners were limited by their "background of physiology, physics and philosophy" and by their "crass ignorance in regard to the causes of diseases and their means of remedy."[77] At worst, Chinese medicine was perceived as superstitious, arcane, and even harmful. According to F.L. Hawks Pott in 1913, "In nothing perhaps is [China] more bigoted than in its own ancient system of healing."[78] Most disturbing to Dr. Frazer Smith was the Chinese belief

> that all diseases are the work of evil spirits, and that these spirits must be driven forth to effect a cure. There is scarcely anything more weird than the procedure they follow in driving out the demon. An exorcist is engaged at a good price, who comes with a large number of his followers carrying cymbals, drums and horns, together with some of their idols ... What with the clanging of cymbals, the beating of drums and the roar of so many voices shouting out their incantations, the wonder is that anyone recovers ... If, as too often happens, the patient dies, then another evil spirit gets all the blame.[79]

Christians were not unfamiliar with the idea of demon possession. New Testament scriptures are filled with examples of Christians driving out evil spirits who were thought to cause a myriad of ailments in their human hosts. Yet Canadian medical missionaries were more inclined to look for scientific causes and effects. They considered the rational science of medicine to be a "saner method of dealing with disease" than Chinese superstitions and traditional rituals.[80] To North Henan missionaries, Chinese beliefs about evil spirits were rooted in the religion of Daoism. Murdoch MacKenzie wrote that the effect of Daoism was to bring Chinese into "bondage with demons, and to innumerable spirits of the dead." He criticized practices such as burning mock money made of yellow or white tinsel in the shape of ingots "to ward off imaginary evils" as an enormous waste.[81] Some Chinese beliefs, such as the understanding that "invisible agencies" cut off queues (long single braids worn by men) and kidnapped children, may have seemed bizarre to MacKenzie, but beliefs such as this had a direct impact on the relationship between the Chinese and early Canadian missionaries. Just as missionaries thought the Chinese had peculiar rituals, the Chinese believed that "the barbarian doctor" had strange and potentially harmful practices. The *yanggui* (foreign devils) were believed to bewitch people and to capture children and gouge out their eyes for medicine. Jonathan Goforth agreed with MacKenzie's perception in his comments about 1893, a year of anti-Christian riots: "They say that we kidnap these little ones and scoop out their eyes and cut out their hearts to manufacture our medicines ... [a mandarin made a proclamation] warning parents to keep a sharp eye on their children."[82] Goforth took such claims to mean that the Chinese were amazed by the efficacy of foreign medicine; such efficacious medicine must contain something precious. At the same time, missionaries reported that fear and dislike of foreigners seemed to seethe beneath the surface of every interaction. Even the most cordial and polite interactions could erupt into violence, and curious crowds could turn hostile – shoving and kicking, unsheathing knives, or showering the missionaries with "clods and bricks."[83] In the mission narrative, danger always lurked. This narrative of danger was central in the early mission record, and was closely related to the narrative of survival that came to characterize the Presbyterian mission in Henan as a whole, including missionary nursing.

One particularly poignant example of the danger/survival narrative is described in Dr. James Frazer Smith's memoirs. Shortly after the Canadians were established in Anyang (1894), a group named the "Blood Spilling Guild" rushed into the compound yard brandishing knives, their faces and hands smeared with their own blood. According to Dr. Frazer Smith, this group attacked missionaries MacVicar and MacGillivray and held them for five hours. Frazer Smith, returning from a trip, describes unwittingly stumbling into the middle of the commotion and being told that the guild was demanding monetary compensation for the life of a man killed in the Canadian yard. Frazer Smith was taken to the "dead man," who was smeared with blood and lying on a plank. After feeling the man's beating heart and recognizing the ruse, Frazer Smith indignantly "gave him a smart tap on a very responsive part of his person which made him squirm and cry out"; the attempt at extortion was abandoned.[84] In this narrative, Frazer Smith renders himself a champion of sorts, whose knowledge of illness, injury, and death thwarted the enemy. After the missionaries survived an attack by bandits during the Boxer Uprising, the danger/survival narrative that came to characterize missionary work in Henan was set.

The Boxer Uprising and "Our Thousand Miles of Miracle"

From the perspective of Canadian nurses at the North Henan (later North China) Mission, missionary nursing was a dangerous and uncertain profession. Periods of growth and progress were punctuated by local and national disturbances that brought the mission to a standstill – and nurses expected it to be that way. From the beginning, the North Henan Mission was thought of as a dangerous mission field. In 1888, CIM founder Hudson Taylor warned Jonathan Goforth of the anti-foreign nature of Henan, stating "Brother, if you would enter that Province, you must go forward on your knees."[85] According to Rosalind Goforth, "go forward on your knees" became a slogan for early missionaries. There were advantages to working in a dangerous field. Church audiences at home were eager to hear stories of mission adventures; stories of hardship, illness, and pain underscored valued characteristics such as courage and self-sacrifice, and pointed to God's providential care. The dramatic events of 1900 crystallized the Canadian view of China as an inherently dangerous field and of the missionaries as having God's protection and favour.

The Boxer Uprising *(Yihe Duan)* of 1900 was named after a violent movement in China against non-Chinese commercial, political, religious, and technological influence in China. A number of anti-European secret societies had been formed, the most aggressive of which was the "Righteous and Harmonious Fists" *(I-ho-ch-uam)*, dubbed by Westerners as the "Boxers." To the Canadian missionaries, the Boxer Uprising would be remembered as an attack on them and their Christian message. All told, the Boxer Uprising claimed the lives of 188 Protestant missionaries, 22 Roman Catholic priests and nuns, and thousands of Chinese.[86] The Boxers were defeated by foreign powers: a combined group of twenty thousand British, Japanese, Russian, American, and French troops "liberated" Tianjin on 14 June and Beijing on 14 August 1900. A peace treaty known as the Boxer protocol required the Chinese to pay indemnities for damages and ensured Chinese dependence on foreigners for years to come.

On 28 June 1900, the missionaries decided to evacuate their mission because of rumours of increasing anti-foreign violence. The month-long journey by cart and boat from Henan to Shanghai, later called "Our Thousand Miles of Miracle" by Rosalind Goforth, was, by all accounts, a frightening experience.[87] Yet far from discouraging the missionaries, the series of tragic events along the journey was eventually interpreted as evidence of God's provision. That is, five of the fifteen adults sustained serious injuries in an attack on their caravan, but it was "a miracle" that none were killed; many of the group received minor injuries, but it was a miracle that their unattended, dirty wounds did not become infected; John Griffith and nine-year-old Paul Goforth went missing one night (and were given up for lost), but by a miracle the two were reunited with the group. Furthermore, it was a miracle that, in the frantic search for Griffith and Goforth, the group inadvertently prevented another attack on their lives. Finally, although four of the missionary children died of disease in the summer of 1900, it was a miracle that no one died from violence.

According to various later mission reports, rumours of "bands of Boxers crossing the river" intensified during the spring and summer of 1900; the "political situation was becoming daily more threatening ... the very air felt electric."[88] In Anyang, there was a rumour that a roving band of fifty or more men was planning to march on the mission station, with the purpose of "destroying the property and massacring the foreigners,"[89] and there was talk of an impending attack in Chuwang.[90] On 5 March 1900, Rev. W. Harvey Grant *(Ge Wende)* travelled from Chuwang to Huilong in response to a letter dispatched by Miss Margaret MacIntosh and Mrs. Martha MacKenzie indicating that a mob was threatening them, and asking that help be sent promptly.[91] Rev. Grant found everything quiet, but escorted the ladies back to Chuwang. In April, Dr. Malcolm took his second wife Eliza to the coast after she became "inconsolably depressed" and "on the verge of a nervous breakdown" following the birth of her second baby.[92] Her fragility was later attributed to the nervous anticipation that was affecting everyone to various degrees: Eliza was simply the "first to succumb."[93] Still, the missionaries stayed on.

On 25 April 1900, a reported two thousand Boxers attacked Roman Catholics near Baoding, north of Anyang. And on 1 June 1900, Boxers reportedly killed Reverends Robinson and Norman of the British Society for the Propagation of the Gospel.[94] Although, as Margaret Brown later suggested, the "Boxer and Big Sword Societies were growing very bold and outrageous," the missionaries stayed.[95] In retrospect, their decision to stay appears foolhardy, given all the purported signs of trouble. Yet Murdoch MacKenzie and Rosalind Goforth would later explain that they felt obliged to remain with the Chinese Christians, who were also under threat but could not escape,[96] and Margaret Brown would suggest that Chinese officials in Henan were showing themselves to be friendly and helpful.[97] Once they decided that their presence might "endanger the lives of their native brethren," the missionaries felt free to leave.[98]

On 10 June 1900, all postal services to Henan were cut off. Within a few days, the Henan missionaries received belated telegrams from the American Consul in Zhifu urging them to escape south because the northern route toward the treaty port of Tianjin was unsafe.[99] Shortly afterward, on 20 June, missionaries received the startling news that Drs. Wallace, McClure, and Menzies and their families had all been murdered en route to Beidaihe. While the message proved to be false, the missionaries decided to leave. The group of Canadian evacuees was composed of six young children and seventeen adults, including nurse Margaret MacIntosh and two Chinese Christians.[100] On 28 June, the group began a two-week journey across Henan into the province of Hubei by a caravan of ten large farmer carts "resembling gipsy wagons" with coarse straw mats and quilts as awnings to protect them from the scorching sun. On 8 July, having just spent an uneasy night at Hsin-tien, the group headed out into the streets with their cavalcade of carts. According to John Griffith, one of the missionaries,

The whole street was densely packed with a mob seething with scarce-suppressed excitement ... One could judge that not fewer than ten thousand were out to see what was going to happen to the fugitive "foreign devils." During our passage along the street an ominous silence reigned; but once outside the town gate it soon became apparent what had been prepared for us. On one side stood a group of more than one hundred villainous looking men armed with swords and other weapons ... no sooner had the carts entered into [a short stretch of deep road ahead] than, with a wild yell, the attackers rushed upon us with a volley of heavy stones ... followed by a rush with swords.[101]

All told, five men in the group were seriously injured. Dr. Leslie's wrist and knee were slashed and broken, and he had a serious wound on his instep. Rev. Griffith had gashes to his palm, fingers, and forehead, and MacKenzie had a sword cut on his head. Rev. Goforth was struck on the back of the neck and head with a two-handed sword, and his left arm was slashed to the bone. Cheng Pi-Yueh, one of the Chinese Christians who accompanied them from Henan, received at least two sword wounds. After the attack, robbers searched the carts and stripped them of any valuables, with the robbers "slashing the cart ropes, dragging off and smashing open boxes and trunks and fighting each other for the contents."[102] Most of the group spent the day at the roadside, where they were "exposed to the taunts and jeers of a curious and ribald mob."[103] Dr. Dow bound up Dr. Leslie's wounds with her underskirt. The Goforths, for some reason, went by themselves to a nearby village where, according to Rosalind Goforth's account of the events, Jonathan collapsed in the street surrounded by his weeping children: "As my husband sank to the ground apparently bleeding to death, the [village] women all began to weep. This moved the [village] men to pity ... they gathered around seeking to help... [one man] quickly returned with the palm of his hand piled up with a fine gray powder with which he filled the great open wound at the back of the head, instantly stopping the flow of blood."[104] Murdoch MacKenzie found the Goforths and brought them back to the rest of the group, which then pushed on to the nearby city of Nanyang (still in Henan), where "the Roman Catholic fortified refuge outside Nanyang was being besieged at this time, and the threats were that our party was to be murdered at that spot in order to terrify the Catholic Mission people."[105] Having been refused a place to stay in Nanyang, the Canadians hired an escort of a dozen foot soldiers and headed out in the early hours of the morning, only to notice that John Griffith and nine-year-old Paul Goforth were missing. After two hours of frantic searching, "Mr. Goforth said that we must go on as the whole party would be in danger if we waited."[106] The group arrived safely in Sinyeh thirty hours after their violent attack and fell asleep on the *kang* (brick bed) and earthen floor of an inn. Griffith and Paul Goforth showed up at midnight, barefoot and shirtless. Griffith later reported that he had taken Paul off their cart after becoming suspicious of the Chinese escort accompanying the Canadians out of Nanyang; Griffith had seen some of the guards whispering together and putting swords up their sleeves, and he intended to follow the carts from a distance. The pair got separated from the caravan, but followed a river and eventually caught up with the rest of the group.

On 10 July 1900, the group travelled safely from Sinyeh to Fancheng, arriving in Shanghai on 27 July, where they met up with Dr. and Mrs. McClure. The unanimous opinion of the group was that all women and children should return to Canada for their safety – except Dr. Margaret Wallace, who was accepted to work at the British Weihaiwei (Weihai) Military Hospital (at Weihai, Shandong – not to be confused with Weihui, Henan) as a "nurse."[107] Arrangements were made for early furloughs, and Margaret MacIntosh, who was due furlough in 1902, travelled back home to Toronto. After a rest of just three months, MacIntosh took up deputation work in Canada, sharing her missionary experiences with local congregations. Her return to China was delayed by a year due to her ill health.[108]

However the missionaries viewed their experience at the time, their realization that a number of missionaries and Christian Chinese were killed in China that summer no doubt catalyzed their collective perception that they had miraculously survived. When the Conference of Mission Boards in New York reported on 15 September 1900 that sixty adults and children from three American missions perished in the Boxer violence, the Canadians' escape "appeared a veritable miracle of God."[109] Just as the Canadian Presbyterian periodical *Westminster* hastened to publish the story of the missionaries' "miraculous escape" on 1 September 1900, subsequent missionary memoirs emphasized eleventh-hour provisions, dramatic reunions, and startling individual missionary tenacity.[110] The sad reality is that not everyone actually survived the ordeal: four Canadian children died in a two-month period. Florence Goforth, the seven-year-old daughter of Jonathan and Rosalind, died of meningitis on 19 June 1900; the baby of James and Elizabeth Slimmon died on 10 July, one day after the missionaries arrived in Fancheng; and two other children – the Menzies' six-month-old son and the McClures' youngest daughter – died shortly after the families returned to Canada for furlough in August 1900.[111]

Through the events of 1900, failure and loss were viewed through a lens of victory and survival. Furthermore, the sense of loyalty (God's loyalty to the missionaries; missionary loyalty to the Chinese; Chinese Christians' loyalty to the missionaries) contributed to the missionaries' collective sense of purpose and protection that would see them through crises still to come.

Missionaries learned that, if they could survive the Boxer Uprising, they could survive anything. The other message was that the violence could happen again – which it did. Over the next five decades, missionaries in Henan would evacuate again three times, in 1927, in 1938, and in 1947.

Summary

Despite its enthusiastic beginnings, in terms of nursing progress, the North Henan Mission was arguably further behind in 1900 than it was in 1889. Compounding the unanticipated loss of nurses Harriet Sutherland and Jennie Graham was the unforeseen loss of nursing's original supporter, Dr. James Frazer Smith. It fell to Margaret MacIntosh to carry the "nursing lamp" alone. It is not surprising that nursing development virtually stopped after 1894, given all the barriers to nursing. For example, the Presbyterian WMS became disenchanted with hiring nurses, MacGillivray protested the presence of single women in Henan, missionary physicians displayed no interest in nursing assistance, and the mission officially valued evangelism over medical service. In addition, Margaret MacIntosh was personally inclined toward evangelistic teaching. Without a hospital to work in, other nurses to collaborate with, or a physician to assist, her shift to full-time evangelistic work was inevitable. Furthermore, it is possible that MacIntosh's experience with the deaths of her friends Dr. Lucinda Graham and Mrs. Christina Malcolm repelled her from close contact with potentially contagious patients. Finally, there were times when sheer survival demanded MacIntosh's full attention, particularly during the Boxer Uprising. Thus, while Canadian nurse Louise Clara Preston later criticized MacIntosh for the lack of nursing progress in North Henan, there seems to have been little to support its development at the end of the nineteenth century.

The events experienced during the Boxer Uprising set the tone for the North Henan Mission during the upcoming decades, and arguably influenced the expectations and attitudes held by missionary nurses who arrived after MacIntosh. That is, those who lived through the "thousand miles of miracle" came to see their experiences as evidence of God's provision, protection, and divine favour toward them and their missionary endeavours. To the missionaries and their supporters, the greatest proof of God's protection was that none of their group was fatally wounded during the Boxer Uprising – even though four children died during the same period. Perhaps the most important result of the Boxer Uprising for the Canadian missionaries is that they came to see themselves as survivors. Sixty years later, Dr. Percy C. Leslie made the interesting observation, "my wife who had been a semi-invalid when we started our long uncomfortable journey had become strong and self possessed ever since the tragic attack made on us."[112] Tragedy, hardship, and pain were not to be feared or avoided. When the second generation of nurses began to arrive after 1914, they came with an assurance that, although the work could be arduous and dangerous, they could count on God's protection and intervention. Nurses looking for personal growth and meaningful work could find it in China, regardless of whether they achieved any significant professional accomplishments.

2
Visions Interrupted, 1901-20

> Measure thy life by loss and not by gain ...
> He who suffers most has most to give.
>
> – Jonathan Goforth, Sermon in the Hospital

Picking up the Pieces

When some of the Canadian missionaries returned to Henan in September 1901 – a year after their dramatic exodus – officials at Chuwang and Anyang unexpectedly welcomed them. The Canadians found themselves guests of honour at feasts and official calls. This first group of Canadian returnees found that, although their houses needed considerable repair, their Anyang property had been relatively well protected and many of their personal belongings had been safely preserved. Chuwang and Sincheng did not fare so well. The chapel and the small hospital at Chuwang lost doors and windows, the dispensary lost its wooden floor, the two residences were beyond repair, and the contents were entirely gone.[1] Taking advantage of the promised Boxer indemnity, the missionaries made a claim for money to refurbish the site.[2]

Missionaries not only found unanticipated support by the Chinese, but they also enjoyed increased financial support from the homeland. The eyes of the world had been on China during the Boxer Uprising. Canadian Presbyterians who may not have paid much attention to their China missionaries before 1900 took notice now. In Toronto, Bloor Street Church requested permission to support Dr. James and Davina Menzies over and above their regular offerings; St. John's Church made a similar request for Rev. T. Craigie Hood.[3] Backed by enthusiastic financial promise, the missionaries began to reconstruct the mission stations. By April 1902, more missionaries had returned to Henan, including Dr. Jean Dow, Minnie Pyke, Mrs. Davina Menzies, and Mrs. Menzies' three-year-old daughter Jean. Margaret MacIntosh, who had not been well, delayed her return to Anyang until November 1902.[4] (See Figure 4.)

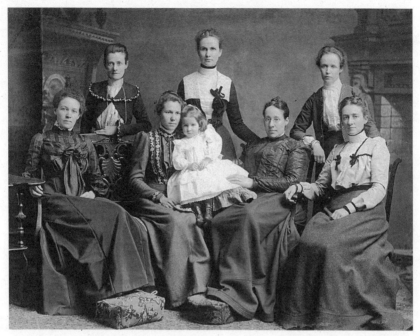

Figure 4 Female missionaries, c. 1903. *Left to right, standing:* Margaret MacIntosh, Jean Dow, Eliza Malcolm; *seated:* Martha MacKenzie, Davina Menzies, Jean Menzies (child), Rosalind Goforth, Minnie Pyke.
UCCVUA 1999.001P/2502

The Noisome Pestilence

By mid-1902, the Henan Mission was "buoyantly hopeful."[5] It now occupied three prefectural cities: Anyang, Weihui, and Huaiqing. Dr. Dow and Miss Pyke were "rejoicing" that Miss MacIntosh was sufficiently recovered to "join them and help to seize the wonderful new opportunities opening up for women workers."[6] The three women moved in together at a residence built for single missionary ladies at Anyang, and enjoyed a sense of companionship, if not single-mindedness. Perhaps not surprisingly, Margaret MacIntosh did not work with Dr. Jean Dow when the latter began a women's hospital at Anyang. Instead, she "did a lot of traveling in the rural areas in training women in Bible School and general evangelistic work."[7]

For the Henan missionaries, personal exposure to communicable disease quickly took precedence as their most pressing concern in 1902. In July, a cholera outbreak reached Anyang, and Dr. James Menzies recommended that the missionaries boil their water, buy no fruit and only minimal vegetables, and eat nothing uncooked. The missionaries agreed, but found it difficult to convey these precautions to their Chinese cooks. Dr. Menzies was also concerned about the missionaries' regular exposure to the seventy

Chinese construction workers and the crowds of patients and their friends. Despite his private fear of contagious disease, Menzies wrote that the Canadian missionaries were used to contagious disease and that "in the noisome pestilence He preserves us."[8] Dr. Menzies was not the only one concerned about contracting disease. Dr. William Malcolm and his second wife Eliza were exposed to tuberculosis on their journey from Tianjin to Henan in September 1902. Not only were the boatman and his family coughing, but the boat was infested with mosquitoes, lice, cockroaches, and "very large rats."[9] The Malcolms attempted to protect themselves with mosquito nets, which kept the rats from running over their faces. After their arduous journey (which also included the sinking of their boat and a subsequent rescue by the Goforths), the Malcolms arrived in Henan on 16 September 1902 with mixed feelings about returning to China. Their trouble, as it turned out, was only beginning.

Within days of the Malcolms' arrival, a telegram sent from the Henan Mission at Huaiqing announced the death of Rev. T. Craigie Hood from cholera on 19 September 1902. Shortly afterward, little Wallace Goforth and his sister Constance fell ill with dysentery. Wallace recovered, but Constance died, a day before her first birthday. She was the fifth Goforth child to be buried in China.[10] Dr. Malcolm expressed concern about the Goforths' Chinese-style house – presumably because it was dark and airless – and blamed the Goforths' cook for the illness in the household. And like Dr. Menzies, Dr. Malcolm faulted the Chinese construction workers for carrying disease into the mission compound.

The Canadians' experiences of illness, death, and violence influenced some of their subsequent decisions about new construction at the mission stations. They built large, airy, foreign-style houses with the hope of diminishing risk of communicable disease (see Figure 5). They placed walls and gates around their expanding compounds in attempts to control the entrance of those people with contagious germs, as well as to prevent the entrance of those with violent intentions. According to Dr. William McClure's son Robert, who was born in 1900 as a Boxer exile and reared in Henan, the walls and gates of the compound served as protection against anti-foreign riots.[11] At the time, little thought was given as to the effect these decisions would have on the Chinese.[12] Later, the walls and foreign-style buildings (not to mention the restorative summer holidays at coastal resorts) came to symbolize – and amplify – the disparity between foreign missionaries and their Chinese neighbours.[13] But in the early 1900s, such protective measures seemed both prudent and necessary.

A year after the deaths of Craigie Hood and Constance Goforth, the missionaries were again faced with serious illness. The newly arrived Rev. Harold M. Clark *(Jia Zhenbang)* contracted cholera while still en route to Henan via the coastal city of Tianjin, and Dr. Malcolm's son was seriously ill. Dr.

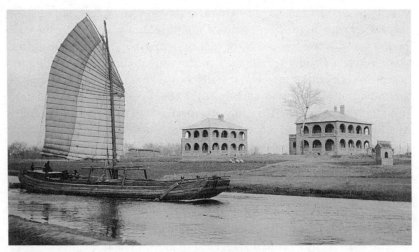

Figure 5 Missionary homes at Weihui, along the Wei River, 1915.
Mary Struthers McKim private collection

Malcolm and Dr. Menzies successfully treated Dr. Clark with "numerous injections of brandy, to which the heart and pulse responded," attributing Clark's survival to the fact that he was "a total abstainer."[14] Dr. Malcolm found himself at a crossroads. Having experienced the death of his first wife and the nervous breakdown of his second, he consulted with the others about what to do about his ill son. He agreed with their opinion that he return to Canada with his family. Dr. Malcolm reluctantly resigned and took his family back to Canada. There his son later died.[15] Despite the ongoing and serious threat of illness in Henan, it would be another twelve years before an additional nurse was appointed to the mission.

Early Hospitals and Dispensaries
The Henan Mission maintained a policy of having a dispensary and hospital at each large station where missionaries resided. Before 1894, Dr. Frazer Smith had expressed his concern about the risk posed by having "hundreds of diseased people with no knowledge of contagion or infection, crowding into the small yard where the staff with little children lived."[16] Self-protection, he thought, demanded separate buildings for in-patients ("bed patients") and outpatients. An early priority was the construction of dispensaries, which were typically connected to chapels by a waiting room.[17] In Sincheng, the chapel itself doubled as a "hospital" where relatives "did the nursing."[18] Before 1900, overnight patients stayed at hostels, found a room with friends, or rented a room at one of the inns. They were fed and cared for by family members. In-patients who required special care, such as post-cataract patients, were kept within the compound, staying either in the "street chapel" or in one of two small rooms "fitted up" especially for this purpose.[19]

In 1903, Dr. McClure moved with his family to Weihui.[20] According to his son Robert, the original hospital was primitive and built within the compound walls. It was composed of "Chinese-style buildings" because "that was the type of building that the Chinese were accustomed to living in." "Chinese-style buildings" were typically a series of small, square rooms built around a centre courtyard. Each building could have a different function: one might serve as a kitchen while others served as bedrooms. To Dr. Robert McClure, "the theory of that type of hospital is extremely good. The idea is that you don't bring the person into a strange environment; you bring them into an environment something like he would have himself. Largely his relatives prepare his meals for him so that he is fed the things that he would get at home [and] the cost of feeding the patient is kept at a very low, low rate."[21]

Over time, although the Canadians still made regular medical trips into the countryside, more patients travelled to meet them at the mission compound. After 1900, patients would come to the dispensaries and primitive hospitals over long distances, as far as one hundred miles on foot. They made the pilgrimage as a last resort after traditional medical measures had failed.[22] In early 1903, little medical work was being done at Weihui, and none at Huaiqing. Dr. McClure (Weihui) was occupied in Tianjin attending to Rev. Clark until October 1903, and Dr. Menzies (Huaiqing) was preoccupied with construction plans. The medical work at Anyang, however, increased steadily. More than seventeen thousand patients were treated at Anyang in 1903 (the average number of patients per day was forty-eight). Six new buildings had been erected, and the old buildings were transformed into a bright dispensary and a chapel, and a separate women's hospital. There was an increasing number of in-patients and, according to the physicians, surgical work made considerable advances. For example, for the first time, a person consented to an amputation at the wrist and knee, while another consented to a partial tongue amputation. Most of the surgery was of the eyes. Dr. Leslie reported that out of the 177 operations he performed that year, 86 were on the eye. (See Figure 6.) In 1904, Dr. Menzies began his medical work at Huaiqing, and Dr. Malcolm joined Dr. McClure at Weihui. Dr. Malcolm "plunged at once into medical work," reportedly providing 11,125 treatments and performing 135 operations that year. At Anyang, the annual number of patients treated increased to more than 23,000 (averaging 63 per day), plus an additional 1,125 treated by Dr. Dow at the new women's hospital.[23]

The Canadians were not the only Protestant missionaries expanding their medical work in 1904. That year, forty-one international mission societies, including the Henan Mission, reported operating 318 "dispensaries or hospitals" in China.[24] Most of the hospitals were small and relatively unsophisticated "native-style" hospitals where patients stayed in shelters in which

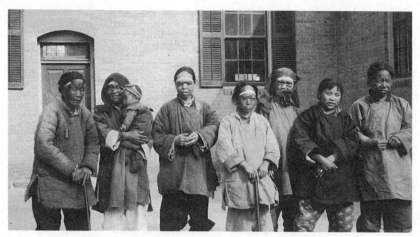

Figure 6 More patients for eye treatment, c. 1915-30.
UCCVUA 1999.001P-2395N

their families cooked and cared for them.[25] The oldest missions ran most of the hospitals: twenty belonged to the London Missionary Society (est. 1807), twenty-six to the American Presbyterian Board (est. 1845), and eighty-five to the China Inland Mission (est. 1865). By 1910, there were forty-seven mission societies administrating 435 hospitals and dispensaries in China.[26]

The subject of separate hospitals for women was controversial for the Henan missionaries. When the mission asked for two single women workers in 1903, it stressed that they were to be for evangelistic and *not* medical work. The members of the Weihui station reportedly felt that "it would be a useless and unnecessary expense to open women's medical work at this station, and the majority of the Missionaries in the field, including the ladies at Anyang Fu, sympathise with them in this view."[27] Rev. W. Harvey Grant and his wife Dr. Susan (McCalla) Grant did not see a need for separate women's work. Having come from India where women's hospitals were absolutely necessary for the women "shut in zenanas," Rev. Grant was impressed with how freely Chinese women moved about. Dr. Jean Dow, however, remained committed to the idea of a separate hospital for women, and worked at the women's hospital at Anyang until her death in 1927. Subsequent missionaries criticized Dow's commitment, since "excellent medical work for women was being done in both Weihui and Huaiqing for many years in one General hospital without even a woman doctor."[28] This was a complete reversal of opinion from the 1890s, when the Henan Mission vigorously endorsed the Western ideal of separate women's work for women. Why the change in sentiment? Possibly the initial, collective opinion of Jonathan Goforth, Thomas Paton, and Hudson Taylor – that only female missionaries could access Chinese women – was erroneously based. Since most of the

American and British missionary experience to that point had been in cosmopolitan treaty ports such as Tianjin, the idea that men's and women's work should be separate may have been accurate for urban communities, but not for rural Henan. Whereas upper-class, urban Chinese women were secluded, rural women in China's interior were not.[29]

As committed as Dr. Dow was to women's medical work, there is no evidence that she ever appealed for a nurse for her hospital. Nor did Dr. Percy Leslie, Dr. James Menzies, or Dr. William McClure ever appeal for one. To Margaret Brown, the "Henan medical folk did not seem to place a high value on the contribution of nurses [despite the fact that] Dr. Frazer Smith ... had set them a fine example."[30] In 1888, Dr. Frazer Smith had a vision of a thoroughly equipped hospital, moderate in size, staffed with three doctors and at least two graduate nurses. A quarter-century later, the sole WMS nurse busied herself with evangelistic work, and Frazer Smith's vision was still not realized. Although the original medical missionaries never did endorse nursing service, some of the younger medical missionaries began to ask why nursing services were so lacking. The issue was formally raised in 1909.

Recognizing a Need for Modern Nursing Services
In May 1909, Dr. William J. Scott, a Henan missionary for three years, reported to the Henan Presbytery on the Huaiqing medical work, stating that he "deplored" the deficiency of nursing facilities there.[31] According to Dr. Scott's son, both Dr. Scott and his colleague Dr. O. Shirley McMurtry were "shocked" to discover that "what was called a hospital in Henan" was "totally lacking in nursing service."[32] Their request to improve medical facilities – in part via a financial grant from McMurtry's father – was favourably received at first. Rev. Jonathan Goforth and other elders later objected to the scheme, however, on the basis that it would undermine the evangelistic priority of the mission. The Henan Presbytery turned down the money, stating that it could not accept a grant that would be meant for materialist and non-religious purposes. The young physicians subsequently quit China because of the Henan Mission's refusal of the money, plus its negative attitude toward modern medicine. Years later, Dr. McMurtry was still bitter. He told his son that Goforth and some of the older missionaries perceived medical treatment as "just bait to bring in people for salvation."[33]

The Henan Mission's rejection of the young physicians' plan in 1909 may have been a symbol of its unswerving devotion to what it saw as the greater Christian ideal of preaching and teaching, rather than a rejection of modern medical progress per se. The first generation of missionaries, led by Goforth, was firmly committed to the idea of evangelism first. One notable exception was Dr. William McClure, who, "as one of the few liberals" in the mission, was "completely polarized [from Goforth] in theology." McClure saw the practice of medicine as his main focus. At the same time, he was content with the old Chinese-style hospitals, and it was "not his piece of cake to design a new modern hospital with modern nursing services and that sort of thing."[34] The second generation of medical missionaries, on the other hand, was committed to both the primacy of medical practice and the idea of building modern hospitals and providing state-of-the-art medical service. While Henan medical missionaries before and after 1900 perceived a strong relationship between Jesus' preaching and healing ministry, the younger missionaries coming out to China saw alleviation of physical suffering as a priority, and were keen to capitalize on advances in modern science to achieve the goal of health for Henan. The subsequent, subtle shift in emphasis from evangelism to medicine can be traced back to the mindset of the post-1900 group of missionaries.

For some, like Drs. Scott and McMurtry, it seemed ludicrous not to take advantage of new science, technology, and funding sources. For others, even if they came to China with the idea of evangelizing, the reality of the physical needs of the population stirred a desire to respond in more temporal, pragmatic ways. This is exemplified by the explanation given by Rev. Andrew Thomson *(Tangshan)* for his active support of a hospital project in Daokou in the 1920s. Thomson, who arrived in Henan in 1906, later defended his controversial action by saying: "But, you say, why not be satisfied with your evangelistic work without taking on the responsibility and burden of attempting to run a hospital? I have with more or less devotion been giving my life to preaching and teaching. But how far can you go in teaching the life of Jesus without coming up against the sick folk of Galilee?"[35]

Although there had always been a difference of opinion and personality in the Henan missionaries, the rift that formed between the older and younger generations of medical and nursing missionaries would eventually grow into a fissure. For the time being, the conservative Henan Presbytery stood firm. It could not justify accepting McMurtry's grant money in 1909. It *could,* however, request new nurses – provided that the nurses' function was primarily evangelical, since evangelism was still the "sole purpose for bringing out a nurse."[36] In its next list of needed recruits, the Presbytery requested five female evangelists, "two of them with nurses' training." As it was, no nurses responded to the appeal.[37] Among those who *did* respond, however, was Miss Margaret R. Gay *(Gai Magu)*. Gay was appointed to Henan as an evangelistic worker in 1910. Thirteen years later, she took up nurses' training at the Vancouver General Hospital, and subsequently worked as a missionary nurse in Henan until 1941. As will be seen, her story exemplifies the shift from evangelism to service at the North China Mission. Through her progression from evangelistic missionary to professional nurse, Gay found a way to integrate and embody both evangelistic and nursing ideas.

In October 1911, China was in the midst of another national crisis – the "First Revolution." After the Boxer Uprising in 1900, the Chinese government under the Manchu Qing Dynasty was considered hopelessly enfeebled and out of step with the rest of the world.[38] The Empress Dowager Cixi Taihou, who had ruled China for forty-seven years, died in 1908, leaving two-year-old Aisin-Gioro Puyi to ascend the Qing throne. A series of anti-dynastic movements in 1911 culminated in the overthrow of the Qing Dynasty. Dr. Sun Yat-sen was elected first president of the new Republic of China. The political turmoil did not directly affect the missionaries in North China. They were preoccupied with another threat – the pneumonic epidemic. Medical missionaries from all over North China offered their services to the government and, according to Yuet-wah Cheung, helped to get the epidemic under control. The epidemic was stopped.[39] Western medicine, Cheung asserts, was officially recognized in China after its worth was proved during the pneumonic epidemic, which signalled a turning point in the Chinese attitude toward Western ideas.[40] Dr. Robert McClure stated that suddenly it was a great thing to be Western: "[The Chinese] began to wear Fedora hats. They began to wear long-john underwear in the wintertime I remember. It was the mark of the modern man and to show that you had it, you wore it [over top of other clothes] ... Those fellows felt absolutely 'the last word in modernity.'"[41] As Western ideas gained popularity in China, missionaries reported a new level of acceptance.

The Second Generation of Nurses: McNeely, Gay, and Ratcliffe

The focus of the Henan Mission was changing. While the older missionaries valued evangelistic practice, the newer missionaries were not so interested in direct preaching and soul winning.[42] The 1911 revolution opened up new opportunities for medical missions in general and for nursing in particular. The Christian Medical Association of China published an article entitled "The Work of Medical Missions in 1911," which had a section on nursing that stated: "This has undoubtedly been the weakest side of Medical Mission work. Raw material for nurses, male and female, has been the only material available for each centre started ... Experts are needed for teaching, and efforts are being made on all sides to better present conditions. Social conditions now permit of lady nurses coming to China as matrons both to men's and women's hospitals."[43] The Henan Mission's opposition to medical endeavours in China may have been unique, but its disinterest in nursing was not. In 1911, the China Medical Commission had found that only one in two hospitals had a nurse and that there were only 140 nurses in all of China. Western missionaries had founded the Nurses Association of China (NAC) in 1908 with Mrs. Hart as the first president and Miss Maude Henderson as the secretary, but they accomplished little during the first three years. It was Miss Nina D. Gage, a graduate from Wellesley College in

New York City, who gave new impetus to the NAC in 1912. The NAC was first and foremost a missionary organization. Its "theology" was "stated in seven words: For God so loved that He gave."[44]

American missionary nurses had been keenly involved in the development of professional nursing in China from the beginning. Miss Elizabeth McKechnie (later Thompson), the first trained nurse to come to China, arrived in Shanghai in 1884.[45] Five years later, American and British missionaries were providing nurses' training, mostly in coastal cities. In 1912, the Americans were again at the forefront of nursing development in China. Nina Gage called a meeting in Kuling, where the new nursing association drew up a constitution. The NAC aimed to raise the standard of training, adopting a uniform course of study, uniform examinations, and uniform rules governing candidates for the association's diploma for nurses in China. Miss Gage was elected president of the NAC in 1914 and later became president of the International Council of Nurses.[46] The purpose of the NAC was to set a standard for nursing schools in the country, formulating a curriculum and holding certificate examinations. It also planned "a great national conference to be held at regular intervals to discuss plans for future development."[47] Because no term for "nurse" existed in Chinese, Elsie Mawfung Chung, a 1909 graduate of Guy's Hospital in London and the first Chinese nurse to be trained abroad, consulted with sinologues to come up with an appropriate term. Under her recommendation, *hu-shih*, a term meaning "caring scholar," was adopted by the NAC in 1914. Suddenly nursing seemed a viable profession.

In 1913, the China Medical Missionary Association (CMMA) met in Beijing, where the association expressed the purpose of medical missions in China. Medical missionaries were not to be considered as a "temporary expedient for opening the way for the Gospel, but as an integral, co-ordinate and permanent part of the missionary work of the Church."[48] The group of medical missionaries envisioned a cadre of union medical colleges at Shenyang, Beijing, Jinan, Chengdu, Hankou, Fuzhou, and Guangzhou, where different mission organizations could work together to "bring blessing and healing to the souls and bodies of the people of China and to give young men and women training in Medicine and Surgery."[49] Not only were nurses considered "indispensable" in all hospitals associated with medical colleges, but it was thought that a foreign-trained nurse should be present in every large hospital in China. The Henan Presbytery discussed a report from the CMMA meeting, and approved of the "idea" of entering union medical work with an established medical college. The Presbytery later chose the Shandong Christian University ("Qilu" University) at Jinan rather than the Peking Union Medical College (PUMC) in Beijing, not only because it had a long-standing relationship with Qilu, but also because courses there would be taught in Chinese, whereas the PUMC planned to teach in English. As a result of the CMMA report, the Henan Mission pressed the FMB to appoint more doctors, and sent cost estimates for a new modern hospital at Weihui. Ironically, by the time the Henan Mission was ready to consider expansion of its medical work in this way, Drs. Scott and McMurtry had already resigned, in 1912 and 1913, respectively.[50]

After the "Christian Medical Association of China" (apparently an alternate name for the CMMA) prepared a pamphlet in 1913 that urged mission boards to have at least one foreign-trained nurse in each hospital, the Henan Mission appealed to the Foreign Mission Board (FMB) for a fully qualified Canadian nurse – but not for hospital work.[51] This nurse was to care for missionaries and their families, who, in turn, would pay the Henan Mission for her services. Any spare time she had might be spent in the hospital. In response to the request, and on the recommendation of the Woman's Missionary Society (WMS), the FMB appointed Miss Mary Elizabeth (Maisie) McNeely to Henan in 1914. McNeely started her tenure with language study, along with other new Henan missionaries, including Rev. H. Stewart Forbes, Dr. Ernest B. Struthers, and Miss Sadie Lethbridge.[52] McNeely became engaged to Rev. Forbes. She resigned from the WMS in 1916 and transferred to her husband's board, the FMB. Although she was no longer officially a WMS missionary nurse, McNeely Forbes remained involved in nursing work at Henan until 1940 by occasionally volunteering her nursing services. The Henan Mission, now keen to have a nurse, sent a request to the FMB for McNeely's replacement before she even married. None was ever sent.[53] Nursing progress was thwarted, once again.

It was not only medical missionaries who perceived a need for expanded medical service in Henan in 1914. Non-medical missionaries such as Rev. Andrew Thomson also felt burdened by the presence of illness around them. Similarly, evangelistic worker Margaret Russell Gay was daunted by the medical needs at Wuan, a small mission outstation where she worked from 1914 until 1920 (see Figure 7). There had been a fledgling Canadian hospital at Wuan, but its two physicians had to leave for health reasons, and it was closed. The empty hospital haunted Gay, who later wrote,

> We passed the [hospital] buildings day after day, knowing that inside were beds, drugs, instruments, equipment of every kind, but neither nurse nor doctor to carry on any work of healing for the many thousands in all that countryside who looked to our Mission for help in time of sickness. I traveled through the towns and villages in that region, but never could ask any sick person to come back with me to the Hospital. Never could I offer anything in the way of medical care, yet people would be carried many miles, arriving at our houses asking for help that they thought would surely be there.[54]

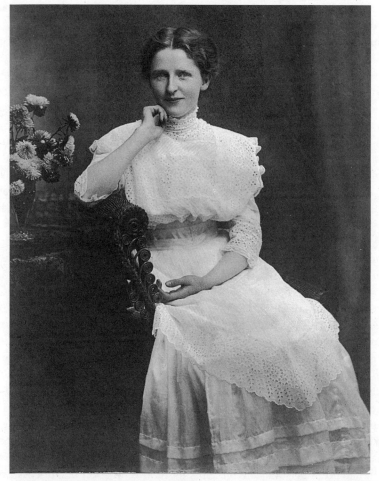

Figure 7   Margaret Russell Gay, c. 1910.
UCCVUA 76.001P-2110

Eventually Gay acted on her desire to learn more about nursing by entering nurses' training at the Vancouver General Hospital. In the meantime, she sent to the Evans' Bookstore in Shanghai for "books on Nursing." These books, whatever they were, were deemed "helpful," but not enough. She later sent for "a correspondence course in nursing" from the United States, but it is unclear what came of this.[55] As will be discussed later, it was not until her furlough in 1922 that Gay was able to pursue her nursing dream.

Margaret Gay's decision to shift from a focus on evangelism to a focus on nursing is a benchmark in the development of nursing services at the Presbyterian Mission in Henan, and stands in sharp contrast to Margaret

MacIntosh's decision to pursue evangelistic opportunities over nursing service. Unlike the appointment of the first three nurses in 1888 and 1889 in response to requests by the mission (Frazer Smith's desire for an assistant, Goforth's desire to provide care to Chinese women, and the prevalence of missionary illness), Gay's decision to pursue nursing was based on requests by the Chinese themselves. MacIntosh studied nursing in Toronto to lend practical support to her evangelistic work; Gay studied nursing in Vancouver to lend practical support to the Chinese.

The first appeal for a hospital nurse in Henan came from Dr. Fred Auld *(Oerde)* in 1915. Land had been purchased for a large modern hospital at Weihui, and Dr. Auld, who had arrived in Henan in 1910, was making plans for it. He took a tour of eighteen mission hospitals in ten large centres and noticed that most had, or were in the course of making provision for, nursing services. Thus, Dr. Auld requested a Canadian nurse for full-time work in the hospital-to-be at Weihui. He also asked for permission to send a young Chinese man to a school of nursing to equip himself for taking charge of work in the men's wards; the male nurse would work under the direction of Dr. Auld and a foreign matron. The older medical missionaries were divided in their opinion of Dr. Auld's proposal. Dr. Leslie did not agree with it, but Drs. McClure and Menzies seconded a motion to accept it.[56] It is interesting that Dr. William McClure seconded the motion since he had no personal interest in developing a new modern hospital with modern nursing services. He realized, however, "that these hospitals must come to China."[57] Two months later, Dr. Auld specifically requested that trained nurse Mrs. Jeanette C. Ratcliffe *(Yao Xiuzhen/Rao Xiuzhen)* be appointed to the position of matron of the new Weihui Hospital. The appointment was made.[58]

Ratcliffe would become a key figure in Henan nursing over the next quarter-century (see Figure 8). For all her public accomplishments, however, Ratcliffe's personal life remains mysterious. Mission documents extol her professional work, and fellow missionaries describe her as "well-loved," but the silence surrounding her pre-Henan life is striking.[59] How did Ratcliffe come to the Henan Mission in the first place? She was born in St. Catharines, Ontario, in 1876, which would have made her thirty-four years old when she came to Henan in 1910 as the matron of the school for missionaries' children. Evidently Ratcliffe volunteered her services: the WMS did not actually appoint her until after Dr. Auld's proposal in 1916, and her home church (First Presbyterian) did not designate her as a missionary until 1918. Oddly, even her mission records do not list her maiden name; her biographical file simply calls her Mrs. J. Ratcliffe.[60] Mrs. Ratcliffe was a widow before coming to Henan.[61] Some clues to Ratcliffe's background come from the work of Ruth Compton Brouwer in her study of Canadian Presbyterian women in Central India between 1876 and 1914.[62] In a table listing Western Division missionaries at North Henan, Brouwer lists a Jeannette *McCalla*

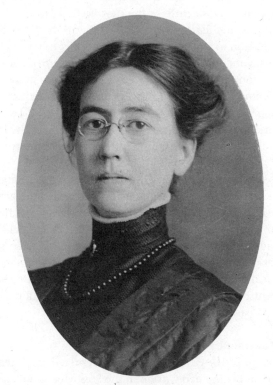

Figure 8 Jeanette C. Ratcliffe, c. 1910.
UCCVUA 76.001P-5373

Ratcliffe. Elsewhere, Brouwer notes that the "McCalla" sisters went to China.[63] It thus appears that Jeanette Ratcliffe was the sister of Dr. Susan (McCalla) Grant, who married Henan missionary Rev. W. Harvey Grant in 1902, while they were both serving in India.[64] It seems reasonable to speculate that Jeanette Ratcliffe, after suffering the death of her husband, came to Henan at the invitation of her sister. She occupied herself as the matron of the small boarding school for missionary children, which would have included some of her own nieces and nephews. Since Ratcliffe was trained as a nurse, the opportunity to become the first matron of the new Weihui Hospital must have seemed propitious.

Ratcliffe had already completed nurses' training and one year of university when she came to China in 1910.[65] When she was appointed as the Weihui Hospital matron in 1916, there was not yet a hospital. As Ratcliffe awaited its construction, she took a furlough to Canada, where she completed a postgraduate course – possibly in administration – at Toronto in 1917. Afterward, she spent time on staff at Qilu, the Shandong Christian University Hospital at Jinan. Although everyone seemed to be in agreement with the idea of having Ratcliffe as the new Weihui Hospital matron, not everyone supported her desire to further her education. When Ratcliffe first requested permission to work at Qilu, the Henan Mission was divided: nineteen voted in favour, and thirteen expressed disapproval. Some felt that Ratcliffe should come directly back to Henan for language study, while others agreed to her going only if Henan missionaries did not require her nursing services for themselves. Eventually, the Presbytery and WMS board approved of her plans, and for a year Ratcliffe was "Acting Matron of the Hospital and Nurses' Training School [at Qilu] during the absence of the regular Matron on furlough."[66]

The time seemed ripe for developing nursing services and nursing education in Henan. In 1918, one of the graduates of the mission's girls' school at Anyang entered nurses' training, possibly at Qilu. This is the first record of a North Henan girl entering the nursing profession. That Ratcliffe was dedicated to her nursing work was apparent not only in her keen preparation, but also in her particular and significant contribution to the development of professional nursing in Henan. It is a tribute to Ratcliffe that her final accomplishment before retiring in 1940 was the completion of a book on communicable disease for nurses, written in Chinese.[67]

The Great Movement Forward, Interrupted

In the autumn of 1916, Henan missionaries entered the Great War. The British minister in Beijing had written to the Presbyterian mission at Henan asking for missionaries to volunteer for service in France because of their knowledge of the Chinese language. Doctors were needed to staff a Chinese general hospital, while non-medical men would be in charge of Chinese labourers recruited in North China to work in France.[68] Rev. Andrew Thomson's son later wrote, "Thirty-two missionaries wrestled with their consciences and priorities. Each had chosen the difficult, all-absorbing life of a missionary and its demands of language, health, physical stamina and spiritual strength. Now, they faced a call to defend their King and country, which appeared to be in mortal danger. In the end, fourteen missionaries, including most of the medical staff, went off to France. Thus, the Great War took precedence over the Great Movement Forward in Henan."[69]

The male missionaries left Henan for France in the summer of 1917. Meanwhile, a "second nurse" had been appointed to the mission.[70] Miss Janet Lillian Brydon, a graduate of Victoria Hospital in London, Ontario, arrived in Henan after the doctors had already left for France.[71] Brydon was born in Eramosa Township, Ontario, in 1886, and received her First Class Teachers' Certificate from the Faculty of Education at Kingston. She tried teaching but found it was "not her calling." After hearing an address by Dr. Waters of India, Brydon decided to give her life to the church. She took nurses' training at the Victoria Hospital, followed by a public health course. Brydon

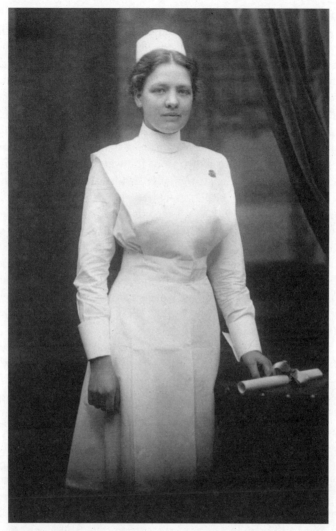

Figure 9 Janet Lillian Brydon, Victoria Hospital, London, ON, c. 1910.
WCMA ph 14851

graduated in 1916 with India as her goal. Her two older sisters were also nurses. To the Brydons, intelligence was a gift from God; to ignore it would be ungrateful to Him.[72] After spending a year at the Presbyterian Deaconess Training School in Toronto, Brydon applied to the WMS to become a missionary in 1917. Rather than India, she was sent to China (see Figure 9).[73] She was designated at the Barrie Hill Church in Eramosa, Ontario, on 13 July 1917, and was presented with a Bible and a "purse of gold."[74]

By the time Brydon arrived in Henan, the development of nursing was no longer a priority. Dr. James Menzies and Dr. Isabelle McTavish *(Mei Xiuying)* had remained behind in Henan, but the departure of the others for France slowed down any significant medical progress. Brydon stayed in Huaiqing to study Chinese, even though by that time, new Henan missionaries typically took their first year of language study in Beijing. Staying in Huaiqing allowed Brydon to "give first aid to missionaries if any occasion arose."[75] Brydon spent her first three years "on the staff of the hospital at Huaiqing," but nursing progress seems to have come to a standstill as the missionaries waited for the physicians to return from the war.[76] Most of the Canadian missionaries returned to Henan well after Armistice Day on 11 November 1918 (and as late as 1921). Little was written about the Henan Mission during the years 1917 to 1919. Perhaps records were scarce because the usual chroniclers were off at war. Or maybe the experiences of war and the simultaneous Spanish influenza pandemic were, as Dr. Bob McClure once said, "too complicated" to write about.[77] Finally, the reason the missionaries did not reflect much on the events of 1918 and 1919 may have been that the "great tragedy" of 1920 subsequently overshadowed other reminiscences.

The Menzies Murder

On 17 March 1920, missionaries Janet Brydon and Sadie Lethbridge were alone in the WMS house at Huaiqing, in the "Ladies Compound," preparing for their duties the next day. According to later accounts, their servants were all attending a wedding feast in the Chinese quarters of the "other" Henan Mission compound on the other side of a small road (the two compounds were connected by an overhead brick bridge). At 10:00 p.m., Sadie "viewed with satisfaction her box, ready packed for the long-delayed evangelistic tour in the country" and tucked a roll of twenty silver dollars into the box.[78] At the same time, nurse Janet Brydon prepared for bed. Suddenly, a loud sound of crashing glass brought them rushing into the hall; each thought the other had fallen and broken a lamp. As the sounds continued, Brydon and Lethbridge looked over the second floor railing and saw men breaking into their front door below. Panic-stricken, each fled to her own room, and slammed and locked the door. Looking for a hiding place, Lethbridge went out onto the verandah outside her bedroom, climbed over the railing, and "clung precariously" to the outside of one of the huge brick pillars, her toes gripping an inch-wide ledge as she hid from the robbers. Brydon's room did not have a verandah. She extinguished her lamp and went through the French window onto the flat roof of the kitchen "just as the robber's axe crashed in her door."[79] When a lighted lamp revealed Brydon, she began to call loudly for help. Brydon was surrounded and forced back inside, where the robbers made her open locked drawers while they demanded money and ransacked her room.

From her position clinging to the pillar, Sadie Lethbridge saw Janet Brydon being forced back into her room. Lethbridge called for help. Within minutes, she heard the sound of footsteps running along the walk on the other compound, where the married missionaries lived. Lethbridge saw a figure on the bridge that connected the two compounds, standing and listening. In a subdued voice, Lethbridge called out to the figure. She recognized Dr. James R. Menzies' voice when he reportedly asked, "What's the matter?" Lethbridge responded that there were "many" robbers. After telling Lethbridge that he was not armed, Menzies disappeared from her view. Lethbridge heard Menzies call loudly for the men inside to hurry out. Then she saw two men grapple on the lawn below her – Menzies and a man who had apparently been below the bridge standing guard for the robbers. Lethbridge watched as the intruders rushed out of the WMS house and surrounded Menzies and the other two. She saw flashes and heard two shots. The band, numbering about twenty, hurried off, with twenty-five silver dollars, a gold watch, and a fur garment.[80]

Lethbridge returned inside and, finding Janet Brydon unharmed, went out with her to the lawn where "Dr. Menzies lay moaning in great pain."[81] While Brydon knelt down beside him to administer some nursing care, others appeared and assisted Menzies into the house on a stretcher. He had two wounds – one in the shoulder and one in the abdomen. Menzies knew he was dying, and after stating that his will and money were in the safe, he "requested morphia." Menzies' medical assistant reportedly "rushed out to the dispensary while Mr. [Rev.] Slimmon prayed," but before the assistant returned, Menzies had died.[82]

At the time of Menzies' murder, many of the Henan missionaries were gathered at Weihui for a Presbytery meeting. They received a telegram from Huaiqing stating that Menzies had been shot, but did not know until they arrived in Huaiqing on the next train that he had died.[83] The Henan missionaries were shocked. This was the first time in the perilous history of the mission that the tragedy of a violent death had occurred. Menzies, who had been close to retirement after twenty-five years in China, had become a martyr. Not surprisingly, much was made of the fact that Dr. Menzies had chivalrously come to the aid of the two single female missionaries. The April 1920 edition of the *Henan Messenger* – a weekly newspaper previously edited and occasionally printed by Menzies himself – was dedicated in memoriam to Rev. James R. Menzies, M.D., D.D. Chinese and Canadian friends and colleagues filled the entire issue with articles extolling his "unwavering devotion to duty," "courage," "Christ-like habit," and "selflessness, " which led Dr. Menzies to make "the supreme sacrifice," giving his life for another: "Greater love hath no man than this," they wrote, "that a man lay down his life for his friends."[84] Menzies would forever be remembered for his sacrifice.

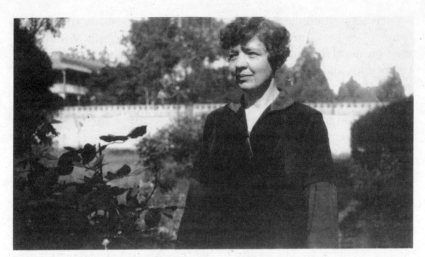

Figure 10 Janet Brydon in a China garden, c. 1920s.
Howard Parkinson private collection

Janet Brydon and Sadie Lethbridge had two very different reactions to
Menzies' death. Brydon moved forward with her nursing work, rarely men-
tioning the incident. In all Brydon's records reviewed, there is only one
mention of her participation in the tragedy. In 1993, Rev. Doug Brydon
recalled that Brydon had been "one of two nurses in charge of running a
hospital in Hunan [sic] ... when the director of the hospital was killed during
a bandit raid on the hospital."[85] One can only speculate on the effect this
experience had on Brydon. It is a testament to her tenacity that she continued to work as a nurse in Henan for two more decades, until 1939.[86] (See
Figure 10.) Sadie Lethbridge did not fare so well. According to her friend
Margaret Brown, Lethbridge "never really recovered from the shock of that
night."[87] As those around her venerated Dr. Menzies, saying, "the Doctor
had died for the ladies," Lethbridge reproached herself, wondering how things
might have been different had she not called or had she warned him of the
guard at the gate. Lethbridge cringed at the thought of facing Mrs. Menzies
and the family, who were in Canada at the time of Menzies' death.

While the Henan missionaries mourned, Mrs. Davina (Robb) Menzies and
her three daughters were unaware of his death. Mrs. Menzies had gone home
to Toronto for her daughters' schooling, and she was in poor health herself.
Her oldest daughter, Jean – who was in her first year of nurses' training at
the Toronto General Hospital – had just interrupted her schooling because
of an attack of rheumatic fever. On 24 March 1920, Canadian newspapers
reported that a J.R. Menzies had been killed in "Sichuan." It was not until
26 March, nine days after Menzies' murder, that the Menzies women received a long telegram from Huaiqing confirming the tragic news. Menzies'

funeral service, conducted in Chinese, had already been held in Henan, on 22 March.[88] On 28 March 1920, a memorial service for Dr. Menzies was held at the Bloor Street Church in Toronto. The church, which had already pledged $30,000 toward the building of a "Bloor Street Hospital" at Huaiqing, promised to build an "even better" hospital than it had planned; it would now be called the "Menzies Memorial Hospital."[89] Three years later, Jean Menzies and her mother Davina returned to Henan as missionaries themselves.[90]

Sadie Lethbridge died four months after the attack on Dr. Menzies. She continued to be "haunted" by her participation in the tragedy and was transferred to Anyang for a "change in scenery."[91] Lethbridge started feeling unwell, and on 28 June, Dr. Dow diagnosed her with dysentery. It was hot in Anyang. Some days reached a sweltering 108 degrees Fahrenheit in the shade. Although missionaries usually escaped the heat by heading to mountain or coastal resorts in the summertime, Lethbridge's illness kept her in Anyang, where her attendants cared for the bedridden Lethbridge on the residence verandah. She died on 28 July. To the Henan missionaries, Lethbridge's death was directly related to the emotional trauma she had suffered.

All told, four Canadians died in 1920. Added to the missionaries' grief in 1920 were the deaths of one-year-old Donnell Clark (23 March, of "convulsions") and eleven-year-old Hedley Auld (31 October, of dysentery). The dysentery at Weihui was "of a peculiarly virulent nature," and two weeks after Hedley's passing, one of her schoolmates also died.[92] The school for missionary children – which boarded missionary children from other parts of North China – was temporarily closed. Dr. Dow and Janet Brydon came to Weihui to offer their medical services. The missionaries believed that it was the Chinese workmen constructing the new Weihui Hospital who had brought the disease into the compound. Dysentery-carrying flies "were everywhere" because the workmen were "careless about sanitary arrangements."[93] Mrs. Jeanette Ratcliffe became ill and was sent home to Canada to recuperate.

Ratcliffe's departure at the end of 1920 left Janet Brydon and Margaret Mitchell as the two main missionary nurses in Henan (Margaret MacIntosh was now classified as an evangelistic worker). Margaret Mitchell was a Scottish nurse "with experience in South China" who had recently joined the mission.[94] Two others, Isabel Leslie *(Lei Runtian)* and Eleanor May Galbraith, were on their way to North Henan in 1920. Little is known about Isabel Leslie's background, except that she was born in Dundee, Oregon. Leslie, who arrived in Henan in 1921, went on to work in Henan for the next nineteen years.[95] Galbraith was born at Lorneville, St. John County, New Brunswick, in 1896. She took nurses' training at the Rhode Island Hospital, and was designated by St. Andrew's Presbyterian Church in St. John, New Brunswick, on 28 July 1920. She sailed for China on 26 August 1920, arriving about a month later. Galbraith had only just begun her language study when she resigned to be married to Rev. H.T. Bridgman of the South Presbyterian Mission (United States) on 25 December 1920.[96] Little else is known about her. Thus, although there were six WMS nurses associated with the North Henan Mission in 1920 (MacIntosh, Ratcliffe, Brydon, Mitchell, Galbraith, and Leslie), it would be Janet Brydon and Margaret Mitchell who would usher in the era of modern nursing in North Henan, at Weihui.

Summary

The period immediately following the Boxer Uprising was a pleasant one for the Henan missionaries. Not only did they enjoy a relatively peaceful existence with their Chinese neighbours, but they also enjoyed a new level of acceptance of their presence and the Western knowledge they possessed. Medical missionaries across China took advantage of the opportunity to expand medical services, and the Canadians at North Henan were no exception – at least, as far as the practice of medicine went. While there was considerable interest in the development of staffed hospitals and dispensaries, the missionaries were not in agreement as to how elaborate these should be. Some, like Jonathan Goforth, did not agree with the movement toward increased medical service, believing that this would take attention and resources away from evangelistic service. Others, like the young missionary physicians Dr. Scott and Dr. McMurtry, were eager to modernize the existing hospitals to become more like Canadian hospitals, complete with state-of-the-art equipment and round-the-clock nursing service.

While Scott and McMurtry's ideas proved premature, it was not long before national events in China triggered the very changes they were aiming for. When China became a republic after the 1911 revolution, the Chinese were becoming more interested in Western ideas. After medical missionaries successfully responded to an outbreak of pneumonia that same year, Western medicine gained acceptance in China. The Canadians at Henan became eager to develop new, modern hospitals. Dr. Dow organized the women's hospital at Anyang to complement the work of the general hospital there, while plans were laid to build new, multi-level, Canadian-style hospitals at Huaiqing and Weihui. Yet until 1916, the development of nursing was largely overlooked. Mrs. Ratcliffe, a trained nurse, was hired as the matron of the mission school in 1910. Maisie McNeely was hired in 1914, but her role was to take care of missionary families. Whatever her role might have become, Miss McNeely resigned within two years to be married. The FMB did appeal for more missionary nurses, but the nurses' primary function was to be evangelistic workers. Nurses in Canada did not respond to the appeals. Margaret Gay came to China as an evangelistic worker in 1910, but turned to nursing after being confronted with the health needs of the rural population in Henan.

It took the persuasive powers of the post-1900 missionaries to put nursing on a modern and directed path. Dr. Fred Auld considered the recommendations of the Christian Medical Association in China and, after making a careful study of what was going on in the large hospitals of other missions, concluded that Henan needed to move beyond what was largely an out-patient practice to organized in-patient services. The association recommended foreign nurses as hospital matrons. Dr. Auld found the solution in the person of Mrs. Jeanette Ratcliffe, a widowed graduate nurse who was already living at Henan.

Mrs. Ratcliffe was as meticulous as Dr. Auld in her preparation for her new role. While she waited for the construction of the hospital to be completed, Ratcliffe sought postgraduate education at Toronto, as well as hands-on experience as the acting matron at the Qilu university hospital at Jinan. She also studied the Chinese language. At about the same time, a second nurse was hired, Janet L. Brydon. As it turned out, Brydon's work was interrupted by the advent of the Great War: from 1918 to 1919, most of the male missionaries – including physicians – were helping with the war effort in France. In 1920, the Henan Mission was finally ready to move forward with nursing development: Ratcliffe and Brydon were prepared. Then came the murder of Dr. James Menzies.

That Menzies was killed while coming to the aid of Brydon and her housemate Sadie Lethbridge made the tragedy all the more poignant. Brydon responded, it seems, by focusing on her nursing work. In response to the outbreak of dysentery that plagued the Henan Mission during the summer of 1920 and killed both Sadie Lethbridge and Hedley Auld, Brydon moved from Huaiqing to the centre of the epidemic, at Weihui. After Ratcliffe left Weihui for Canada to recuperate from an illness (possibly dysentery), Brydon accepted the increased responsibility of planning the new nursing service at the as-yet-unopened hospital.

Canadian nursing at the Henan Mission during the first two decades of 1900 was influenced by both external and internal factors. Externally, the development of nursing was "controlled" by the national milieu and Chinese attitude toward foreigners and their Western ideas. It was also controlled by the desires of other missionaries, particularly the all-male Presbytery, which held the power when it came to recruitment decisions. The Presbytery, in turn, was influenced by the priorities and perspectives of Protestant missions as a whole in China. When other missions pushed for expansion and national coordination of medical and nursing services, the Canadian Presbytery acquiesced. Finally, the establishment of the NAC signalled to medical missionaries and prospective missionary nurses that foreign nursing leaders were poised to take seriously the role opening up for them.

Internally, the second generation of nurses showed a commitment to the vision of modern nursing and medicine. Ratcliffe, Gay, and Brydon, in particular, exemplified the drive and tenacity necessary to respond to the health needs of those around them, the resilience to bounce back from personal tragedy, and the mental and physical vigour to withstand the challenges of the day.

3
Modern Nursing at Last, 1921-27

Opening a training school, graduating nurses, doesn't it sound easy?

– L. Clara Preston

Canadian Interest in "Our China Missionaries"

During the 1920s, nursing in China was well on its way to becoming a well-organized, professional workforce of Chinese and foreign nurses. In 1920, a school of nursing was opened in the new Rockefeller Foundation–sponsored Peking Union Medical College (PUMC) in Beijing. Equipped with the best facilities and a first-class faculty and staff, it introduced the first joint bachelor of science–nursing program in China. That same year, the first professional nursing journal in China, called the *Quarterly Journal for Chinese Nurses,* was published by the Nurses Association of China (NAC). And on 22 May 1922, the NAC was admitted into full membership of the International Council of Nurses.[1] The trend of nationalization in China during the 1920s was reflected in the increasingly Chinese membership of the NAC. Over the next ten years, the NAC membership would grow to six thousand members working at two hundred nursing schools around the country.

This was a propitious time for Canadian missionary nursing. By 1921, construction of the new hospital at Weihui was well underway. It was to be the first of three modern hospitals in North Henan, at Weihui, Huaiqing, and Anyang. Of these, Weihui would be "the most modern and up-to-date [hospital] in the province and one of the finest in the country outside Shanghai and Beijing."[2] The Weihui Hospital had two sections: the dispensary (or outpatient department) and the hospital proper (or in-patient department). The new dispensary opened in 1920 – three years before the new hospital – and included four hostels (two for men, two for women) capable of accommodating 250 patients.[3] The dispensary also had a consulting room;

a surgical dressing room; an eye, nose, and throat room; a dispensing room; and a chapel each for men and women. The dispensary hostels were to be used by patients suffering minor ailments or convalescing from more serious illness; hostels could also accommodate patients' friends and relatives. Food was available for a reasonable price in a "comparatively clean" kitchen, supervised by medical staff.[4] The response was encouraging. Patient numbers increased by 40 percent after the new dispensary opened, and before the main hospital building was even completed. Construction of the Weihui Hospital was painstakingly slow, and a lack of funds delayed work on the main building.

The total cost of the hospital project to the mission was $58,614.52, of which the Woman's Missionary Society (WMS) paid $17,697.00.[5] Other funding came from the Forward Movement Peace "Thankoffering Fund," and gifts from the Chinese. In addition to the cost of the hospital was the cost of a nurses' residence, for which Mrs. Geo Bingham donated the requisite $4,000.00 in memory of her late husband. It is remarkable that the WMS contributed so much to the cost of nursing in China – not only to the salary, outfitting, and travel of Canadian nurses, but also to this particular building project. The road to nursing in Henan was paved by Canadian tea socials, bake sales, and Sunday-school collections.

Churchwomen across Canada saw it as their duty to do what they could to financially support the cause of "our missionaries in China."[6] This was true of the Methodist and Presbyterian missionary societies before church union in 1925, as well as afterward. For example, records of United Church (formerly Methodist) WMS minutes from Alberta describe special donations during 1925-26 that included $30.00 from the Westlock Ladies Aid toward the Chengdu Hospital (Sichuan) and $40.00 from the Calgary Central Auxiliary in "support of a child in China." Similarly, at the Alberta WMS provincial branch meeting in 1928, one delegate noted, "[President Mrs. Hencher] told us about the children in one of the Ruthemian WMS school homes in her District, whose self-denial equaled those of Miss Jack's school in China. They abstained from dessert for a week, thereby saving 25 [cents] a piece for WMS Thankoffering."[7] The creativity and dedication of Canadian women to missions in general is striking; pennies added up to thousands of dollars. Also striking was the generosity and support of individual congregations toward Canadian nurses. Churches that "designated" specific missionary nurses from their congregations took seriously the pledge to support them; just as the nurses solemnly dedicated themselves to China, the church members solemnly dedicated themselves to the nurses. Here, too, the churchwomen showed creativity. At nurse Louise Clara Preston's home church at Stratford, Ontario, churchwomen raised money for her work in Henan by making a quilt: supporters paid ten cents each to have their names embroidered on it.

The churchwomen in Canada saw themselves as valuable partners in the work of their missionaries to China. Not only did they raise funds, they also took a studious interest in the progress of China missions. For example, the First United Church WMS of Lacombe Presbyterial kept records of how many stations, outstations, schools, colleges, hospitals, dispensaries, missionaries, and Chinese workers there were in China.[8] And the Evening Auxiliary of Central United Church studied publications on China missions and listened to "scholarly reviews" of study books such as *Fourth Daughter of China, Serving with the Sons of Shuh,* and *China Rediscovers Her West.*[9] The Canadian churchwomen also took a keen interest in lectures by missionaries who were on furlough, where they were told of the state of affairs for Chinese women and children and how the Chinese required Canadian help. According to one WMS group, "China owes a great debt to Christian Missions – for her schools which 236,000 of Chinese children (Protestants) attend: and 100 hospitals besides asylums for Insane, Blind and Lepers of whom China is said to have 400,000 ... many of these foreigners [i.e., the Chinese] have lived in poverty, ignorance and dirt in their native country and have to be educated to need of proper living conditions, medical care and education. Hospital work provides [the] best 'open door' for this instruction and for the gospel teaching."[10] Given how reliant the Canadian missionaries were on the support of the Canadian church, the importance of nurturing the missionary-home church relationship can hardly be overstated. If the churchwomen were to continue to invest their time and energy into the work of the China missionaries, they had to have confidence that this work was worthwhile – even if their perception of the work was not always accurate or up to date.

It is interesting that the WMS supporters in 1926 continued to emphasize medical work as a gateway through which to share both the Christian Gospel and the gospel of soap and water. If the new generation of medical and nursing missionaries did not see it as part of their role to preach and to teach, why did the homeland supporters continue to perceive medical work as primarily evangelical? Perhaps the answer lies in the subtle change of wording in the publications. Whereas early mission reports referred to the evangelistic work of *persons* (i.e., physicians), contemporary mission reports referred to the evangelistic work of *institutions* (i.e., hospitals). In the 1920s, it was no longer necessary for the physician or nurse to directly preach or teach, as long as someone else in the hospital system assumed this task. At North Henan, for example, it was Chinese medical assistants who gave Gospel presentations to outpatients and in-patients.[11] And just in case patients were somehow missed or overlooked, they would at least be aware of the hospital's mission, since it was printed on all the registration cards. Each new patient at the Weihui Hospital was given a card that read, "This hospital is established for the purpose of making known, by the ministry of healing,

Christ, the Great Physician and Saviour of the world."[12] A shift from direct to indirect evangelism had begun.

Another reason that supporters in the homeland continued to perceive medical work as evangelistic was that some medical missionaries *did*, in fact, directly evangelize. By the early 1920s, a number of the older generation of physicians and nurses were still on the mission field and still committed to the idea of direct evangelism. For example, Dr. Jean Dow – who had been at Henan since 1895 – incorporated evangelism into her medical practice throughout her career. After her death in 1927, fellow missionaries paid tribute to her singular evangelistic efforts: "[Dr. Dow] set one forenoon of the week free from all operations and, herself and assistants going to different wards and yards, would preach and teach that half day to insure that among the crowds none came and went without hearing the Good News."[13] Mission supporters in Canada were thus assured that their investment in China missionaries was worthwhile. Even if medical and nursing missionaries were no longer expected to be evangelists, they were expected to be unambiguous representatives of the Christian faith. Mission supporters back home could be content with the knowledge that, by supporting their missionaries, they, too, were active partners in the cause of Christian missions in China.

The "Scientific Efficiency" of Henan Hospitals

Despite their ambitious plans to expand and improve medical and nursing service in Henan, the Canadian Presbyterian mission's progress lagged behind that of other missions. According to a report entitled "An Enquiry into the Scientific Efficiency of Mission Hospitals in China," presented at the China Medical Missionary Association (CMMA) in Beijing in February 1920, Henan hospitals rated near the bottom of the scale.[14] While the report does not differentiate between various Henan hospitals, there were as many as seven missions operating some form of hospital in Henan during this period; presumably all were included in the report.[15] The CMMA report was an analysis of statistics from 192 mission hospitals in thirteen provinces of China. In terms of modern facilities, equipment, and staffing, Henan was archaic when compared with other missions and the new hospital ideal. In the CMMA study, Henan hospitals were found sorely lacking in most areas, including hospital buildings, outpatient dispensaries, hospital accommodations, building materials, ventilation and airspace, accommodation of patients' friends, diets and kitchens, water supply, bathing facilities, laundries, sanitary systems, laboratories, facilities for specialization, nursing arrangements, and scientific work. Mission hospitals in Henan were a long way from modernization. The standards of comparison give some insights not only into the facilities at Henan, but also into what was considered to be state-of-the-art medical and nursing care in 1920:

1 Henan hospital buildings were of mostly "pure Chinese style" or "modified Chinese style" instead of the multi-level "foreign-style;"
2 Henan had some of the poorest outpatient facilities (that is, without easily and regularly cleaned floors, walls, and furniture, and without laboratory facilities or a darkroom for ophthalmic investigation);
3 Henan had a low proportion of beds per foreign or foreign-trained physician: the average was forty-three; Henan had thirty-one;
4 Henan used poor building materials – of particular concern was the lack of "rounded corners" in the wards and operating rooms;
5 Henan hospitals were poorly ventilated and did not have much "air space" for patients; most of the adverse reports about ventilation came from Henan, which was also one of only two provinces reporting the ongoing use of paper (rather than glass) windows;
6 Henan hospitals did not provide protection of patients from infection and from insect-borne disease. Apparently Henan had no isolation wards or courtyards, nor did it have any screens or nets to protect patients from disease-carrying flies and mosquitoes;
7 Henan hospitals allowed patients to bring their friends in to live in the wards with them;
8 Henan patients did not follow controlled diets;
9 Henan hospitals did not have running water, and patients were not bathed on admission;
10 Henan hospitals had inadequate (or no) laundry accommodation;
11 Henan hospitals had no drainage system and used "ordinary Chinese latrines," or *mao-fangs,* rather than septic tanks. Latrines were to be emptied daily;
12 Henan had some laboratory facilities, but these were not used regularly. Henan did not have facilities to study or grow bacteria;
13 Henan reported no X-ray equipment; and
14 finally, Henan was not involved with research work, did not base treatment on pathological investigation, and had no post-mortem examinations.

On a more positive note, Henan did score well in a few areas: it provided clean bedding for patients and was among the few hospitals that employed more than one physician. And, needless to say, the Henan mission had the lowest average expenditure of all the provinces surveyed.

One of the most interesting aspects of the CMMA report was the section entitled "Nursing Arrangements." Since the arrival of the first American missionary nurse in China in 1884, the development of nursing in China had always been closely linked with medical missionary work.[16] By 1920, some training of Chinese nurses had begun in Beijing, Shanghai, Fuzhou, and Guangzhou, but it would be another ten years before Chinese nurses would acquire leadership roles held by foreign nurses.[17] In 1920, there was a serious shortage of qualified nurses all across China. The CMMA believed that the best way to fill the nursing void was with foreign graduate nurses who would, in turn, train Chinese nurses. According to the CMMA report, only 48 percent of the 192 hospitals surveyed had a trained foreign nurse (or nurses) on staff, and 38 percent had no nurse at all: "In other words, in one third of all these hospitals there is no sort of skilled nursing whatever, and in 60% of them there is no more than can be attempted by a single graduate nurse."[18] Out of all the provinces, Henan was among the worst staffed, having few foreign *or* Chinese nurses. Henan also had the largest proportion of hospitals with no skilled nursing at all. Although 41 percent of the hospitals surveyed had training programs for Chinese nurses, Henan had none. Furthermore, Henan had one of the "worst records" for leaving the care of patients to their own friends and of having no regular system of night nursing. If the Canadian Presbyterian mission in North Henan were to take seriously its development of medical services, it would have to pay close attention to the development of nursing services as well.

The Arrival of Louise Clara Preston

According to the CMMA report, by 1920, it was "no longer necessary to perpetuate the older methods [which are] frankly opposed to every idea of hygiene and good nursing, or of scientific methods of diagnosis and treatment."[19] Nor was it "necessary" to continue to allow patients to bring their friends in to live with them for moral support. When Louise Clara Preston arrived in China in 1922, the old style of hospital was still in existence at Anyang. Although she valued modern medicine and fully supported the development of modern hospitals, Preston would also come to miss some of the advantages the older hospitals had over the new ones: "The patients felt more at home, it was easier for women to finance, it took less administration, and gave the staff more time to teach patients how to read and give lessons in hygiene. It was amazing the number of cures and the results we had in spite of conditions."[20]

Louise Clara Preston *(Peng Hu Shih)* is among the most noteworthy Canadian missionary nurses at North Henan (see Figure 11). Her career in China spanned a quarter-century, ending only when the North China Mission permanently closed in 1947. The year 1922 was a watershed year for nursing for three reasons: the Canadian mission opened its school of nursing at Weihui, Chinese members joined the NAC for the first time, and the NAC joined the International Council of Nurses.[21] The timing of Clara Preston's interest in China missions was auspicious not only for these reasons, but also because two of the WMS nurses at Henan had recently resigned. Both Eleanor Galbraith (Bridgman) and Margaret Straith (Fuller) married fellow

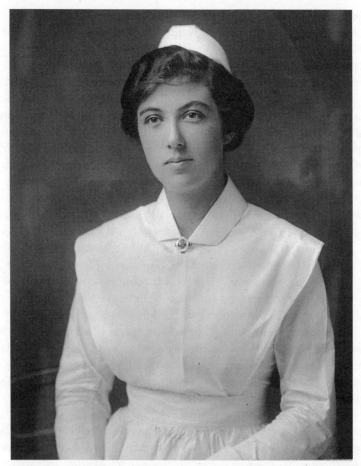

Figure 11   Louise Clara Preston wearing an RVH graduate pin, 1922.
UCCVUA 76.001P-5282

missionaries within months of their arrival in China – Galbraith in 1920, and Straith in 1921.[22]

Louise Clara Preston was born in Boissevain, Manitoba, in 1891, and studied at a business college at Stratford, Ontario, before taking the nurses' training course at the Royal Victoria Hospital in Montreal. She graduated from the Royal Victoria, was appointed to Henan, and was designated by the Knox Presbyterian Church in Stratford – all in quick succession. Preston crossed the Pacific from Canada with Mrs. Jeanette Ratcliffe, who was returning to China after an extended illness, in 1922.[23] During her tenure in China, Preston became intimately involved with the development of nursing education and services in Henan, despite being evacuated from Henan four times due to national political instability – during the Nationalist advance (1927), the Anti-British Movement (1939), the Second World War (1941), and the Civil War (1947).

Clara Preston was thirty-one years old when she joined the WMS as a missionary nurse. According to her family, Clara was engaged to be married before she entered nurses' training in 1919, but her fiancé, who was away at war, died of the Spanish Flu on the boat when returning to Canada. In her memoirs, Preston did not directly refer to a fiancé, but wrote, "Then followed the war years [the First World War]. How easy to write that sentence, yet what volumes it speaks. First this friend, then that friend, cousins, neighbours, and then my youngest brother Jeffrey. So many dreams of youth shattered."[24] Assuming that Preston was engaged at one time – and considering that she did not enter nurses' training until later in life – it would be easy to conclude that her decision to become a missionary was borne out of a sense of loss and a need to revision her future. Preston intimated, however, that becoming a missionary was a long-time dream: she and "a friend [had spent] many, many hours talking and planning how we could prepare so we could offer our services for the foreign field."[25] Her suitability for a nursing career was confirmed to Preston during her experience as a volunteer in the homes of ill families during the Spanish Flu epidemic in Stratford in 1918. Although the worst of the epidemic was over within two weeks, Preston had witnessed much anguish and suffering. In one family alone, the mother and four children died within days of each other. Preston found herself drawn to the families she helped through "scrubbing floors and washing diapers and bathing the baby until they were able to carry on," even while she herself slept in a bed made of "three chairs put together in the kitchen."[26] The experience would prove to be an invaluable preparation for missionary life. Preston turned to her religious beliefs to sustain her, writing that "the ninety-first Psalm had been my Bible reading for the day and it seemed a definite promise of help and protection."[27] Turning to the Psalms for solace in the face of threat would come to characterize Preston's nursing work in China.

If being an unmarried, religiously devout woman was not enough reason to pursue her dream of becoming a foreign missionary, a precedent for missionary work had already been set in Preston's family. Her aunt, E. Augustine Preston, had been a WMS missionary in Japan since 1888. Clara visited "Aunt Gussy" in Kobe en route to China.[28] Still, Clara's parents were hesitant to see her become a missionary – she had to "win them to [her] point of view."[29] When Clara Preston started her nurses' training in Montreal, it was with the understanding that she would become a missionary.

At the Royal Victoria Hospital in Montreal, Quebec, Clara Preston came to value "modern" or scientific medicine, with its emphasis on efficiently designed buildings (where attention was paid to ventilation and cleanliness, and where nurses could take care of patients in large wards), state-of-the-art equipment (such as X-rays and laboratory materials), and scientific diagnosis and treatment (where technology such as the microscope was used to assist in diagnosis, and decisions for treatment were based on scientifically tested theories). To Preston, modern hospital nursing was where she could fully experience and express her Christian faith: "There is an interesting book called, 'Jesus Christ and the modern Hospital' and to me it is the place where I find Christ nearest and can say 'does not our heart burn within us as we work with Christ in our hospitals.' The modern miracles performed each day – things we did not dream possible."[30] Given how much Preston valued modern medicine, it is not surprising that she fully supported the modernizing efforts being made by the Henan Mission at Weihui. Yet it would be a few more years before a new hospital was built at Anyang, where Preston was stationed after her arrival in 1922. Although she found nursing care to be hindered by poor buildings, inadequate equipment, and a lack of trained help, Preston also came to treasure her experience with the old-style mission hospital – realizing afterward that she had borne witness to a passing era in China.

The Demise of the Old-Style Hospital

In 1922, Anyang had two old hospitals: a men's hospital run by Dr. Percy Leslie, and a women's hospital run by Dr. Isabelle McTavish and Dr. Jean Dow. At first, the Henan Mission planned to amalgamate the two hospitals in order to save money, personnel, and space. But the two female doctors at Anyang could not be persuaded to allow their hospital to be combined with the men's hospital into one new general hospital, insisting instead on a new women's hospital "for some reason, sentiment or otherwise."[31] It should not be surprising that Dr. Dow was loath to give up "her" hospital. Considering that women could not hold authoritative positions in the Presbyterian Church and local Presbyteries, and that women often deferred to men in hospital hierarchies, Dr. Dow's position as the head of her own hospital for more than twenty years was unique, if not enviable. Out of respect for Dr. Dow, the Henan Presbytery reluctantly agreed to build a new women's hospital beside the men's in Anyang. It also agreed to buy more land upon which to build a house for the female doctors and nurses. Thus it was that Clara Preston started her missionary nursing duties with the expectation that she would become supervisor of nursing at the new women's hospital. Since Dr. Dow had not shown interest in graduate nursing services during the previous twenty-two years, it is likely that her younger colleague, Dr. McTavish, influenced her to support the appointment of Clara Preston.

Like other old-style hospitals in North Henan, the old Anyang women's hospital had a chapel, a dispensary, and an operating room. In-patients stayed in small single-story buildings that faced each other around a central courtyard. "Regular" patients slept on *kangs* (brick platforms) covered with straw matting, over which they spread quilts. "Bedpatients" used hospital beds made with hospital sheets, a quilt, and a pillow. One of the buildings was used as a kitchen. The mission supplied a number of portable stoves for patients and their friends to cook their meals; patients supplied their own coal and food. During the winter, patients cooked in their own rooms for extra heat. This posed a problem for the doctors, who worried that patients might fall asleep with their stoves on and be overcome by coal gas – a problem they resolved by poking holes in the paper windows for ventilation. A "poor woman of the lowest classes" swept the courtyards and kept the latrines clean, while a scavenger paid the hospital a monthly sum for the privilege of carrying away the human excrement ("night soil") to fertilize his gardens.[32]

Since there were no graduate nurses in Anyang before Clara Preston, Chinese women were used as medical assistants. These assistants, who were "preferably young widows with unbound feet," gave "anaesthetics, helped with operations, dispensed simple drugs, wrapped up powders, sterilized dressings, and helped with the outpatient's dressings."[33] They carried dressing trays across the open-air courtyard into patients' rooms – a delicate feat if it happened to be rainy or wintry. In addition, the Chinese assistants – who would be on call at night – gave "intravenous injections," watched the seriously ill, bathed the newborn babies, and spent "hours teaching the patients the Gospel of Christ."[34]

Poor lighting and heating made it difficult to do efficient work, and in the summertime, flies were a menace. Even if the windows were screened, the doors had matting curtains that were opened wide on hot days, and flies easily entered patients' rooms. Preston recalled caring for a young wife who had been beaten by her husband because of infidelity. The patient was raw from her hips down and had open sores on her body. Preston and the others lifted their patient twice each day into a galvanized tub, afterward dressing her wounds. Preston's best nursing care was no match for the "flies and maggots" that were attracted to the open sores, however, and eventually the woman was carried home on a wooden Chinese bed to die. It is no wonder Preston felt so strongly the need for "screened wards and more convenient working quarters."[35] To Preston, the promise of modern hospitals and nursing service would be a relief after having experienced "knowing the fear of fires when oil lamps had to be used; the fag of insisting on clean bedpans when there was no running water; seeing the mud and water that always seemed to come in with the water carrier; and finding the tanks empty just when you needed water the most and no man in sight to carry it."[36]

The situation at Weihui before 1923 was much the same. At the old-style hospital, patients brought their own bedding and huddled together in rows on the brick *kangs* in their "small, dark, dingy rooms," or slept on brick floors, or in the courtyard under the stars.[37] No routine bathing was possible, "even for those who had not had [a bath] for decades." After operations, patients continued to wear the same dirty clothes and use the same dirty bedding – in response to which Dr. R. Gordon Struthers *(Di Ruwen)* quipped, "It is perhaps well to draw a veil over that bedding and clothing and bury its entomological contents in a decent silence."[38] While Preston would have to wait until 1926 for the opening of a new hospital at Anyang, the Weihui Hospital was ready in 1923. The new Weihui nursing school had already begun in 1922, before the hospital was officially opened. The opening of the new Weihui Hospital ushered in a new era of missions at North Henan. By then, it had been almost ten years since Dr. Fred M. Auld first received approval of his plans and estimates for the new hospital at Weihui.

The New Weihui Hospital and Nurses' Training School

On 8 November 1923, the main building of the new Weihui Hospital was finally opened, to much fanfare. (See Figure 12.) Its opening symbolized the new, prominent place of medical work in mission policy. According to Henan missionary Margaret Brown, "the change in purpose came so gradually as to be almost imperceptible. Medical work was no longer to be a mere means to an evangelistic end. It was in itself to be a living expression of the Christian Gospel and must, therefore, maintain the highest standards. It was the age of the Social Gospel, and Medical work could be a strong arm of this Gospel."[39]

The grand opening of the new Weihui Hospital included both morning and afternoon services of dedication – one held in the church, and one in

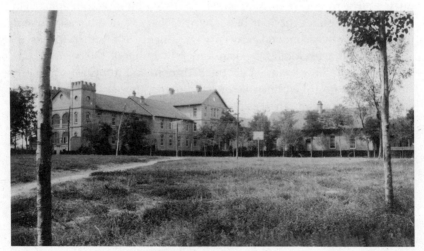

Figure 12 Weihui Hospital, 1920s.
Mary Struthers McKim private collection

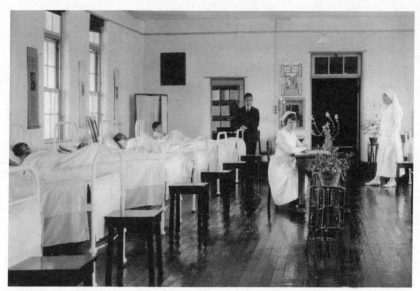

Figure 13   New hospital ward at Weihui, c. 1924, with Jean Menzies sitting.
UCCVUA 1999.001P-1938

one of the large hospital wards. About two hundred guests attended, mostly officials, scholars, and merchants. It was a building to be proud of. The hospital had four great, bright, airy public wards of sixteen beds each, as well as room for two additional large public wards in the basement, if required.[40] (See Figure 13.) One of the wards was designated for children and, interestingly, one for missionaries. No longer would the Henan Mission request a nurse to care for missionaries; they could now be accommodated by the hospital. Besides the four public wards, there were private and semi-private wards to accommodate twenty-six patients. Altogether, there were about 90 beds, with room for expansion up to a total of 130 beds.[41]

Patients were now admitted via the bathroom and furnished with clean clothing and fresh bed linen before heading to the wards, where nurses would care for them. The design was based on contemporary Canadian hospitals and included a main kitchen, "diet kitchens" (run by Dr. Auld's wife May, who was a dietician), X-ray and operating suites, surgical dressing rooms, sterilizing rooms, bathrooms, an office, a waiting room, and a verandah for all patients.[42] Nurses had their own charting room and a lecture room to use for nurses' training. Hospital staff and patients were not the only ones to benefit from the hospital construction: since such a modern facility would require electricity and running water, the entire missionary compound was fitted with electric lighting and modern sanitation.

A unique feature of the new hospital was the training school for nurses – the first one in North Henan. Mrs. Ratcliffe was the principal, and Miss

Margaret Mitchell her assistant. The school had actually opened the previous September (1922) under the leadership of Miss Janet Brydon, while Mrs. Ratcliffe was on illness leave in Canada. When Ratcliffe returned to Weihui, Brydon returned to the old hospital at Huaiqing. The Weihui nursing school had strict standards of admission. It was important to choose students of the right age, educational standards (three years of high school), physical fitness, and financial backing – not to mention a "Christian spirit."[43] To Mrs. Ratcliffe, the objective of the nursing school was "to give a training which would, first, open the eyes of the nurses to the physical and spiritual ignorance and misery about them; second, make them feel their responsibility towards these conditions; third, teach them how most effectively to relieve and banish them."[44]

The Henan Mission credited Mrs. Ratcliffe for conceiving the possibility of a nursing school and making her vision a reality. The ideals of nursing were considered inseparable from the ideals of Christianity, and Ratcliffe's vision was expressly a Christian one. As such, nurses' training in North Henan had a dual purpose – to contribute to the development of the nursing profession in China and to stimulate nursing students and nurses to a deeper, more mature Christian faith. To Ratcliffe, the former could not be accomplished without the latter. Her vision was similar to that expressed at Qilu and reported by Margaret Brown, where "the founding of the nursing profession by Christians was an even greater achievement than the introduction of modern medicine; medical schools ... would have come sooner or later anyway. But young women would not have taken up nursing without the example set them by Christian women of the West."[45] According to Margaret Brown, to appreciate what the nursing school at Henan meant, one must understand that educated girls in China were reared to think that menial work was beneath them: "To care lovingly for filthy patients was a new idea and required the Grace of God in the heart. To see rich and poor alike placed in clean beds and waited on in the same way revealed the revolutionary idea of service."[46] As missionary nurses saw it, there were many cultural barriers to overcome in order to successfully introduce Western nursing into China. That is, some of the core concepts and values of nursing were unfamiliar to the Chinese or even at odds with traditional Chinese culture. These included the value of service (including menial labour), caring for strangers, and caring for someone of the opposite sex. Chinese culture valued filial piety as well as loyalty to extended family and friends. Caring for the sick was a family responsibility: it was not acceptable to be cared for by strangers or to care for ill strangers. This posed a problem for Canadian missionary nurses, to whom the concept of practical sympathy and self-denying love to ill and injured *strangers* was at the core of nursing – and at the core of Christian service. In order to minimize cultural differences and to maintain the Christian vision of the nursing school, the Henan

Mission taught in Chinese, and accepted only Christian students into the nursing school – namely, graduates of the mission schools who had made public professions of their faith.

Another method used to minimize cultural differences was the training of both male and female nurses. Out of respect for traditional Chinese mores, which demanded strict separation of the sexes, the school accepted both male and female students so that nurses would care for patients of their own sex (see Figure 14). The training of both male and female nurses at Weihui is interesting, considering that nursing in Canada at that time was essentially a female profession. As previously discussed, Henan missionaries in 1888 believed that it was necessary to appoint female missionaries because it was culturally inappropriate for male physicians to care for female patients in China. Yet when Dr. Jean Dow fought the amalgamation of her women's hospital into a general hospital, the Henan Mission downplayed the need for separation of the sexes in medical care. Thus, while it was common practice for male physicians to care for female patients, it was considered inappropriate for female nurses to care for male patients. At the Weihui Hospital and training school, male nursing students cared for patients in the men's wards, while female nursing students cared for women and children.

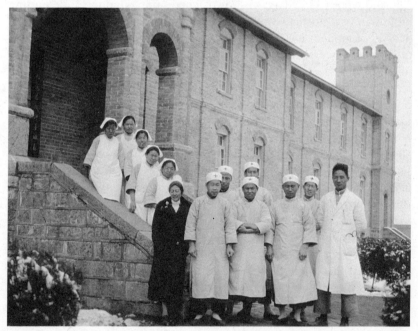

Figure 14 Mrs. Ratcliffe and staff at Weihui before the 1927 evacuation. Note the male instructor and six male nursing students.
UCCVUA 1999.001P-1957

To Mrs. Ratcliffe, nursing was a valuable profession for both men *and* women in China, even though it was not considered so in Canada. She expressed pleasure that nursing seemed to have "taken hold of the interest of many of our young people, [equipping both men and women] for a life of useful service."[47] At the same time, Ratcliffe was not convinced that males were as good at nursing as females. Despite her interest in educating both men and women, she believed that women "naturally [possessed] more aptitude for the work than the men."[48] Her accommodation of men in nursing was related to her acceptance of Chinese cultural norms.

Although all the Weihui students were Canadian mission school graduates who had been exposed to – if not acculturated in – the worldview of the Canadians, there were still cultural barriers to overcome. That is, Chinese students and their Canadian instructors had disparate views on illness causation, personal hygiene, and the importance of precise measurements (time, medication amounts, and patients' vital signs). The nursing instructors found it difficult to turn their students from the philosophy of *cha pu tao* ("not much difference") to one of exactness – "that medicine to be given at four must not be given at a quarter to five, or that a tablespoonful of medicine must not be given when only a teaspoon was required."[49] For a culture accustomed for centuries to estimate the time by the sun, the idea of prompt and accurate efficiency was new. Yet teaching precise measurement was relatively easy in comparison with teaching Western values and cultivating Christian virtues.

To the Henan missionaries, a nurse's temperament and moral fibre was of central importance; only those who displayed a "fine Christian character" were to be admitted into nurses' training.[50] This ideal was an adaptation of the expectations of nursing schools in Canada, which, while open to non-Christian students, nevertheless promoted Christian ideals about morality and character. In China, the Canadians were not the only ones emphasizing character, however. In 1925, Nina Gage, former president of the NAC and present dean of the Hunan-Yale school of nursing at Changsha, reported to the International Council of Nurses that "certificates of character are evidently required by all ... In China, students are required to have a 'bondsman' to answer for the good behaviour of the student."[51] Although there must have been many aspects of administering the nursing school that gave Ratcliffe personal gratification, she identified the "development of character" of the nursing graduates as giving her "great satisfaction."[52]

In the first year of the new four-year nursing program at Weihui, eleven pupils enrolled, but only eight were accepted for training – five women and three men.[53] The students were all graduates from the Henan Mission schools. One student, Miss Chou, was the granddaughter of Chou Lao-Chang, the first Christian convert in North Henan.[54] The Chinese Church (an organization separate from – but supported by – the Henan Presbytery) took a special interest in the nursing school. Its members proposed that all applicants for admission into the school of nursing be first recommended by their congregations. Furthermore, the Chinese Church requested that all fourth-year students attend summer classes for evangelists and be examined by a committee appointed by the Chinese Presbytery, in addition to taking their regular nursing examinations. Although it is not clear whether all these proposals were implemented, the proposals themselves highlight how important it was to both Canadian missionaries *and* the established Chinese church – the Church of Christ in China – that nurses be practising Christians. Modern nursing was taking root in Henan, and the first generation of Chinese nurses would be shaped and supported by both Canadian and Chinese Christians.

Registration with the NAC

In January 1922, Janet Brydon joined ninety other nurses from all over China for the NAC's biennial conference in Hankou. This was the first year that Chinese nurses were in attendance at the week-long conference, and the first year that Henan was represented. Organizing the conference was no small matter. The nurses travelled by train and riverboat; some from Guangzhou were two weeks en route to Hankou. They were billeted with local missionaries, and they travelled by "steamlaunch, cab or ricksha [sic] [through] rain, ice, snow and slush" to visit Hankou hospitals, and to gather for large meetings.[55] According to Brydon, the most important decision made at the conference was to have "sectional groups" of the NAC (presumably by region). She returned to Henan invigorated: "It was a mountainheight [experience], for from it we came back to our work with a broader vision of what came before and of what may be ahead, a better idea of problems we *shall* have to face and *may* have to face, a strengthened resolve and a fuller consciousness that we are one of many, all working for a sure goal, even though isolated and in places where pioneer work has to be done."[56] Since there were no government schools of nursing in China, the NAC acted as the governing body for the nursing profession until the 1930s. The NAC translated and prepared textbooks, set examinations, acted as a "placement bureau" for graduates, edited a nursing journal, and looked after the biennial meetings for China.[57] It also set the standards for accreditation: if nurses graduated from an accredited school, their credentials were recognized all over China. By 1923, the NAC had adopted standards that ranged from curriculum requirements (for three- or four-year programs) to the style of nursing cap worn by Chinese nurses (foreign nurses wore the cap of their alma mater).[58] The NAC inspected prospective schools, registering them if the standards were met. The Henan missionary nurses were keen to have their school at Weihui accredited.

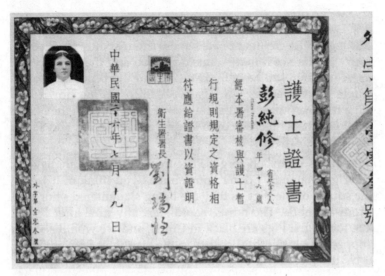

Figure 15 Clara Preston's NAC certificate, 1930s.
L. Clara Preston, *Flowers amongst the Debris*

Although the NAC was historically composed of foreign nurses, its aim was to have an increasing number of Chinese nurses in leadership positions. The addition of two Chinese nursing instructors to the Weihui staff in 1924 reportedly increased Henan's chances at achieving registration with the NAC. One of the (unnamed) instructors was a "fine Christian graduate male nurse," and the other was Miss Yang, a former mission pupil and teacher at the Weihui children's school who had just graduated from the nursing school in Jinan – presumably at the Shandong Christian University. The addition of these Chinese tutors "gave the school a new prestige," and the Weihui school of nursing was admitted into the NAC in the fall of 1924 (see Figure 15).[59]

With the new hospital and nursing school well underway at Weihui, the Henan Mission turned its attention and resources to Anyang. According to the social gospel that came to characterize the Henan Mission, medical work was to be of the highest standard possible. Medical care would gain preeminence, even though every facility in the mission was to be offered evangelistic workers, and physicians and nurses would take part in conducting regular devotional services with missionaries and staff. Medical missionaries had much to live up to. In the early 1920s, the Rockefeller Foundation had made the very best in Western medicine available to the Chinese through the new PUMC. The Christian Medical Association of China was concerned that unless hospitals attained a high standard, there was a "danger of an unfavourable attitude being taken towards a Christianity represented by hospitals so far below recognized standards."[60] There were to be three types of hospitals in China: teaching hospitals linked with a medical school, long-established hospitals that would serve as models in the surrounding area, and pioneer hospitals, where "superstition and prejudice [toward Western medicine] still had to be broken down."[61] Henan laid ambitious plans for the second type of hospital, without knowing all that would be involved in maintaining such an institution. This change in focus made more than a few missionaries nervous. For example, Dr. Percy Leslie did not like the mission's new policy of large, modern hospitals. He was concerned that they would be too costly in terms of human and financial resources, and that medical care would overshadow evangelistic work. Thus, after twenty-seven years as a Henan missionary, Dr. Leslie retired to Canada in 1924.

When Clara Preston arrived in Anyang after her language study in Beijing, plans for the new women's hospital had already been laid, under the direction of Dr. Jean Dow and Dr. Isabelle McTavish. The women's hospital was to be built next to the men's hospital so that the two could co-operate. By this time, the mission at Anyang was spread over two compounds – the eastern compound was a twelve-minute walk from the hospital compound. Every day, Clara Preston would walk from the eastern compound to the hospital compound to inspect the hospital progress and participate in final decisions. She wrote, "We all helped to plan cupboards, where the window would go – how we could put the furniture to best advantage, and how the work could be carried out most conveniently."[62] Equipping the hospital was by trial and error: "A back-rest, bedside table and stool, mattress, cradle, baby's bassinet, electrical baker seemed so simple as we used them every day in our training days."[63] Preston also helped out by going to the store to buy screws and hinges for the construction workers. She was intrigued by the lack of modern machinery, inadequate tools, and lack of paintbrushes (the hospital was painted by using silk waste soaked in the paint and rubbed in by hand). It was slow but steady progress. By 1926, the hospital was ready, and Preston moved in.

Mishkids and the Menzies Memorial Hospital

In all the excitement at Weihui and Anyang, the Huaiqing Hospital became neglected. In fact, it had been closed since 15 July 1920.[64] After Dr. Menzies died in March, Rev. Slimmon took over the supervision of the hospital, but within four months, the Henan Emergency Committee closed it, pending the appointment of a new Canadian doctor. Various attempts were made to secure physicians (first Reeds, then Baird and Struthers) but furloughs, language study, and illness thwarted the plans. By 1923, there was still no physician. When Dr. Reeds returned from his furlough, he was discouraged to find the hospital progress stalled and funds from the Forward Movement exhausted. Believing that the Henan Mission had a moral obligation to construct the new Menzies Memorial Hospital as promised, Dr. Reeds went ahead with plans for the new building.

The Bloor Street Presbyterian Church in Toronto – Dr. James R. Menzies' church – was keen to see medical work at Huaiqing continue. The congregation's desire to support another physician to replace the martyred Dr. Menzies was realized in the person of Dr. Robert (Bob) McClure, son of pioneer Henan physician Dr. William McClure. As both a "mishkid" (missionary kid) and a physician, Bob McClure was the ideal candidate for the Henan Mission.[65] Bob McClure *(Loa Ming-yuan)* had intended to become a missionary at some point, but was actually on his way to graduate studies at Harvard when Rev. Dr. George Pidgeon called him to the vestry for a discussion. According to McClure, Dr. Pidgeon said, "'Bob, our missionary in China has been shot by bandits, how would you like to go out and take his place?' And I was a postwar generation. Toronto was a very quiet place. I felt I had missed all the excitement of war and that sort of thing. And this seemed like a chance for a great adventure."[66] After completing some additional surgery training, McClure packed his bags for China. If it was adventure he was looking for, he went to the right place. Over the next two decades in war-torn China, McClure would have more than his share of excitement.

Dr. Bob McClure was not the only Henan mishkid to return to the Henan Mission that year. Jean Menzies, the daughter of Dr. James R. Menzies, also returned to Henan (see Figure 16). On 17 June 1923, in a moving designation service at the Bloor Street Church, Bob and Jean were "set apart" for mission service in Henan, along with Jean's friend, nurse Coral May Brodie. (See Figure 17.) Jean Menzies was born at Anyang, Henan, on 9 March 1898.[67] She was a toddler during the Boxer Uprising. Jean spent her early childhood at Huaiqing and her school years at Weihui, where she boarded with the McClures.[68] Jean Menzies was like a sister to Bob McClure. In fact, "McClure" was her middle name.

Jean Menzies would have been thirteen years old when Mrs. Ratcliffe became matron of the Weihui school for missionary children in 1911. Missionary kids did not learn Chinese at the school at Weihui, but rather from their Chinese playmates – sometimes to the chagrin of their parents. According to Bob McClure, his father William used to draw a chalk line across the door of their house, and give him a "really good spanking" if he spoke a word of Chinese inside that chalk line.[69] William McClure was apparently concerned that his son was more comfortable with Chinese than English, and that he might have difficulty when the family returned to Canada. Thus, when Bob McClure and Jean Menzies went to language school together in Beijing in 1923, it was not so much to learn to speak Chinese, but to "clean up" their street vernacular and Henan dialect. They also had to learn to write in Chinese.

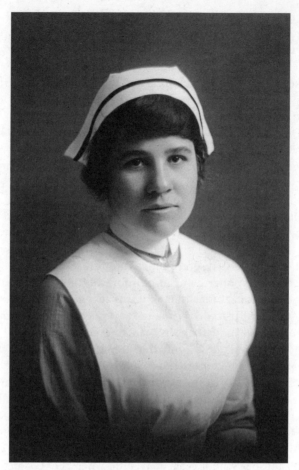

Figure 16 Jean McClure Menzies, 1922.
UCCVUA 76.001P-4615

When Dr. James Menzies was killed in 1920, Jean Menzies was living in Toronto with her mother and two sisters. Mrs. Davina (Robb) Menzies had returned to Canada the previous year to recover from "sprue," a tropical disease.[70] Jean was a first-year nursing student at the Toronto General Hospital when she received word of her father's death. It is not clear whether Jean had always intended to return to Henan as a nurse, but it seems a natural choice, given her parents' dedication to the mission and the growing need for nurses at Henan. As a newly graduated nurse, Jean returned to China with her widowed mother, Davina Menzies. The missionaries at Henan were delighted to have "one of [their] own" return as a missionary in her own right. Jean would be the first of seven Henan "mishkid" nurses – children of missionaries who returned to China after taking nurses' training in Canada.[71]

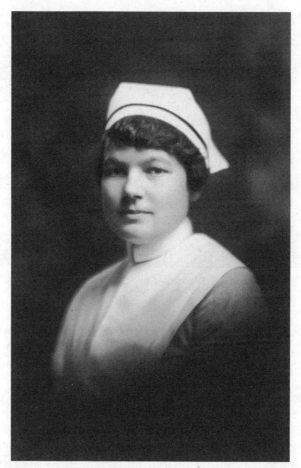

Figure 17   Coral Brodie, 1921.
UCCVUA 76.001P-628

Jean Menzies' friend Coral May Brodie was born on 3 May 1897 at Bethesda, Ontario. Brodie attended Toronto General Hospital School of Nursing, graduating one year before Menzies, in 1921. (See Figure 17.) Brodie took a year of training at the Presbyterian Missionary and Deaconess Training Home in Toronto in 1922, and was ready to travel to China with Menzies and her mother in 1923.[72] After language school, Menzies and Brodie were appointed to Huaiqing, where they were to work under the leadership of Janet Brydon at the as-yet-incomplete Menzies Memorial Hospital. Both nurses were at the old Huaiqing hospital when Dr. Bob McClure first arrived there in 1924.[73]

Retrospectively, one must wonder at the Henan Mission's decision to place Jean Menzies, Bob McClure, and Janet Brydon together at Huaiqing, considering how intimately connected each was to the tragedy of Dr. Menzies'

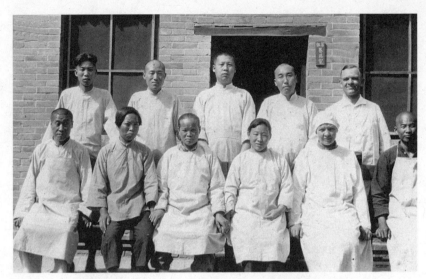

Figure 18　Huaiqing hospital in pre–nursing school days, 1920s.
UCCVUA 1999.001P-1811

murder. Did the mission not foresee the awkwardness of the situation, where Jean would have to work under the leadership of the very woman her father had died to save? McClure's biographer later commented on the bizarre situation: "The nurse at [McClure's] side making ward rounds was the late doctor's daughter [Jean]. The head nurse, Janet Brydon ... was one of the women Dr. Menzies had rushed to aid on the night he was murdered ... There was no escaping Menzies. Everybody around still remembered him as clearly as though he had just left the room."[74] Perhaps the full emotional impact of the scenario did not hit Jean until she actually arrived at Huaiqing. Or perhaps she followed her mother's lead back to their Chinese "hometown." Whatever her reason for going to Huaiqing, Jean Menzies did not stay there long. Sometime in 1924, Jean transferred to the hospital at Weihui.[75]

The Huaiqing hospital staff, such as it was, carried on with medical care while awaiting the construction of the long-promised memorial hospital. They pressed forward with the meagre resources and primitive facilities at hand (see Figure 18). In 1924, they were faced with an onslaught of a new category of patient: wounded Chinese soldiers. They resigned themselves to spreading sawdust on the operating room floor during amputations to collect the "gory" waste.[76]

Rising Nationalism and Anti-Foreignism
By the end of 1924, the nursing situation at Henan was better than it had ever been, with Jeanette Ratcliffe, Margaret Mitchell, and Jean Menzies at

Weihui, Clara Preston at Anyang, Janet Brydon and Coral Brodie at Huaiqing, and Isabel Leslie at the small station at Wuan.[77] In addition, long-time evangelistic worker Margaret Gay was in Canada taking nurses' training at Vancouver General Hospital, with plans to return to China in 1926. It was a heady time for the nurses as they moved forward with plans for modern hospitals, schools, and registration with the NAC. Once again, however, the winds of political change were blowing, and the Henan nurses found themselves propelled off course.

The years 1924 to 1927 were a period of upheaval and redirection, for the Presbyterian mission in North Henan and for China as a nation. The Presbyterian Church of Canada was going ahead with plans to amalgamate with the Congregationalists and the Methodists into one United Church of Canada by 1925. Under the new union, three Canadian missions in China were restructured as United Church missions: the Presbyterian mission in North Henan became the North China Mission; the Methodist mission in Sichuan became the West China Mission; and the Presbyterian mission in Guangzhou became the South China Mission. Almost all the missionaries at the North Henan Mission agreed with the church union (only one or two voted against it). Being part of one United Church provided opportunities for collegiality among Canadian missionary nurses: United Church missionary nurses became part of a Canadian family spread thousands of miles apart in China.

The political changes in the Presbyterian Church were significant, but it was political changes in China that had the most direct impact on the Canadian missionaries during this period. China was in upheaval. After the overthrow of the Qing Dynasty during the First Revolution, President Sun Yat-sen worked to mould China into a unified republic. Yuan Shih-kai betrayed the republic by trying to set himself up as emperor, and the nation rose in rebellion against the idea. Yuan died in 1916, and chaos followed. The country was divided into spheres of interest, with various warlords fighting each other for territory. Parliament was set aside as warlords struggled to increase their spheres of influence. Bandits ruled supreme in a large portion of the interior, particularly in Henan.[78] Dr. Sun Yat-sen died on 12 March 1925, without achieving his vision for a unified China.[79]

Although accustomed to living in a volatile environment, Canadians in North Henan in 1925 were nervously anticipating the eruption of serious trouble. After Sun Yat-sen's death, anti-foreign nationalism had become palpable – particularly among China's student population. This surge of nationalism was fuelled by three separate incidents in which foreigners opened fire on Chinese demonstrators – in Shanghai, Guangzhou, and Wanxian.[80] After the "May 30th Incident" in Shanghai, missionaries at Huaiqing detected an upsurge of violent nationalism. As one Chinese general advanced toward Huaiqing with the goal of taking control of the coal mine railway and the Yellow River away from local warlords, wounded Chinese soldiers from both sides began to show up at the mission hospital. The medical and nursing work escalated – as did the threat of banditry. According to Dr. Bob McClure, many of the local bandits were army deserters who kept their weapons and ammunition with them when they broke ranks. Patients admitted to the mission hospital were required to surrender their firearms for the duration of their stay, but McClure carried a concealed gun just in case.[81]

At Anyang, Clara Preston also noticed a rise in anti-foreignism after the May 30th Incident. To avoid trouble, the missionaries quietly disbanded their summer theology school, but by the end of June, some of the Chinese church elders advised the Canadians to send as many as possible away for summer holidays. This was not easily accomplished. Clara Preston and Minnie Shipley accompanied Margaret MacIntosh to the train station; sixty-eight-year-old MacIntosh rode in a rickshaw across muddy roads in the rain, with Preston and Shipley alongside. As Preston wrote, "it was so hard going that [Miss MacIntosh] twice felt she couldn't make it but we urged and encouraged her to try. When we arrived at the station the students were there with banners with anti British mottoes telling the innocent peasants how terrible the British were, and the posters showed in graphic cartoons how some had been killed."[82] By 2 a.m., there was still no word of the train, so the three women headed to the Canadian hospital compound, which was nearer to the train station than the eastern compound, to spend the rest of the night. As Preston later recalled, "the walk back from the station was an eire [sic] experience. The road was wet and slippery. We tried to carry umbrellas and a lantern to avoid slipping off the road into the dirty ditch on the side. The dogs heralded our approach and at nearly every house or store we passed we saw a door cautiously opened and a face peering out to see why the dogs were barking. In some cases we would see just an eye peering at us."[83] Relieved to be in the shelter of one of the mission compounds, the ladies spent the night; an (unnamed) doctor gave up his bed to MacIntosh, while Preston and Shipley slept on the floor. The train finally arrived the following evening, and the ladies headed north to safety.

The hospital at Anyang was subsequently closed for three months during the summer of 1925. The women had hoped that they could move into their new women's hospital in early 1926, but its opening was delayed until later in the year. (See Figure 19.) When the new hospital finally opened, there was no fanfare like there had been at Weihui three years earlier. Instead, the missionaries simply expressed satisfaction in the expanded opportunities provided them by the new facilities. For example, they took pride in the fact that several obstetrical cases were cared for in the new wards by nursing staff under the direction of Clara Preston, and considered

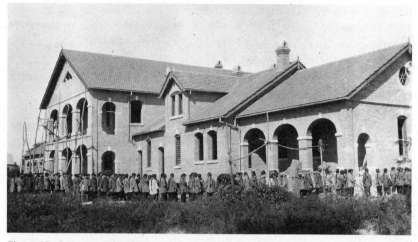

Figure 19 Inspection by Chinese schoolchildren of the new women's hospital at Anyang, c. 1926.
UCCVUA 1999.001P-1666N

the successful outcome of the first major abdominal operation a "cause for great rejoicing."[84]

Like the hospital in Anyang, the new hospital at Weihui noted an increase in wounded Chinese soldiers and civilians. Five times in one month the hospital received men with abdominal wounds, and throughout the spring, there were soldiers in the wards. The doctors were "delighted" to have qualified nurses to care for those with serious abdominal wounds. As tensions in China mounted, Mrs. Ratcliffe ensured that the hospital work carried on "with something like regularity and routine," despite being faced with "the uncertainty of being able to do what was planned."[85] Ratcliffe struggled with the logistics of ordering and receiving supplies, preparing rooms for military patients and refugees, and working with only one physician – Dr. R. Gordon Struthers – while Drs. Baird and Auld were away. The difficult political conditions affected the nurses' training school, but Ratcliffe was determined to carry on.

By 1926, the Weihui nursing school had twenty-three students, most of whom were male: in fact, only four of the eleven third-year students were female.[86] At the end of the school year, three senior nursing students successfully completed their nursing examinations. This marked a milestone in nursing history: North Henan had graduated its first class of nurses.

Wedding Bells and the Case of Married Nurses

As frequently happened, one of the new missionary nurses resigned from the WMS in 1926 to marry a fellow missionary. Jean McClure Menzies became engaged to Dr. Handley Stockley of the English Baptist Mission. They planned to marry in 1926, but Dr. Stockley was "shut up for eight months in the siege of Xian."[87] The siege was lifted in December, so the marriage took place in January, at Weihui. The Baptist Mission gained a missionary wife, but the Henan Mission lost both a missionary nurse and a beloved mishkid.

The nurses who worked at the Henan Mission during the missionary era can be divided into three categories: (1) WMS nurses who stayed unmarried; (2) WMS nurses who resigned to be married; and (3) FMB missionary wives who happened to be nurses. Some of the nurses in these categories were Henan mishkids who took nurses' training in Canada and then returned to China as missionary wives (see Appendix 3: Three types of missionary nurses). Although married nurses were not officially hired for their nursing services, they have been included here because of their contribution at various times to health care. Of the twenty-one WMS nurses in this study, twelve resigned to be married. Of these twelve, ten married China missionaries and remained in China as missionary wives. Although little is known of their contribution to nursing after their marriages, it is clear that some volunteered their nursing services when the need arose. For example, Mrs. Maisie (McNeely) Forbes lived at Henan for another twenty-four years after her marriage to Rev. H. Stewart Forbes in 1916. Maisie made herself available during wartime crises, including helping out in the operating room in 1938.[88] Similarly, Mrs. Elizabeth (Betty) (Thomson) Gale helped out at the nursing school at Qilu University after marrying Dr. Godfrey Gale in 1940, and then became a prisoner of war with her husband and infant daughter from 1941 to 1945.[89] Finally, Mrs. Jean (Menzies) Stockley remained in China for at least sixteen years after her marriage to Dr. Handley Stockley in 1927. From Xian in 1943, Mrs. Stockley aided refugee students from Henan, including one nursing student who had contracted tuberculosis during nurses' training.[90]

In addition to the ten former WMS nurses who remained in China after they married, some of the women who came to China as FMB-supported missionary wives were also graduate nurses. These included Mrs. Christina Malcolm, Mrs. W.C. Netterfield, Mrs. M. Roulston, Mrs. MacKinley, Mrs. Harriet Alexander, and Mrs. Anna Marion (Fisher) Faris. In addition, Mrs. Amy (Hislop) McClure – the wife of Dr. Bob McClure – took two years of nurses' training at Toronto General Hospital, but did not complete her program before coming to China. As missionary wives, these women had no formal obligation to work as nurses, and many kept busy caring for their children. Still, many did offer their nursing skills when the mission was shorthanded. For example, Mrs. MacKinley helped her husband in the operating room in 1931, and Mrs. Alexander became the temporary superintendent of nurses at Weihui in 1946.[91]

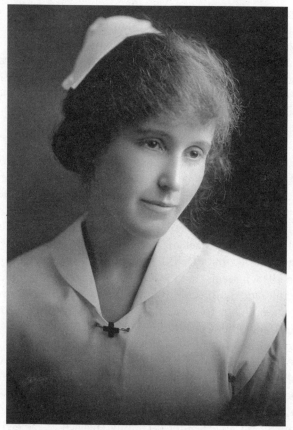

Figure 20 Anna Marion Fisher Faris, 1923.
UCCVUA 76.001P-1832

Marion Fisher (later Faris) made history on 10 May 1923 when she, along with Margaret Healy and Beatrice Johnson, accepted her bachelor of applied science (in nursing) degree at the University of British Columbia convocation. These three women were celebrated as the first to acquire university degrees in nursing "anywhere in the British Empire." (See Figure 20.) Ethel Johns, the director of the new program in 1919, had hand-picked Fisher because she had already taken a year of university (the UBC-McGill program, in 1913). Although she successfully completed her degree, Fisher contracted tuberculosis and, immediately following her graduation, went as a patient to the TB San (Sanatorium) at Tranquille for a year. Fortunately, hers was not an advanced case, and Fisher was able to complete her recovery at Gabriola Island.[92] Marion Fisher married Rev. D.K. Faris, and they were both appointed as missionaries to Henan, where they worked from 1925 until 1937. Although Mrs. Faris was designated as an "evangelistic worker," she did not lose sight of her nursing interest, as evidenced by an article she wrote for the *Henan Messenger* in 1927, in which she described the "sick room in Wuan": "Here we find Agnes Bruce, the 'Pollyanna' of our mission. For months she has been in bed and unknown to herself is always playing the 'just being glad' game. After being 'war-stayed' on Kikungshan for six weeks, there followed a hard journey of days during cold November, but she was 'so glad to be home for Xmas' ... Our prayers follow her and her family as they journey to Canada, where it is hoped she will soon regain her health."[93]

It is difficult to know to what extent married nurses were involved with the care of the sick and injured in Henan, since no formal record was kept of their service. For example, Mrs. Florence (MacKenzie) Liddell lived in China for seven years after taking nurses' training (1934-41), but it is unclear whether she practised nursing there. Similarly, Florence's sister-in-law, Mrs. Dorothy (Lochead) MacKenzie lived in China for six years (1943-49). Although there is record of Dorothy teaching nursing students in Fowling, Sichuan, in 1948, it seems that most of her energies were spent on her husband and children.[94] Both Dorothy and Florence were Henan mishkids who took nurses' training in Toronto, then married China missionaries. Neither fit neatly into the other categories of nurses described.

The daughter of North China Mission missionaries Hugh and Agnes MacKenzie, Florence had always wanted to become a nurse. But she was not certain if she would return to China after studying nursing in Canada – that is, until she met and fell in love with a missionary she met in Tianjin, where her parents ran a boarding house for missionaries under the auspices of the United Church of Canada. After becoming engaged at age eighteen, Florence headed to Toronto General Hospital, along with her best friend and fellow Henan mishkid, Elizabeth (Betty) Thomson. Florence planned to return to China when she had completed her nursing education; her father believed that all women should have some kind of training before getting married.[95]

In 1933, after a lengthy and long-distance engagement, Florence married Eric Liddell – a 1924 Olympic gold medalist who had been with the London Missionary Society since 1925. In 1941, when Florence was expecting their third child, she returned to Canada with her young daughters because of the escalating war in China. Eric stayed in China and subsequently became a prisoner of war. He died at the Weixian internment camp (at Weifang in Shandong province) in 1945, of a brain tumour. Finding herself widowed with three children, Florence went back to work as a nurse in Canada.[96]

Of the twenty-one WMS nurses in this study, twelve resigned to be married, seven had long careers, one resigned due to illness, and one resigned due to the closure of the mission in 1947. Thus, with few exceptions, the WMS nurses either resigned to be married or worked for many years in

China. On average, unmarried Canadian nurses worked in Henan for twenty-five years. These included Margaret MacIntosh (thirty-eight years), Margaret Gay (thirty years, including thirteen as an evangelistic worker), Jeanette Ratcliffe (twenty-five years), Clara Preston (twenty-five years), Janet Brydon (twenty-one years), Coral Brodie (eighteen years), and Margaret Mitchell (seventeen years).[97] These nurses' commitment to China through so many periods of tumult is extraordinary. As it was, all of these long-serving nurses were already appointed to China by the time of the Great Exodus of 1927.

The Great Exodus of 1927

The year 1926 was an historic year for nursing in Henan, with the graduation of three students from Weihui. It was also an historic year for China. Dr. Reeds of Huaiqing described 1926 as a year of "unrest and upheaval, of turbulence and warfare, change and unsettlement, banditry and exaction."[98] That year, Chiang Kai-shek's Nationalist Revolutionary Army headed north from Guangzhou, and there was a growing number of student demonstrations. The Henan missionaries were increasingly on edge as they tried to make sense of reported and rumoured political developments. As Reeds understood it, China was an "armed camp" with two million men in uniform "contending for supremacy;" it was a battle of the North against the South, with Chiang Kai-shek leading the South. To Reeds, China's sudden change from a dynasty to a republic had been a great failure, and the most pressing need was for a central government, with power to govern.[99]

When the Nationalist army seized Nanjing on 24 March 1927, it was with the aim of establishing a new central government. The struggle to unify China was characterized by bloodshed and violence, and the foreigners felt threatened. By the time Chiang entered Nanjing, many foreign missionaries had already been evacuated to the safety of the coastal treaty ports. Yet the Henan missionaries lingered on. Except for comparatively small local skirmishes, the Henan Mission remained relatively isolated from the Nationalist campaign. Besides, the missionaries had crises of their own to contend with, including the death of Dr. Jean Isabel Dow on 17 January 1927. For Henan, Dr. Dow's death meant the loss of a "precious gift to China."[100] For Margaret MacIntosh, Dr. Dow's death meant the loss of an "intimate and tender relationship" that had spanned thirty-two years. At age seventy, MacIntosh decided it was time to retire.

For the missionary nurses at Huaiqing, Anyang, and Weihui, there was more than enough work to keep their attention. Clara Preston had been in Beijing helping to nurse Dr. Dow in her illness and accompanied her remains back to Anyang by train. Preston noticed some "unrest and tension in the air" during the spring of 1927. In a letter to friends in Canada dated 19 February 1927, Clara Preston described her day-to-day nursing experiences at the newly opened women's hospital in Anyang:

Our children's ward is full (3) beds [sic]. The first boy came from the village where the people were massacred. His mother was shot before his eyes and he himself is badly shot in the thigh and leg. He has nightmares and bad dreams poor boy! ... In the next bed is a poor thin boy with kala azar and he has bronchitis. He coughs a great deal, he sure was dirty when he came in. He calls me his adopted mother. In the cot is a small girl who was also shot at that place. Her temperature to-day was 104. She is badly shot in the leg and thigh. A number of women and children were in a group and the soldiers shot right into the group. In another room we have an old woman the soldiers shot through the breasts, she is 70 years old.[101]

Despite the rising political tension, the missionaries did not expect to have to leave Henan. When a telegram arrived from Tianjin on 1 April 1927, asking the missionaries to "All leave at once," it "came like a bolt out of the blue."[102] The missionaries scrambled to pack for the journey north. Huaiqing missionaries travelled by train, in third-class compartments without heat or windowpanes; cold wintry air blew in for two days. There was room for only four or five to sit down at a time, and baggage was stacked high in the aisles. Soldiers lay in the deep overhead luggage racks, from where they spat at those sitting below. When it came time to disembark, the crowds were too dense to press through. The Huaiqing missionaries squeezed themselves – and their baggage – through the train windows onto the platform below.

At Anyang, the Canadians called the Chinese hospital staff together to inform them of their plans to evacuate. While Preston and the others took inventories and gave away supplies in preparation for their departure, they were disconsolate, realizing that "the work of years for the older missionaries had to be closed in three days' time. What mingled feelings we all had – when could we return – who would look after the sick – where would our staff go ... Only those who have seen their work grow and then have to be laid aside know what that means."[103]

Preston and the others boarded a train for Tianjin, taking along a lunch of cold toast sandwiches and soup inadvertently made with sour milk ("our cook was away, and the second boy tried so hard to help").[104] In Tianjin they met up with the other Canadians, as well as numerous other foreign refugees and slept with as many as fifteen to a room. The Henan missionaries (ninety-six of them) later camped out in three unfurnished houses in a compound known as Mimosa Court. They had one dining room between them. American Marines loaned army cots to the group, and the missionary men used boards to make tables and benches.[105] Those who were due furloughs were given permission to leave for home; Preston was among this group, and she returned to Canada. Others waited out the storm in Tianjin. A deputation from the home church in Canada that had planned to meet with the Henan missionaries had already reached China, and was keen to

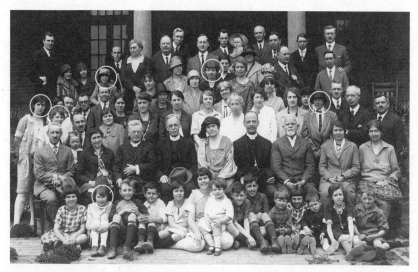

Figure 21   Historic last meeting of the Henan Presbytery, Tianjin, 1927. *Highlighted faces, left to right, back:* Florence MacKenzie, Mary Boyd, Marion Faris, Janet Brydon, Jeanette Ratcliffe; *front:* Dorothy Boyd.
UCCVUA 1999.001P-1602

meet with the missionaries. Thus it was that the Henan missionaries formally met for the last time as Presbyterians while refugees in Tianjin. A group photo taken to mark the historic meeting shows Janet Brydon, Jeanette Ratcliffe, Marion Fisher Faris, and three mishkids who would go on to nurses' training before returning to China as missionaries themselves: Florence MacKenzie, Mary Boyd, and Dorothy Boyd (see Figure 21).

The year 1927 would be remembered as the year of the Great Missionary Exodus. In total, 8,300 Protestant missionaries were evacuated; 3,000 never went back to their missions.[106] The Henan Mission lost twenty of their ninety-six missionaries, including missionary nurse Margaret MacIntosh.

Summary

By the early 1920s, the necessary support was in place for the development of nursing in North Henan. WMS supporters in Canada provided funding and moral support, the CMMA provided scientific evidence of the need for nursing in China, the NAC and the International Council of Nurses provided a national and international professional network, the Church of Christ in China provided a link between the mission and prospective nursing students, and the Henan Mission provided human resources to establish modern hospitals. In addition, graduate nurses – both Chinese and Canadian – responded to the call for nursing leaders: two Chinese instructors came on staff at Weihui, and six Canadian nurses were appointed by the WMS (Leslie,

Galbraith, Straith, Preston, Menzies, and Brodie). For all intents and purposes, modern nursing was poised to take root in Henan.

As China struggled to redefine itself through revolution, warlord rule, and the Nationalist advance, the need for nursing care seemed more poignant than ever. Along with the anticipated illness and injury care came an increased number of wounded soldiers and civilians. Paradoxically, the same events that triggered an increased need for nursing care also triggered the interruption of nursing services. When the Canadians evacuated Henan in 1927, nursing services were still in their infancy, largely dependent on foreign nurses and, therefore, not sustainable. Once again, nursing services at North Henan came to a standstill.

4
Golden Years, 1928-37

The City and Country need the help of many graduate nurses and we hope it is just the beginning.

– L. Clara Preston, 1936

Winds of War

The Nationalist Army reached North Henan while the exiled missionaries waited at Tianjin. In August 1927, the army began its occupation of Anyang, Weihui, and Huaiqing. It looted homes, schools, and hospitals at every Canadian mission station except Wuan. Although Tianjin had seemed a safe haven, there was growing concern that it might also come under attack. Thus, all the missionaries due furlough within the next two years were ordered back to Canada. Clara Preston returned to Montreal, where she took nursing courses at McGill University. Some missionaries who remained in China also took further education: Dr. R.G. Struthers and Dr. Reeds took postgraduate courses at Beijing. Others were allocated for work at mission sites in the northeastern provinces, Shanghai, Japan, and Taiwan. Janet Brydon was among those who went to the northeastern provinces to work with the American Presbyterian mission. A small Canadian contingent remained in Tianjin, including the Forbes, the Boyds, the Griffiths, and the Grants.[1]

In May 1928, Coral Brodie was "temporarily" sent to the Shandong Christian University Hospital in Jinan. Her appointment at Qilu was supposed to last only until her services were again required in Henan, but she remained there for eleven years.[2] A cordial, interdependent relationship between Qilu and the Henan Mission (now called the "North China Mission" [NCM]) had begun a few years earlier, when the Canadian missionaries chose Qilu over the Peking Union Medical College as the university with which their medical work would be affiliated. Other NCM missionaries had already moved to Qilu to work as professors and on the hospital staff. These included Dr.

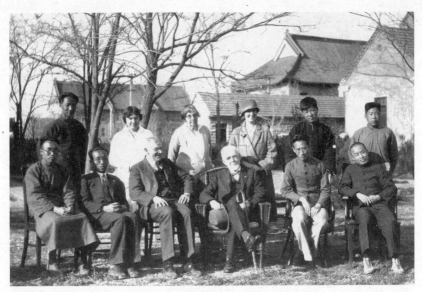

Figure 22   Canadians living in Jinan, 1930s. Qilu Campus, Shandong Christian University. *Left to right, standing:* Janet Brydon, Mrs. Mitchell, Margaret Struthers; *seated in middle:* Rev. R.A. Mitchell, Dr. William McClure.
Mary Struthers McKim private collection

Ernest B. and Margaret Struthers, and Bob McClure's parents, Dr. William and Margaret McClure (see Figure 22). The relationship between the NCM and Qilu would continue throughout the duration of the missionary era.

When Brodie arrived in 1928, Jinan was a battleground. The Nationalist army from the south had ousted northern Chinese soldiers from Jinan on May Day. The Nationalist troops were not the only army occupying Jinan. Japanese troops had also arrived from Japan, ostensibly to protect the interests of Japanese civilians living in Shandong. Fighting broke out between the Japanese and the Nationalists. It was not until 1929 that the Nationalists gained control of Shandong province.[3] The hostilities at Jinan in 1928 foreshadowed the coming Sino-Japanese War (1937-45). Throughout the troubles in 1928, the Qilu University hospital stayed open; it was filled to overflowing with wounded civilians and soldiers. It was no small feat for the university hospital to continue treating patients, considering the very real threat posed by the Japanese to patients and staff alike in 1928. NCM missionaries were exposed to the horror of war crimes at Jinan. On or around 11 May 1928, shortly after Brodie arrived at Qilu, Dr. E.B. Struthers was asked by the Swastika Society (the Chinese Red Cross) to investigate and report a gruesome incident at a Chinese military hospital. His findings were ghastly: "We found that in the operating room and on all the wards everyone in bed or running around had been bayoneted, usually in the chest. We counted 115 corpses including a priest who had crawled under the table. There was also a patient who had climbed into a boat [?] thinking he might escape being seen. The raid, said to be in revenge [against the Chinese] for fighting against the Japanese, took place at about 6:00 a.m. when some of the patients had begun to prepare breakfast. Nearly all were done in as they lay in bed."[4] Dr. Struthers' shocking report is corroborated by a letter written on 29 May 1928 and circulated to "a list of friends," in which a certain W.B. Djang from the Shandong University in Jinan recorded what he saw "with my own eyes" of Japanese atrocities on and around the campus. Djang wrote of the indiscriminate shooting of Chinese refugees by Japanese hiding in the southwest corner of the Qilu campus, the robbing and looting of Chinese staff homes on campus, and the murder of wounded soldiers:

> In the West suburb there is a public hospital in which there were about 70 wounded soldiers under medical care. Early in the morning on May 11, a band of Japanese soldiers broke into it from a neighboring house and murdered all the patients in their sick beds and all those who waited on them. The people living in the immediate neighborhood were attacked and 57 of them also killed by the Japanese with bayonets. Of these were two Taoist priests whose temple was nearby, and one Christian old gentleman ... I saw some of these victims with my own eyes when the Red Swasticus [sic] were carrying the dead bodies out for burial.[5]

What makes this incident particularly troubling is that it occurred three years before the Japanese invaded the northeastern provinces in 1931, and almost ten years before the Japanese began their violent invasion of the rest of China in 1937. Yet the international community turned a blind eye. Dr. Struthers wrote up the incident but was unable to find anyone willing to bring it to the attention of the League of Nations. W.B. Djang similarly attempted to get the attention of the international community. At the same time, Djang expressed doubt that the "truth" of the incident would be publicized. He outlined eyewitness accounts during the Nationalist takeover of Jinan, and the apparent overreaction of the Japanese: "It is hard to believe the [sic] for the protection of 2,000 nationals Japan would send 12,000 to this city and 28,000 to this province." He also stated that he believed the international media would turn the incident around to appear that the Japanese were defending themselves against Chinese aggression. His prediction that "the Japanese would have undoubtedly broadcasted [Chinese defense] as signs and proofs of the anti-foreignism of the Chinese" foreshadowed claims made by NCM missionaries ten years later that the Anti-British Movement of 1939 was actually instigated by the Japanese. Djang was infuriated by the Japanese. He was also frustrated by the indifference of the international community to events in China, and its willingness to uncritically accept the Japanese version of events: "Yes, the truth will no doubt triumph when, after two or three hundred years, some unbiased Oxford or Harvard professor of history endeavors to sift the gold out from the dross ... The policy of China is still one of peaceful negotiation and non-resistance, although many people are getting tired of it and would like risk rather than roast ... many are wavering between Maccabeanism and Christianity. The contest between the Gospel and the Gun almost exhausts the patriotic Christian."[6]

Brodie was at Qilu at the time of the murder of Chinese patients at the public hospital. Many years later, Brodie told her family of a deeply disturbing incident whereby the Japanese bayoneted all the patients under her care – she was likely referring to the event described by Struthers and Djang. Although Brodie did not work at the public hospital where the murders took place, and although it is doubtful that she was an eyewitness to the massacre, she was profoundly disturbed by the incident. This (and possibly other) acts of Japanese aggression left a deep and lasting impression on Brodie, who subsequently "had no good thing to say" about the Japanese.[7] Coral Brodie remained at Qilu for the rest of her China career, until 1939.

Vandalism and Looting at the NCM at Henan

In early 1928, representatives from the NCM who were still in exile at Tianjin decided to tour Henan to see what kind of damage had been done to the mission stations during the Nationalist takeover. At Anyang, they were refused entrance to both the hospital compound and the eastern compound; the Nationalist 30th Army occupied both (see Figure 23). When they were later granted permission to inspect the compounds, the NCM cadre found "all houses had been looted, from cellar to attic, of clothing, beds, bedding, sewing machines, dishes, cutlery, bicycles, in fact of everything the soldiers

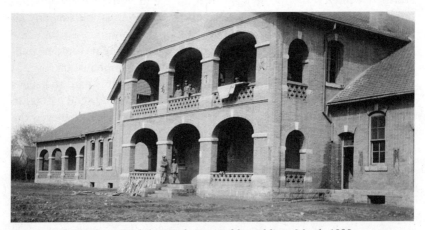

Figure 23 Anyang women's hospital occupied by soldiers, March 1930.
UCCVUA 1999-001P-1668

fancied. Heavy furniture had been stripped of drawers and mirrors and badly damaged. Pianos and heavy organs had been maliciously smashed to fragments with hammers ... Furnaces, pipes and glass windows were destroyed. Doors and shutters were torn off and burned as fuel. The Foreign cemetery had been desecrated and the basements of hospitals and houses used for latrines."[8]

The NCM inspectors found a similar situation at Weihui. Of the eleven missionary houses, one had been burned with all its contents and the others looted of everything. The missionary children's boarding school had been burned to the ground. And the new Weihui Hospital had been completely looted, with windows and furnaces smashed. At Huaiqing, the compound had been raided six times, but it was not as badly damaged as the other stations. There were personal losses from the homes, and the Huaiqing hospital lost most of its equipment, bedding, and mattresses. Altogether, the damage to the mission stations was estimated at Cdn$121,600.[9]

The damage could have been worse. At Weihui, a Chinese caretaker managed to hide 85 of the 120 hospital beds, as well as two sterilizers and the "balopticon."[10] Still, repair expenses were daunting – particularly in light of the unfavourable exchange rates with Canadian currency.[11] The missionaries were later asked to write up lists of their personal losses so that they could seek reparations from the Chinese authorities. Submissions by nurses Ratcliffe, Brodie, Preston, MacIntosh, and Mitchell came to Cdn$1,408.50.[12]

At the time that the NCM was trying to find funds to help repair its damaged property, Canada was entering a severe economic depression. As a result, the United Church of Canada found its income seriously reduced; the church had to take drastic measures to try to make ends meet. By 1932, missionary salaries had been cut by 15 percent, and travel to and from Canada was reduced. Furloughs were postponed, and children over the age of fourteen were not allowed to return to China at the mission's expense. All China boat and train travel was to be done by cabin class or tourist class.[13] The Chinese sympathized with Canada's financial concerns. News of grave economic conditions on Canadian farms stirred Chinese generosity: out of their meagre incomes, Henan Christians collected Ch$149.81 for "our fellow Christians suffering famine" in Saskatchewan.[14] Canada had supported famine relief efforts in northern China in the past, and to the NCM missionaries, this act of reciprocal giving signified China's understanding of the spirit behind Canadian humanitarian efforts in Henan.

Funding would continue to be problematic through the Canadian Depression years. The NCM missionaries agreed to reduce their hospital budgets and to charge patients for services. While some of the missionaries reconciled charging patients as a prelude to Chinese self-sufficiency, others worried that some patients would not receive the care they needed if charged. The mission secretary, W. Harvey Grant, urged the Canadian home board to find ways to support charitable work since "until now we have been able to say that no person needing the help of the Christian hospital has been turned away from our doors simply because he or she could not pay for treatment."[15] It was important to the Canadians that they be able to treat impoverished patients:

> A few days ago, three Kala Azar cases came into the clinic, one was able to pay for his treatment, the other two could only produce one or two dollars for a course of ten treatments for which the cost of medicine was fifteen dollars ... one of them had come over ninety miles [for treatment] ... Almost daily, cases of ill-nourished under-fed children are seen for whom a little cod-liver oil to supplement their poor food is a necessity, but the cost of a bottle would be more than the father of the family could earn in a week.[16]

The NCM would never enjoy the same level of financial giving that it had experienced in the years immediately following the Boxer Uprising. Despite diminishing financial support from the home church in Canada, however, the NCM proceeded with plans for medical and nursing expansion. The mission would soon be supporting two modern hospitals and nurses' training schools (Weihui and Anyang) as well as new Chinese medical staff (three doctors and five graduate nurses) in addition to its regular missionary staff. The missionaries continued to seek creative ways to keep costs down but, ironically, it was diminishing evangelistic costs that helped to offset the growing medical costs. That is, between 1923 and 1933, the NCM had lost a sum total of eleven missionaries – ten of whom were evangelical workers. Thus, in a very tangible sense, the NCM was becoming "less an evangelistic mission" than a medical one.[17]

Reopening the Hospitals
By the fall of 1928, the situation at Henan was settled enough for the missionaries to return. Finding the hospitals in "shocking condition," the medical and nursing staff opened up clinics at Weihui and Huaiqing while the rehabilitation of the Weihui Hospital got underway. Repair of the Anyang hospitals was put on hold because there were no physicians available: Dr. Netterfield had resigned, and Dr. McTavish was temporarily in Canada for family reasons. Clara Preston was still on furlough.[18] The mission at Huaiqing was also short-staffed, with Dr. Bob McClure and Dr. Robert Reeds still away. Dr. R. Gordon Struthers' imminent furlough meant that not only were plans for the new Menzies Memorial Hospital delayed, but there was also talk of closing the existing Huaiqing hospital, too. Thus, between 1928 and 1931, most of the mission resources went to restoring the medical work at Weihui. Much to the relief of the cash-strapped mission, a doctor and nurse from Canada volunteered to work at Weihui for two years without salary: Dr.

MacKinlay performed tonsil, appendix, and gall bladder surgery while Mrs. MacKinlay, a graduate nurse, assisted him in the operating room.[19]

By 1931, Huaiqing and Anyang were ready to re-establish nursing services. The NCM forwarded a request to the United Church Woman's Missionary Society (WMS) in Canada for Clara Preston's return – if not permanently, at least for a period of two to three years so that Janet Brydon could go on furlough.[20] Preston had been working in a London hospital in Canada and was eager to return to Anyang to help in the rehabilitation of the hospital. Meanwhile, the NCM requested an additional two nurses, preferably one with graduate education in public health. Allegra Doyle and Georgina Menzies responded to the call for nurses. Both were recently graduated nurses and were accepted despite the fact that neither had extra public health education. Georgina was a mishkid, born to Dr. James R. and Davina Menzies in 1906, and a sister to former Henan nurse Jean (Menzies) Stockley. Georgina Menzies and Allegra Doyle graduated together from the Toronto General Hospital training school for nurses in 1929.[21] They travelled to China with another recently graduated Canadian nurse: forty-five-year-old Margaret Gay was returning to Henan after an absence of almost ten years.[22]

Margaret Gay: Planting a Bit of Vancouver General Hospital (VGH) in the Orient

The story of Margaret Russell Gay is central to the story of missionary nursing in Henan. Gay's life in China from 1910 to 1945 embodies the various tensions inherent in missionary nursing, and through her choices and experiences we see how nurses found a place for themselves within certain dichotomies that characterized missionary work. For example, rather than envisioning nursing as *either* evangelism *or* service, Margaret Gay saw missionary nursing as *both*. While her contemporaries downplayed direct evangelism, Gay perceived evangelistic aims as that which differentiated missionary nursing from other forms of nursing practice. Nursing skills were a natural and necessary extension of evangelistic work. In China, people in the villages approached her for help with their illnesses. This was, to Gay, irrefutable evidence of a need for practical nursing skills. Once Gay decided to pursue nursing studies in 1922, she immersed herself in the culture of modern hospital nursing practice in Vancouver, and came away with a model for illness care that stressed efficiency, orderliness, and, most of all, cleanliness. Together with her colleagues at the hospitals at Weihui, Anyang, and Huaiqing, Gay strove to develop a system of nursing that she was absolutely convinced was necessary for the well-being of the people of Henan.

Margaret Russell Gay was born at Toronto in 1886. She was appointed to Henan as an evangelistic worker in 1910, but after seeing the health needs of the rural communities where she worked, she desired to learn "a little of how to take care of sick people, even very simple procedures that [she] might

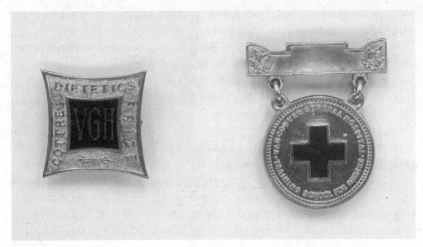

Figure 24   Margaret R. Gay's VGH nursing pins, including VGH Cottrell Dietetic Prize.
Irene Pooley and Muriel Gay private collection

learn in about three months time in a hospital somewhere."[23] Gay decided to look into possibilities when in Canada on furlough in 1922, realizing that her prospects for education were slim since most nursing programs would not accept a thirty-six-year-old probationer. While in Vancouver, Gay asked her friend Mrs. J.S. Gordon if she knew of anyone who might be able to tour her around VGH so that she "would be able to judge similar institutions by comparing them with the Vancouver General which [she knew] was one of the best in Canada." Mrs. Gordon "did not even wait to finish the meal, but rose at once and went into the library to phone Marion Fisher," who was just completing a five-year B.Sc. degree in nursing at the University of British Columbia (associated with VGH).

Marion Fisher – who later married Rev. Don K. Faris, with whom she went as a missionary to Henan in 1925 – showed Margaret around VGH. After insisting that Gay meet the nursing superintendent Miss Ellis, Fisher told the latter of Gay's desire to learn "a little about the care of the sick." Much to Gay's surprise, Miss Ellis asked if she would like to study for a few months alongside the young VGH probationers. "You could stay longer," Miss Ellis said, "or drop out at any time." Margaret Gay entered nurses' training at VGH on 16 July 1923.

Neither Miss Ellis nor Miss Gay envisioned how successful Gay would be at her nursing studies. Both had been concerned that Gay might not be able to handle the workload since she had "a severe nervous breakdown in China."[24] As it was, Gay "missed not one day" of the three-year program. Not only did she become a registered graduate nurse (RN) but she also graduated at the top of the class, with a 90.2 percent grade point average for twenty-six examinations.[25] In her final RN exams, Gay was ranked fifth out of 135 students, and at her graduation, Gay was awarded both a VGH nursing pin, and the VGH Cottrell Dietetic Prize (see Figure 24).[26]

As a student, Margaret Gay showed her capabilities as a writer in a humorous article entitled "Scrubs," published in the 1926 VGH yearbook. In it, Gay described the journey from probationer to graduation, emphasizing the centrality of cleanliness and hygiene in nursing practice. In the days before antibiotics, the "gospel of soap and water" was the most vital aspect of nursing care – a gospel that Gay and the other Canadian nurses brought with them to China. Excerpts from Margaret Gay's composition read:

For scrub we must – the ward must shine –
Beds must be white, and all in a line;
In service room too, we must scrub away,
Till instruments are all in bright array ...

There's another sink in the big O.R.,
Where gloves and masks and needles far
Beyond all count do accumulate;
For something to clean you need never wait ...

You soon will find that the nurse who can clean
Is the one whose days are most serene.
For all must be spotless in that place
Where life and death may be running a race ...

The more germs scrubbed and boiled away
The better the chances, so they say,
For wounds to heal in the long, hard fight
To bring back health. Can it be right

To do less than our best in so great a task?[27]

The centrality of cleanliness, sanitation, and hygiene to modern nursing practice in Canada during this period cannot be overstated. The obsessive attention given to scrubbing, boiling, and disinfecting during nurses' training in Canada was brought over to China – an arduous task considering the different cultural ideals. The reasons for cleanliness were to combat germs and to provide a soothing environment. In 1926, Cora E. Simpson of the Nurses Association of China described the centrality of cleanliness to early missionary nursing:

The popular idea at home as well as on the field at that time seemed to be that the hospitals were places in which "to heal and to teach." There are different methods of carrying out this idea. A patient will be much more likely to believe your message after he or she has had a nice warm bath, been fed and cared for by a clean, intellectual Chinese nurse ... it is not necessary to have a "pig nest" or dirty patients and slack scientific medical work with no nursing in order to do good evangelistic work in the hospitals.[28]

Simpson recalled that "we were told China did not need nurses and had no place for them." A "morning in the clinic proved different," however: trained nurses used to spending considerable effort on cleaning and disinfecting would respond to dirt and grime not only with repulsion, but also with a sense of duty. They found ways to ensure that standards of hygiene were at least attempted, if not met, in China:

How many of us have had someone paddle the hand in our precious sterile water we had taken hours to prepare and then the operation had to be delayed while more was prepared. I well remember our "linen" the doctor told me consisted of "two towels." But after a moment's thought she said: "No I guess it is really only one for I tore it in two to wrap twins in." You can imagine the feelings of a nurse fresh from the spotless halls of the home hospitals as things like this met her the first few days and months.[29]

At VGH, Margaret Gay was indoctrinated with the gospel of soap and water, light, and fresh air. During her three years as a nursing student, Margaret Gay held onto her dream of returning to China. Her classmates described Gay as one of the "brilliant ones of the year," whose "aspirations [circled] around China and its missions." Her ambition? "To plant a bit of VGH in the Orient."[30] But Gay's years at VGH were not without difficulty. One incident in particular tested – and proved – Gay's resolve.

While the VGH nursing students were in the lecture hall awaiting their guest speaker one evening, a tragedy was unfolding on the "foreign ward," a men's ward occupied by Chinese, Hindu, Mexican, and Japanese patients. A disgruntled patient had discharged himself earlier in the day after becoming annoyed at a nurse for giving him what he thought was the wrong pill. He made good his threat to return, somehow managing to enter the ward during evening visiting hours. As the ex-patient sat visiting with his former roommates, Anne Roedde, a second-year student nurse, passed by with a tray of medicine. The man jumped up behind Roedde and slit her throat with a razor blade, killing her in front of the other patients. Upon hearing of the trauma, Margaret Gay's thoughts turned to the "little fair haired girl [who was asked to] take over the care of that ward for the remainder of the evening." Gay offered to take over night duty from the young nursing student because: "I was accustomed to Orientals and to the dreadful things that used to happen out in China, bandit raids, etc., and was glad to be able to help. When I went up to the ward and hung my [nursing] cape on the

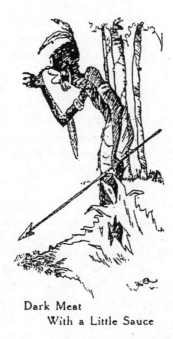

Dark Meat
With a Little Sauce

Figure 25 Cartoon from 1926 VGH yearbook.
Irene Pooley and Muriel Gay private collection

back of the office door, the [frightened] little fair haired nurse threw her arms around me and said, 'You Angel.'"[31] Nursing could be a dangerous profession for young women. Clara Preston had once been punched in the jaw by a male patient in Henan.[32] In Canada, "foreign" (that is, non-white) male patients were considered to be particularly threatening. In an era of Social Darwinism in Canada, where the white race was thought to be at the apex of the evolutionary scale, "foreigners" could be portrayed as subhuman or simply ridiculous. Racist humour was common, even among nurses, as a cartoon from Gay's 1926 yearbook exemplifies (see Figure 25). If working among foreigners was both risky and frightening, missionary nursing was downright dangerous. While her classmates may have viewed Gay as courageous for going to China, Gay viewed nursing as a profession requiring courage, whether at home or abroad. While Gay did not expect all nurses to be capable of withstanding potentially dangerous situations, she did expect it of herself.

After nursing her aging father in Toronto, Margaret Gay was ready to return to China in 1931. She was appointed to Weihui Hospital, where she worked alongside Jeanette Ratcliffe, Isabel Leslie, Dr. R. Gordon Struthers, and Dr. Margaret Forster *(Fu Yinde)*. Here Margaret Gay's roots as an evangelistic worker came to the fore. She did Bible teaching on the men's wards each morning from seven to seven-thirty, taking "great satisfaction and pleasure to be able to combine the nursing with definite evangelistic teaching during the ten years of my stay."[33] Gay's direct expression of her faith to Chinese patients contrasted with that of other NCM nurses, who tended to express their Christian beliefs directly to fellow Christians (for example, Chinese colleagues and students) but *indirectly* to patients (through compassionate service, for instance, and through supporting the direct evangelistic efforts of others). To Margaret Gay, however, direct evangelism was precisely what differentiated "missionary nursing" from other forms of nursing practice.

Communication Breakdown

Although the NCM formally expressed delight at the arrival of Margaret Gay in Henan in 1931, her arrival had actually come as a surprise. There had been a communication error, and instead of three newly arrived nurses (Preston, Doyle, and Menzies), the NCM suddenly found itself with four. The NCM had originally requested the return of Clara Preston, plus two others. Somewhere along the way, "information was received by some individuals that Miss Preston was not coming" so Margaret Gay was appointed in her place.[34] The NCM mission secretary in Henan was irritated by the miscommunication: "It would help considerably if the Mission Secretary could know in advance who will be arriving from Canada, just as I'm sure you would like to know who are returning to Canada before they reach there. It may be, of course, that your letter got lost in the mail."[35]

Indeed, the letter *could* have been lost in the mail. Delays in the mail frequently frustrated communication between mission headquarters in Canada and the NCM in China. Although Henan now had a post office, mail was reliant on railway service; disrupted train schedules meant delayed mail delivery. It could take weeks, and even months, for letters to make the passage between Canada and China. In order to prevent miscommunications, staff would often send brief cablegrams notifying the recipient that a letter was on the way. Cablegrams were also used to send time-sensitive messages, including the arrival and departure dates of travelling missionaries.[36] For mission administrators on both sides of the Pacific, organizing and keeping track of Canadian personnel was a logistical nightmare; mistakes were inevitable.

The confusion over Margaret Gay's appointment can be traced through a series of letters sent back and forth across the Pacific between March and July of 1931. On 27 March, the WMS in Toronto wrote the NCM in Henan of the appointment of Preston, Doyle, and Menzies. On 28 March, Dr. Bob McClure wrote to Henan of his planned sailing date for his return to China with Menzies, and *possibly* Preston. On 27 April, the NCM in Henan acknowledged the appointments of Doyle and Menzies, noting that Preston's appointment was tentative. Finally, on 20 July, Dr. Grant wrote Mrs. Jeanette Ratcliffe that Preston had decided to stay in Canada. According to these letters, it should have been a surprise that *Preston* – not Gay – had returned to China. Apparently Preston's mother opposed her return to China. As Dr. Grant wrote, "Miss Preston agreed to go to Honan [Henan] in opposition to her mother's wish because she felt the need in Honan sufficiently great to justify her doing so. Now that Miss Gay is available [Preston] does not feel that the need is great enough to justify her disregarding her mother's wish."[37] It is not clear why Preston changed her mind and decided to return to China despite her mother's opposition and in light of Gay's appointment. It is possible that Mrs. Ratcliffe urged Preston to return after reading Dr. Grant's comment: "I hope you will be rightly guided. I have no doubt that Miss Preston will respond to the Council's call to an *imperative* need."[38] When *both* Preston and Gay arrived with Doyle and Menzies at Henan in 1931, the NCM had little choice but to make them feel welcome and to find a suitable placement for each.

Restoring the Hospitals

After the arrival of Clara Preston, Margaret Gay, Allegra Doyle, and Georgina Menzies, nursing at North Henan began to advance toward what became its golden period, from 1931 to 1937. Gay headed to Weihui, Menzies to Huaiqing, and Preston and Doyle to Anyang.[39] At Anyang, Preston found herself back at the old hospital buildings in the eastern compound ("East Compound"). Reconstruction of the damaged new hospitals was underway at the hospital compound (now called "West Compound"). Where to start? According to Preston, with sewing.[40] Dr. McTavish bought a sewing machine, and a couple of Chinese women set to work sewing. Before long, "sheets, towels, surgical linen, operating room gowns, etc. were soon being folded away in boxes ready for use as soon as we could start [at the restored hospital]."[41] Then, furniture, doors, windows, cupboards, and floors were made and repaired. Hospital bed frames were brought by boat from Tianjin and painted at Anyang; mattresses were made at the mission, as were bedside tables, stools, desks, and cupboards. Finally, the Anyang hospitals were equipped with "a fine linen room, a good bathroom, a diet kitchen, a surgical dressing room and convenient nurses' office, fine verandahs, adequate flush toilets and large light wards."[42] When the reconstruction was almost complete, Clara Preston became the nursing supervisor of the restored women's hospital, and Allegra Doyle took charge of its operating room.

A Chinese nurse (likely Mrs. Duan) became the nursing supervisor of the restored men's hospital (see Figure 26).[43] Staffing of the hospital was problematic: there were neither male nor female nurses available. Preston and Doyle were already occupied and "our girl nurses had all they could do to look after the women and children's ward."[44] Even if the female nurses had

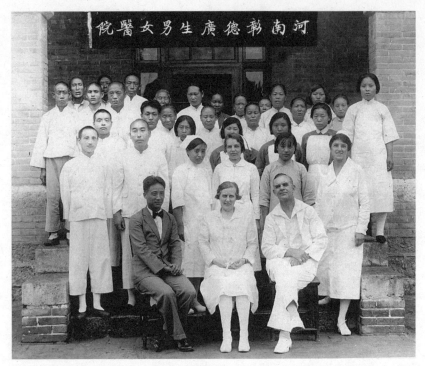

Figure 26   Hospital staff at Anyang, 1930s. *Front, left to right:* Dr. Duan (?),
Dr. McTavish, Dr. Reeds; *second row:* Mrs. Duan (?), Allegra Doyle, unknown,
Clara Preston.
UCCVUA 1999.001P-1657

been available, it would not have been culturally appropriate for females to
provide direct nursing care for male patients since "the community is hardly
ready for girl nurses in the men's ward."[45] Thus, when three boys with no
experience applied for the positions, they were hired.

Although much of the hospital damage had been repaired by the time
nursing services resumed in 1932, it would be another year before electricity and running water were restored. In the meantime, Preston and Doyle
worked around the "fear of fire from upsetting lamps, and the inconvenience of running a laundry, and ward especially, where all the water had to
be carried."[46] Slowly, however, the efforts of both Chinese and Canadian
staff began to pay off. Anyang soon had a good laboratory, trained techni-
cians, experienced dispensers, an X-ray plant, and even telephone service.
The number of staff grew to fifty.

Like Anyang, Weihui was quickly modernizing. Weihui staff believed that
their mission was to make the very best modern hospital facilities available
to the Chinese public. By 1934, the NCM could proudly claim its status as a
medical forerunner in North Henan. The NCM had the "only hospitals with

nursing care," and "every [NCM] hospital [had] a well-equipped laboratory, a qualified dispenser and an X-ray plant ... Our hospitals are open 24 hours a day every day of the year. We are proud that our community expects from us this kind of service, which others as yet cannot supply ... [the Chinese public] are now turning to us for assistance [with] midwifery problems – infant mortality problems – infectious diseases problems, venereal problems – opium addiction problems – all of these are brought to us for our help, and we cannot but respond to the appeal."[47]

Excitement and Innovation

As delighted as the missionaries were with the re-establishment of modern medical services, some were concerned with the fact that many medical needs in the rural villages were not being addressed by the hospitals. Patients had to travel twenty or more miles by farm cart over bad roads to reach the hospitals. Not surprisingly, many Chinese patients preferred to access their local practitioners of Chinese medicine. This disturbed many of the Canadians, who dismissed the work of Chinese doctors as "quackery." For example, in a circular letter from Weihui on 23 November 1932, Norman (the hospital administrator) and Violet Knight wrote:

> Superstition still grips the Chinese to a very large extent, so one can sympathize when they turn to quackery instead of giving us a decent chance ... A woman came to us thinking she was suffering from a "big internal water bag." She had visited a quack who had tapped her for water, but without success, and as a "face-saving device" suggested she visit our institution [at Weihui]. This was the first time she had seen a foreign doctor, who, instead of operating for an ovarian cyst, helped her to give birth to triplets ... the parents were greatly surprised.[48]

Such "superior diagnostic ability" of Canadian doctors may have supported some missionaries' belief that Western medicine should replace Chinese medicine altogether. Ironically, while the Knights described the diagnosis of triplets as a medical success story, all three infants, in fact, died within two days of birth – an outcome no better than what might have been expected without medical intervention.

Dr. Bob McClure seized the opportunity to assist – rather than oppose – the Chinese men he came to affectionately refer to as "my quacks." McClure was sympathetic to patients who "bumped over twenty miles in a springless car to find that all he needed was Epsom's Salts or Santonine [treatment for roundworm]."[49] He also sympathized with the desire of Chinese men who worked years assisting others in hospitals to work independently. In response, McClure established an innovative and impressive system to network traditional Chinese practitioners, Western-trained Chinese practitioners, and the

NCM Huaiqing hospital: the Huaiqing system of rural hospitals and clinics. Here, Western-trained practitioners (all Christian men) would work in small, rural branch hospitals associated with the Huaiqing hospital. These practitioners would either be full medical graduates from recognized medical schools, or men who had taken a six-year NCM course as "dressers." They would refer to the larger Huaiqing hospital but also work in association with traditionally trained Chinese practitioners at private hospitals and clinics. In this way, the Huaiqing practitioners were middlemen in a new and integrated medical hierarchy – responsible to the Huaiqing hospital, responsible for their own patients, and responsive to the desires and needs of neighbouring traditional Chinese practitioners. McClure's system of "barefoot doctors" was one example of his unique, pioneering work. It reflected his singular energy, commitment, and creativity.[50]

The rate of progress of programs and services accelerated beyond the best expectations of the NCM. At Anyang, Clara Preston was overjoyed with the expanding work, but had dreams of her own: "We still keep dreaming on and in our dreams we see – electrical laundry equipment – a trained dietician – a Physiotherapy Dept. – Well Baby Clinics – rural reconstruction work – Social Service and Public Health Workers and evangelists and our own graduate nurses and staff filled with that Abundant Life to give Christlike Service and leadership."[51] Preston also dreamed about a nursing school at Anyang. Nothing seemed impossible. The Nationalist government was supporting the advance of medical work by assisting colleges and hospitals with annual grants for upkeep. To keep up with the changing regulations, Chinese and Canadian doctors were in the process of registering with the Nationalist government at Nanjing – as were the Weihui and Anyang hospitals, and the Weihui training school for nurses. As the NCM nurses sought wider cooperation with others in their profession, they organized the first NAC District Auxiliary.[52]

The First NAC District Auxiliary
In 1934, Chinese, American, and Canadian nurses from five (unnamed) hospitals met together at Weihui for the first time as the first NAC District Auxiliary. Twenty-four nurses from two provinces signed on as charter members. The NAC headquarters at Nanjing informed the group that its auxiliary was the first of its kind in China. (See Figure 27.) The objectives of the organization were "to draw into helpful fellowship the nurses of this district; to improve the quality of our Nursing Service and Nursing Schools; to discover the best methods and do our part in meeting the opportunities of Public Health in this district."[53]

The group of nurses expressed a desire to co-operate with the Nationalist government, who in turn welcomed mission co-operation. For its part, the central government had ambitious plans to coordinate medical services in

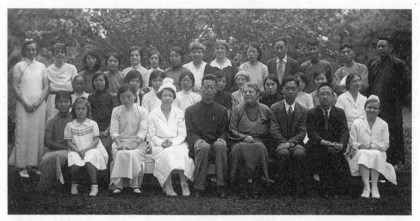

Figure 27 1937 meeting of the first NAC District Auxiliary. Includes Janet Brydon, Clara Preston (last row), Jeanette Ratcliffe (second row), and Anglican nurses Susie Kelsey and Mary Peters (front row).
UCCVUA 1999.001P-2367

China and was attempting to standardize hospitals and schools of nursing. The Weihui training school for nurses actively sought registration. It was "admirably equipped for training nurses," not least of all because of the "phenomenal demand for modern medicine" in Henan.[54] As nursing at the national level became more organized, coordinated, and centralized, nurses at the three NCM hospitals were looking for ways to organize, coordinate, and centralize nursing at the local level in North Henan.

Treatment of Disease and the Kala Azar Success Story

In 1933, Margaret Gay wrote a letter to friends in Toronto, excerpts of which were published in *Canadian Nurse*.[55] In it, she described her life at Weihui Hospital, including the physical surroundings, types of patients, and the school for nurses. In 1933, only half of the main hospital was in use. Downstairs was a men's ward of twenty beds with verandah space for eight more; upstairs was a similar ward for women and maternity cases, plus a small nursery. "Had we sufficient staff," wrote Gay, "we would have the whole hospital open." In addition to the main hospital was the outpatient department, with hostels for accommodating up to a hundred "not very ill" patients. Those who required "real nursing" were accommodated in the main hospital building "no matter whether they can pay or not." For patients who could afford to pay, a "mastoid operation" cost Cdn$1.50, and an appendectomy, "twice that." The hospital cared for patients with a variety of conditions, including asthma, nephritis, pleurisy, gun shot wounds, tuberculosis, "intestinal cases," gastric ulcers, pneumonia, typhoid, and "accidents of all sorts." In addition to these diseases was kala azar.

To Clara Preston, no group of patients was more interesting than "our children with kala azar."[56] Kala azar was a systemic disease caused by a tiny protozoan and transmitted by sandflies; parasites were most numerous in the spleen, liver, and bone marrow. Patients had a dusky appearance, a protruding abdomen (enlarged spleen), an irregular fever, and anemia (see Figure 28). Left untreated, 90 percent of kala azar patients died. Research on kala azar was being conducted in India and South America, and Dr. E.B. Struthers put the research to good use in Qilu after 1920. He began doing spleen punctures on suspected kala azar patients; the presence of Leishman-Donovan bodies on the microscopic smear would confirm the diagnosis. In co-operation with other doctors at Qilu, Struthers began to treat patients with a rather toxic drug – potassium antimony tartrate (tarter emetic). While successful 80 percent of the time, this treatment would take up to eight months. Kala azar patients filled the wards at Henan, and the doctors used the diagnostic and treatment procedures recommended by Dr. E.B. Struthers (see Figure 29).[57] Clara Preston described the regimen for children at Anyang: "Three times a week they would line up to have their temperatures taken, then weighed and wait for the intravenous needle ... One watched weekly miracles as you saw their colour improve, their legs fatten and their abdomen become more normal."[58]

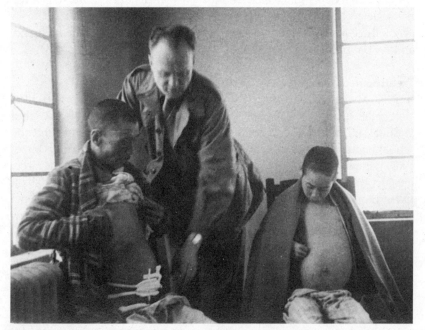

Figure 28 Patients with kala azar, 1930s.
Mary Struthers McKim private collection

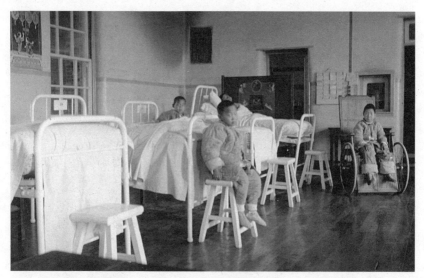

Figure 29 Convalescing kala azar patients, Weihui, 1939.
UCCVUA 1999.001P-1939

To Preston, no group of patients was more grateful, and years afterward, patients would come back to the hospital to express their appreciation (see Figure 30). Over time, new organic preparations of antimony were introduced, and Dr. Struthers tried out their effectiveness at Qilu. Eventually, he found that a cure could be expected in 80-95 percent of the patients admitted, no matter how many years they had been ill. And significantly, the span of treatment was reduced from eight months to three weeks.[59]

Margaret Gay was also pleased with the progress of modern medicine at the NCM. Patients and their Chinese friends were both curious and frightened by the strange surroundings and equipment at the modern Weihui Hospital where Gay worked. When patients were in surgery, friends waiting in the hall outside the operating room would try to peek through a crack to see what was going on. According to Gay, friends and patients would be, "impressed with all the whiteness of everything, and the number of people decked in gowns and masks and looking so queer ... [Patients would] say nothing as they [bent] over for their spinal anaesthetic – we hardly use anything else – and they usually [made] no sound or fuss, just a tight clutch of the [nurse's] hand that [was] keeping tab on the pulse."[60] The difficulty was not in persuading patients to come: "The trouble," Gay quipped, "is they never want to go away, and we have to use all manner of persuasion sometimes to get our beds emptied for new patients clamouring to come in."[61]

At Weihui, the rising demand for Westernized medical care convinced the NCM to open new rooms to accommodate both male and female patients. In 1935, the hospital opened a separate children's ward, an extra

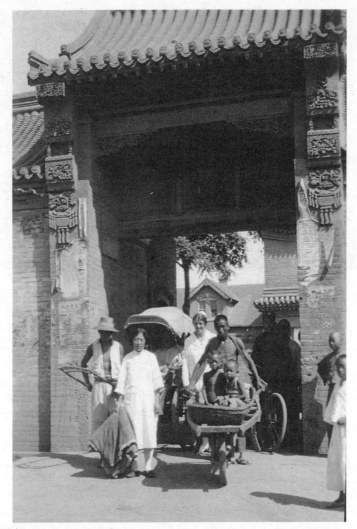

Figure 30   Clara Preston escorting "kala azar sufferers" to the gate,
Anyang, 1930s.
UCCVUA 1999-001P-1704

men's ward, and a delivery room (to relieve pressure from the operating
room) (see Figure 31). In turn, the larger number of patients meant more
nursing staff was needed. Nurses at Anyang and Huaiqing had already begun to contemplate the idea of starting their own nurses' training schools.[62]

Expanded Nurses' Training

As early as 1931, nurses at Anyang and Huaiqing discussed the possibility of
opening new schools of nursing. The Huaiqing hospital was still not as

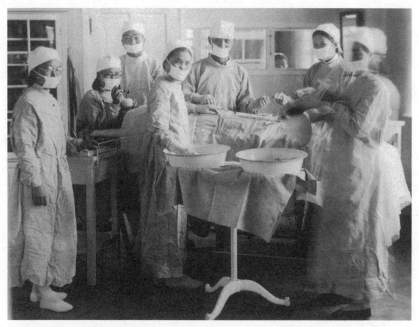

Figure 31   Operating theatre at Weihui, 1930s.
Isabel Struthers Staal private collection

modern as Anyang and Weihui, but it had grown, opening wards in the former NCM industrial school for post-operative and "special investigation" patients. Dr. Bob McClure proposed a scheme whereby each mission station would have its own nurses' training school, but that the three schools would be linked together under one organizational umbrella. The NCM council approved the plan and requested that the NCM recognize the Anyang and Huaiqing hospitals as affiliated with Weihui Hospital. The NAC did not endorse the idea. To the NAC, Huaiqing could not be qualified as a recognized nurses' training school because prospective nursing students did not have high school education (there was no high school in the region). But the NAC did agree that a student who trained in an *unrecognized* school (such as Huaiqing) could qualify for nurse's registration by taking two years in a recognized school (such as Weihui). As a result, the NCM came up with a plan for nurses from Anyang and Huaiqing to take their class instruction at Weihui, followed by practical training back at their home site. In the fall of 1932, students from Huaiqing and Anyang joined students at Weihui for a six-month "central training course" under the leadership of Mrs. Jeanette Ratcliffe (see Figure 32).[63]

Margaret Gay and Isabel Leslie were also involved with teaching at the central training school for nurses at Weihui (see Figure 33). In 1933, they had fourteen students, including three from Anyang. According to Leslie,

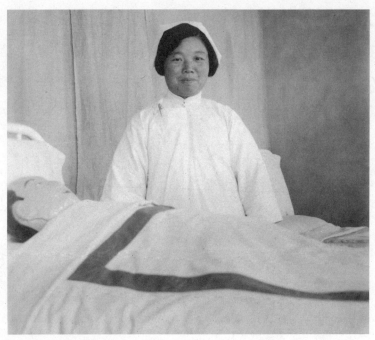

Figure 32   Miss Li (likely Li Shuying) and classroom "dummy," 1933.
UCCVUA 1999.001P-1963N

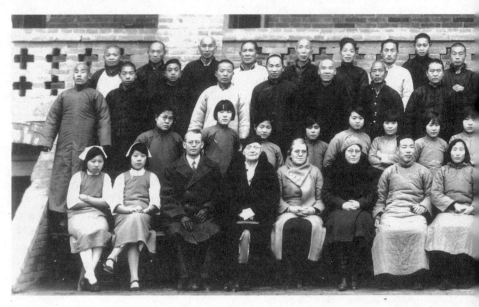

the nursing course was similar to what could be found in Canada: students would take daily classes, followed by putting "theory to practice on the wards."[64] Gay found the work interesting and pleasant "in spite of the fact that one often feels more inclined to do the work oneself than check others up in the doing of it."[65] Isabel Leslie, who was the superintendent of nurses when Jeanette Ratcliffe went on furlough in 1934, felt that the nursing work was "greatly hampered, particularly in interior China, because of the lack of higher education facilities for girls" but that "we do manage to secure some amazingly capable girls who make excellent nurses."[66]

If Huaiqing was hindered by poorer hospital facilities and limited access to secondary education, it was also hampered by a shortage of missionary nurses: Margaret Mitchell left for furlough and never came back and Georgina Menzies left for Anyang to replace the recently engaged Allegra Doyle. Mitchell's departure in 1933 was meant to be temporary, but she had been in poor health during her last term of service. Before Mitchell left Henan for her home in Tarkeness, Scotland, Dr. McClure and Dr. Margaret Forster diagnosed her with an undisclosed illness. She resigned a year later, due to ongoing ill health.[67]

Despite the low staff numbers at Huaiqing, the year 1936 was one of "steady growth and progress in every way."[68] The gap created by the departure of nurses was filled by Janet Brydon and by Mrs. Maisie (McNeeley) Forbes,

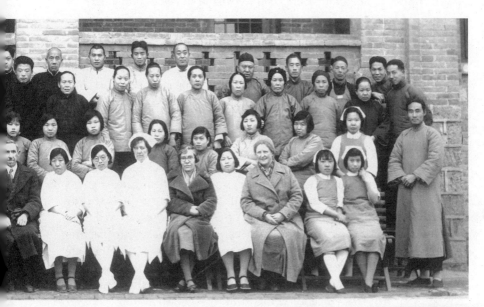

Figure 33 Hospital staff at Weihui, c. 1935–37. *Front row, from centre, left to right:* Dr. R.G. Struthers, Miss Li Shuying (?), Miss Liu Qing Yin (?), Miss Leslie, Violet Knight, unknown, Miss Gay, and nursing students (unnamed).
Irene Pooley and Muriel Gay private collection

who worked part-time. For her part, Mrs. Forbes "[came] to the rescue and ... made a very significant contribution to the care of many of the multitudinous details of running and operating a hospital. Her special work has been to give individual help in their studies to the new members of our staff."[69] Among these new members was a group of married women from the local Chinese congregation. These "sub-nurse standard" students were offered a year of training in the hospital wards and medical programs in order to do "health work" in their homes and communities.[70] Thus, although Huaiqing had neither a high school nor a recognized nursing school, nursing knowledge was brought into the community in creative ways.

Nursing work expanded within the province of Henan, but it was also growing at the Shandong Christian University (Qilu), with which some NCM missionaries were affiliated.[71] In terms of educational opportunities, Qilu was miles ahead of Huaiqing. The training school for nurses had sixty-nine students in 1939, including twenty first-year students, representing six provinces. Coral Brodie's work was almost entirely taken up with first-year students, on the wards and in the classroom. The curriculum had been recently expanded to incorporate a broader public health perspective. In addition to lectures in public health, students gained practical experience at an affiliated rural centre, the outpatient department, a "mother's club" class, a well-baby clinic, and home-visiting services. Like the NCM nurses in Henan, Brodie and the nurses in Shandong were keen to expand nursing's horizons.[72]

First Graduates of the Central Training School for Nurses

Unlike the university-based nursing programs at Qilu and Sichuan, which offered baccalaureate education for nurses, the programs in Henan were basic diploma programs, based on an apprenticeship model. Nurses who successfully completed their apprenticeship took licensing exams and, if successful, could become registered with the NAC ("registered nurses" or RNs). Clara Preston had been looking forward to the day when the Anyang hospital would be staffed with local student and graduate nurses. Like the Canadian system on which it was based, the NCM hospital system relied on resident nursing students to carry on a major part of patient care: students were an important part of the nursing staff. When the first three Anyang students returned from their six months of classroom work at Weihui in 1933, Preston was relieved to have their help as they took their practical training. She took maternal pride in their progress: "How proud they are when they receive their caps and uniforms; how they enjoy the novelty of the ward work; they know the trials of night duty; the awe they feel when they see their first Obstetrical case; the thrill they get when they scrub for their first case in the operating room; and how important they felt on their first call out when they assist the doctor."[73] Finally, in 1936, the first three Anyang nurses successfully completed the four-year nursing program. At the graduation ceremonies, "Miss Chao" (one of the students) gave the valedictory address, while "Miss Li" (likely Li Shuying) gave a farewell message to the graduating class. The nurses were presented with diplomas from the NCM and the NAC, and then enjoyed some refreshments and movies. As Preston wrote, "this has been a dream for years and it hardly seems possible it had really and truly happened."[74] At the end of 1936, the Anyang hospitals had five graduate nurses and sixteen nurses in training – both male and female.[75]

When Jeanette Ratcliffe returned from her furlough in 1936, she was delighted with the developments at Henan in her absence. She was wary, however, of the direction nursing was taking nationwide. Before returning to her duties at Weihui, Ratcliffe attended the biennial NAC meeting in Nanjing – one of the "largest and most representative in the history of the association, Chinese delegates being greatly in the majority."[76] To Ratcliffe, the most important subject under discussion was the registration of the NCM central training school for nurses with the Ministry of Education. With other missionary nurses, Ratcliffe wondered whether registration would interfere with Christian work among patients and students. She also worried about a memorial service held in honour of Sun Yat-sen: "Is it ... a service of worship [and therefore prohibited for Christians], or is it simply a service of remembrance of those ideals through which China hopes to achieve unity and reconstruction?"[77] Furthermore, Ratcliffe wondered whether the proposed curriculum for nursing schools, including public health nursing, sociology, civics, and psychology, would be impossible to attain. State medicine was the aim of the central government, and missionary nurses were expected to keep in line with the aims and ideals of China as a whole. A somewhat disheartened Ratcliffe returned to Weihui – but she was not discouraged for long. At Weihui, the spirit of unity and co-operation temporarily waylaid her concerns. Ratcliffe was impressed by the expansion of nursing work. Under the leadership of Margaret Gay, two new wards had been opened at Weihui, four graduate students were doing routine supervision of the wards, and sixteen new students had been accepted for the upcoming nursing school term. Although she had the able assistance of Isabel Leslie and Mrs. Roulston, Margaret Gay held the ultimate responsibility for both the nursing school and nursing service. Even so, Gay was happy to hand administration duties back to Ratcliffe.[78]

Ward Rounds at Anyang

Georgina Menzies had moved from Huaiqing to assist Preston at the Anyang women's hospital. Menzies' 1936/ 37 report provides a glimpse into daily life on a mission hospital ward.[79] In it, Menzies described seven patients who were hospitalized for long-term treatment of severe burns, gunshot wounds, opium addiction, smallpox, and kala azar. An eight-year-old child and a sixty-year-old woman were shot by bandits. The child had been taken captive after bandits raided his village and was kept in an empty pit, where one foot and hand became frozen. Chinese soldiers eventually rescued him, but he was shot in the elbow during the fight. The woman had also been shot in the arm, but it was two weeks before she was taken to hospital, and "now her upper arm is just pouring pus." One of the "burn cases" was a ten-year-old beggar lad who had lain down by an open Chinese stove during one cold night. His "rags caught on fire, and his arm and side were badly burned before the blaze was extinguished." The opium addict was a twenty-year-old woman whose husband admitted her because of "a new ruling of *shooting* all drug addicts [which] comes into force with the new year."

To Canadian missionary nurses, the missionary hospital was a safe haven – for them and for their patients. Beyond the compound walls lay bandits, filth, poverty, disease, neglect, and abuse. Margaret Gay was appalled by the number of patients with gunshot wounds, "indicating the constant suffering at the hands of bandits throughout towns and villages ... they live in constant fear."[80] In contrast, hospitalized patients were given a measure of protection and love that they may have otherwise lacked. Georgina Menzies described patients who were hospitalized for a long time. The nurses became surrogate mothers to some of the children:

> [Ting Niu is] the pet of the ward! She has been with us over a year now. Her mother and father have both left with promises to come for her later on ... She had multiple abscesses after Smallpox [which] have just recently all cleared up. Textbooks say a child in an institution usually lacks the love and cuddling they receive at home, but Ting Niu gets more than what is good for her. The Nurses all love to cuddle her a bit and teach her new words. She has to learn to walk and talk, as she has been sick for so long.[81]

Menzies found missionary nursing rewarding and purposeful. It gave her the opportunity to exercise Christian ideals of service and compassion. Although Menzies was not opposed to the idea of proselytizing to patients ("we haven't always time to preach to them every day"), direct evangelism was not the most expedient way to share the Gospel: "[We] hope our nurses, by their kindness and willingness to do all they can to ease their pains, act as a living example of a little of what Christ is willing and waiting to do for all of us."[82]

Public Health Work

The year 1936 was characterized by innovation and energy. NCM nurses were encouraged by the interest shown by the new Nationalist government to advance medical care in China, and by the growing local interest in

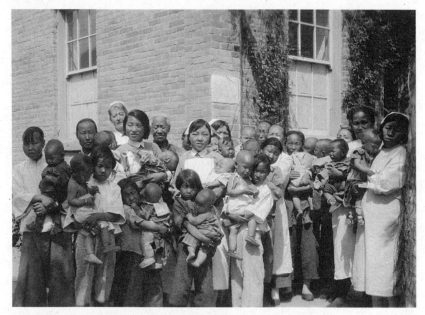

Figure 34 Mrs. Ratcliffe at the well-baby clinic, Weihui, 1930s.
UCCVUA 1999.001P-1880

expanded nursing services. Anyang nurses received requests for public health work, well-baby clinics, rural health programs, and midwifery training. To Clara Preston, "open doors" were everywhere.[83] In response, the Anyang nurses organized monthly baby clinics to teach about the roles of nutrition and cleanliness in illness prevention. Sixty mothers and their babies attended the first clinic, held in April 1936. A room was arranged with benches, chairs, and tables and decorated with "suitable posters."[84] One table held baby clothes, another held books on "child training," while others displayed food for "hygienic baby feeding" of children under two years old. A second room was fixed up for weighing and measuring babies and, significantly for the nurses, for bathing them – some "likely for the first time in their lives" (see Figure 34).

This unprecedented opportunity to share the gospel of soap and water was important to Preston since "good sanitary conditions just do not exist in China."[85] According to Preston, many lifestyle factors contributed to the spread of disease. These included using uncovered wells as the main water supply; dumping garbage into wells and rivers; living in crowded court-yards; allowing children to play among dogs, pigs, and chickens; and leaving food exposed to flies and dust. In addition, although many people received the smallpox inoculation, there was a lack of local interest in preventing trachoma, malaria, dysentery, kala azar, and tuberculosis. While marked progress had been made in China in regard to disease prevention and treatment in the previous hundred years, there was still a long way to go. Preston credited Western medical men and women for leading the way in the progress of medical science but also noted "Chinese doctors and nurses have borne a credible part and are taking an increasing share of responsibility each year."[86]

Among Clara Preston's surviving papers is a ten-page report by the Church of Christ in China Commission entitled "The Work of the Rural Church" and dated July 1937. A section titled "Health" gives insight into the public-health principles and projects that influenced Preston's work. The report stated that the "Church must cooperate in every way with the Government's plan for State Medicine and the Public Health program."[87] The commission recommended four practical public health goals to be accomplished over the following two years: (1) reduce the cost of medical service via health insurance, the training of "lower grade medical personnel," and the use of public health nurses or midwives for common or minor ailments; (2) provide each Christian group in rural areas with a medical kit and training in its use; (3) support "home hygiene," including anti-fly campaigns (fly-swatting, fly-traps, fly-proof cupboards, fly-proof toilets) and healthy children campaigns; and (4) support "maternal hygiene." The Christian church was to take an active role in these strategies – most notably in "home hygiene": "The Church should seek to spread accurate information regarding hereditary and infections diseases, in particular venereal diseases and tuberculosis. Every Christian pastor should urge both parties to seek medical examination before marriage, this examination to include a blood test for syphilis. We request that mission hospitals undertake to supply this service free of charge as their contributions to the Christian home. The Church should make opportunity for demonstrations of Child Care, Home Hygiene, and Child Welfare Clinics."[88] To church leaders in China, public health was an integral aspect of church life. This early version of parish nursing did not have a chance to come to fruition during the chaotic decades that followed the writing of this report.

As awareness of the need for public health services increased, public health efforts expanded at Weihui. For example, Jeanette Ratcliffe's Chinese-language nursing textbook *Communicable Diseases* was published in 1936 and distributed through China.[89] Also, the WMS provided Weihui personnel with a grant to establish a new health centre in the city of Weihui, outside the mission compound. The centre would utilize public health nurses and physicians for work with children and expectant mothers. Interest from the community was encouraging: government schools were inviting public health nurses to give lectures to schoolchildren, and two Chinese nurses (one male and one female) worked virtually full-time in the schools (both village and city). They held clinics in the city and the countryside, and co-operated with the government in immunization campaigns. It is possible that one of the Chinese nurses was Liu Ze, a graduate of the Weihui training school for nurses who received his NAC certificate in 1935.[90] The health centre opened officially in 1937, staffed by two Chinese graduates of the Weihui nursing school, who also had postgraduate courses in public health and midwifery.[91]

In compliance with new Ministry of Education regulations, the face of nursing was becoming increasingly Chinese. Graduate nurses were more prevalent in the NCM, in public health projects around the region, and in leadership positions. At Weihui, in addition to Chinese public health nurses, Chinese graduates worked as "resident nurses" at the district cotton factory and the local normal school. Although one might expect that the Canadian nurses would have been reluctant to give up their own positions of author-ity, the evidence suggests the opposite: they stepped aside with grace and with pride in their nursing colleagues. For example, when a new Chinese principal (Li Su Ying) of the NCM central nurses' training school at Weihui was hired for the fall of 1937, Ratcliffe accepted her new subordinate pos-ition with dignity. Although Ratcliffe had been in charge of the nursing school for twenty years, she focused not on her loss, but on nursing's gain: "All this meant far more than raising standards of education for our nurses, it meant that nursing had won a battle for recognition throughout China, that schools had been standardized, and that the allegiance of educated and high-minded Chinese womanhood had been enlisted."[92] As Ratcliffe reflected on the progress of nursing, she could not have foreseen the tragic events that would eventually lead to her permanent departure from China. Nor could she have predicted that the new health centre – where "proud mothers of a thousand babies had contended for prizes at the well baby show" in the spring of 1937 – would be reduced to "deserted piles of mud and bricks" within a matter of weeks.[93]

Summary

The years 1928 to 1937 would later become known as the Nanjing Decade – a period of moderate peace during which the fledgling Nationalist govern-ment ruled from Nanjing. John Watt describes this decade as "one of the more auspicious periods in the development of nursing in China."[94] He gives four reasons. First, nursing reduced its dependency on foreign mis-sionary leadership – particularly in the NAC. Second, the Nanjing govern-ment's Ministry of Health became interested in the promotion of public health and health education training for nurses. Third, the Ministry of Education established a subcommittee on nursing to register and supervise nursing education. Finally, during this decade, the profession became pre-dominantly the domain of women. Watt observes that nursing education during the Nanjing Decade was principally an urban development, in eastern and southeastern China. It penetrated into the countryside only in a few places singled out for model education and health programs. This point underscores how exceptional the situation was at North Henan. Although the NCM was small and isolated, it managed to successfully undertake some of the same nursing programs as were offered in the larger port cities. Nursing at the NCM flourished between 1928 and 1937, and changed in all of the ways outlined by Watt – except one: it continued as an attractive profession for *both* male and female nurses.

In North Henan during the Nanjing Decade, Chinese males could be found in various nursing positions – as students, graduate nurses, public health nurses, head nurses, and nursing instructors. Although Jeanette Ratcliffe believed that females were more suited to the nursing profession, she nonetheless continued to support the admission of men into the Weihui nursing school (with males sometimes comprising half the number of students) and into staff positions. At Anyang, Clara Preston similarly supported the role of male head nurses and assistants in the men's hospital. At Huaiqing, however, men did not seem to go into nursing services as readily as women. Perhaps this was because there were other options for males interested in medical care. That is, under Dr. McClure's rural system of hospitals and clinics, men were encouraged to enter independent practice as dressers (with six years of training) or doctors. As it was, the NCM missionaries attempted to work within established cultural norms, and displayed a remarkable degree of sensitivity when it came to local values and mores. Although the NCM nurses may have believed that women naturally made "better" nurses, they did not impose this value on the Chinese. For their part, Chinese males continued to enter the nursing profession – one of the few available to men in Henan at the time – and earned their way into positions of leadership as administrators and teachers.

Although the lack of staffing statistics makes it impossible to evaluate the ratio of men in authoritative positions to those in rank-and-file positions, the fact that there were males *at all* at the NCM contrasts sharply with the situation at the West China Mission (WCM) at Chengdu, Sichuan, for example. At the WCM, the all-male student population at the men's hospital training school for nurses was replaced by an all-female student population over a two-year period, starting in 1934. According to Muriel MacIntosh, a Canadian nurse at the WCM, females had never cared for male patients in Sichuan before that time. The entrance of young women into the men's hospital training school in 1934 marked a "new era" of nursing in Sichuan, and by 1936, *all* the students entering the men's hospital training school were female. To MacIntosh, the change from an all-male to an all-female nursing school improved the quality of the nursing care since "it seems to be only the exceptional male who has a real knack for bedside care."[95] If the profession of nursing in China at large opened new doors for young women during the Nanjing Decade, nursing in Henan also opened new doors for young men. Viewed through a twenty-first-century lens, the gender bias underlying the move from male to all-female care at Sichuan may seem a backward move, but at the time it was considered to be forward-thinking and on the cutting edge. This fits with a perception of the WCM as more progressive than the conservative NCM. Now that both were under the auspices of the United Church of Canada, nurses from Sichuan and Henan had the opportunity to share ideas, but few chose to do so – until the closure of the NCM after the Japanese occupation of Henan in 1942 forced NCM nurses to move to the unoccupied premises in Sichuan. As will be seen, these war years brought the differences between the missions into clearer focus.

The Nanjing Decade was characterized by increased governmental involvement in health care. Missionary nurse leaders Jeanette Ratcliffe (Weihui), Janet Brydon (Huaiqing), and Clara Preston (Anyang) viewed governmental interest as a positive stimulus for the development of nursing at the NCM. With unprecedented public recognition of, and support for, modern nursing in China, the NCM nurses enthusiastically took up the task of standardizing the nursing curriculum, meeting registration requirements, and promoting public health. Although Ratcliffe, for one, was wary of how Chinese nursing headship might diminish the heretofore-Christian underpinnings of the nursing profession, she nonetheless supported the movement toward Chinese leadership – even when it meant giving up her authoritative position at Weihui.

As NCM nurses were enjoying more support and recognition within China, they were also losing the attention of Canadian supporters in the homeland. During the 1930s, Canadians turned their attention toward the grave economic conditions at home and the worrisome political developments across the Atlantic. NCM nurses could no longer count solely on the Canadian church for organizational support and direction, and they started to identify more strongly with the nursing profession. They turned to the national and international community of nurses for support and direction. Whereas previously the Canadian nurses had been content to conform to the vision of the NCM hierarchy (the WMS, the Presbytery, and the physicians), now they began to develop independent ideas of what the profession of nursing should look like in China. Still committed to the goals of the United Church mission organization, the nurses also agreed with the goals of the increasingly organized nursing profession, and tried to find creative ways to meet the demands of both.

During the Nanjing Decade, Jeanette Ratcliffe, Clara Preston, Margaret Gay, Coral Brodie, and Janet Brydon emerged as independent, tenacious, creative leaders. They drew on the wisdom of the Chinese nurses and broader Chinese Christian community, sought council from the NAC, and kept abreast of developments at the union universities such as the Peking Union Medical College in Beijing and Qilu University in Jinan. They also made stronger connections with the nursing profession at home, seeking continuing education in Canada and the United States during furloughs. Finally, they increasingly identified with the nursing profession at large, seeing themselves more as *nurse*-missionaries than *missionary*-nurses. They began to rely on – and report to – their Canadian colleagues via the *Canadian Nurse* journal rather than solely through church publications. And when they were in Canada on furlough, they could as likely be found speaking at nursing alumnae events as at United Church functions.

The organizational accomplishments of NCM nurses during this period are remarkable, especially considering the eroding financial base for Canadian missions due to the economic depression in Canada, the threat of Japanese invasion at Jinan, difficult travel and communication, and the resignations of Margaret Mitchell and Allegra Doyle – two of the nine WMS nurses. The NCM nurses restored nursing programs and services decimated in 1927, expanded nursing education beyond Weihui, and extended public health services – all while supporting and nurturing Chinese colleagues into positions of leadership. The church in China supported public health nursing and, it could be argued, introduced an early version of the concept later developed in North America as "parish nursing." As the church sought to improve the health of its members, public health nurses brought their skills to the congregation as community. Yet despite their tenacity, courage, and dogged hope, the NCM nurses would never again enjoy the same level of success achieved during the relatively peaceful Nanjing Decade. For the rest of the missionary era, China would be at war.

5
Scattered Dreams, 1937-40

Everything is very green and the birds sing and flowers bloom, but a wrong note remains.

– Janet Brydon, 1938

Outbreak of the Sino-Japanese War

On 7 July 1937, the news of an outbreak of armed hostilities between Chinese and Japanese forces came with the "suddenness and unexpectedness of a lightning flash."[1] At first, the Canadians were not unduly disturbed at the news of the armed incident at the Marco Polo Bridge at Lugouqiao near Beijing (Peiping) since "clashes between the two groups were not infrequent."[2] Unlike more remote skirmishes, however, this clash occurred at the very gates of China's ancient capital – a bold and taunting move. The Lugouqiao Incident would mark the starting point of the eight-year Sino-Japanese War. Japanese troops began an aggressive campaign to occupy China, beginning with the north. When the Japanese attacked and captured Tianjin, the Canadian missionaries realized how dire the situation actually was.

Clara Preston was on vacation at Yu Ta Ho in Shansi province when the Sino-Japanese War started. She heard news about the Lugouqiao Incident, and talked with other vacationing missionaries about how it would affect them and their work. After each day brought more disturbing rumours, Preston decided to head back to Anyang. Weihui missionary Helen MacDougall accompanied her. While on the train back to Henan, Preston observed hordes of refugees attempting to escape southward to safety. The roads were "black with people, some on donkeys, some riding in rickshas [sic], some on bicycles, and a great many on foot carrying their most valued possessions."[3] Torrential rains periodically delayed the trip back to Henan. At one point, the two women waited for almost a day for washed-out bridges to be repaired. They filled the tedious and anxious hours with conversation and by reading aloud novels by Emily and Charlotte Brontë. The rains continued unabated. By the time the train reached Weihui, the city was under so much floodwater that MacDougall had to be ferried by boat to the North China Mission (NCM) compound. Boats became the normal mode of transportation around Weihui during that wet summer.[4]

By the end of the summer, the hostilities had eased and, except for occasional air raids, missionaries felt safe to continue their work. How long peace would last was anyone's guess, but the North China missionaries "were accustomed to living dangerously."[5] To missionaries at Weihui, the imminent war was the least of their concerns. More pressing was the extreme flooding and resultant famine. Jeanette Ratcliffe wrote in her diary on 15 July 1937: "Water rising fast; nurses' yard flooded; nurses moved to hospital fourth floor. Myself waded knee deep to hospital to get kitchen and laundry moved to main floor." Two months later, Ratcliffe added to her entry: "For two months these useful auxiliary services remained there perched precariously on verandahs whose floors were always sinking and whose ceilings were always falling. 'Tis well the Chinese are an adaptable race."[6] Rain continued to fall on the fields of millet and corn, and by August, the swollen rivers had flooded the fields. To make matters worse, earthquakes weakened the sodden mud houses and shops, and many homes and buildings collapsed. Ratcliffe wrote, "We almost got accustomed to the 'squee-sh' of falling mud houses in the village."[7] The new health centre was destroyed. While Henan was still reeling from these natural disasters, the Japanese began their invasion of the province.

As Japanese armies advanced toward Weihui along the Beijing-Hankou train line, refugees started pouring into Henan from the north. The Weihui Hospital staff watched as retreating Chinese troops marched past the Weihui compound. They began to see more casualties. According to Ratcliffe, "[Japanese] planes carrying bombs droned and roared overhead, and victims were carried into the operating theatre, most of them to die of wounds a little later."[8] Because the Japanese had promised not to target British property, the North China missionaries began to fly British flags. They also painted large Union Jacks on the roofs of all large buildings and on the outside of the Weihui compound wall (see Figure 35).[9]

On 1 October 1937, Anyang was heavily bombed. All single women except Dr. Margaret Forster were sent to Weihui. Clara Preston helped out at Weihui for a couple of months, but then decided to take an early furlough back to Canada with Margaret Gay.[10] The remaining staff at Weihui Hospital filled their days caring for the wounded and for refugees. The Canadians were fulfilling their sense of mission and purpose by such altruistic service. They had little doubt that theirs was valuable work and assumed their Chinese colleagues felt the same way. To the shock and disappointment of the Canadians, Chinese medical and nursing staff began to leave the Canadian

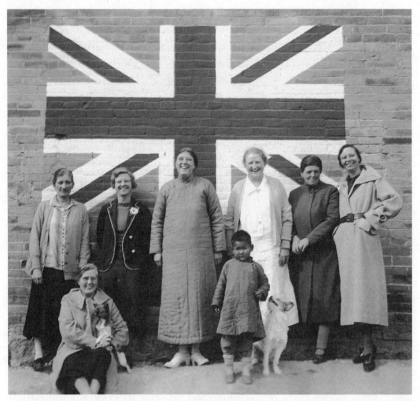

Figure 35 South gate, Weihui compound, November 1937. *Left to right, rear:* unknown, Durrant, Preston, Gay, Warren, McDougall; *front:* McTavish, He Pao Lien's child.
UCCVUA 1999.001P-2484

mission to do medical work elsewhere. To the Canadians, the British flag was a source of pride and protection. Not so for the Chinese, who desired to do something of value under the *Chinese* flag. As much as the Chinese Christians respected the Canadians, and as devoted as they were to the Christian faith, working with Canadian partners limited them. Loyalty to the Christian purpose was immense; loyalty to China was greater. Jeanette Ratcliffe was astonished that most of the Chinese staff abandoned the mission: "The infection of fear spread, and on one never-to-be-forgotten day twenty of our staff left. Within two weeks our staff was reduced to one Canadian doctor, two Canadian nurses and seven Chinese graduates and pupils."[11] By the end of 1937, the Weihui Hospital had lost all of its Chinese doctors and 75 percent of its student and graduate nurses. Some of the student nurses headed south to carry on with their training in a safer place. Most of the graduate nurses found work at national hospitals. For example, five graduate nurses went to Nanjing to work at a military hospital, and four joined the Red Cross staff, where they cared for thousands of wounded.[12]

A skeleton staff at Weihui continued to care for wounded patients, maternity cases, and cholera victims. Despite the war, Weihui graduated three nurses in 1937, and took in a class of ten probationers – not because it desired such a large class, but because these students were refugees and homeless. It was a year of emotional highs and lows, as Ratcliffe wrote to her nursing colleagues in Canada: "And thus a year beginning with such expansion of opportunities, with such planning for better work was all swept away – gone with the wind. Yet, we still treasure the unique privilege of standing with our people in their deep sorrow, of experiencing the loyalty and friendship of Chinese colleagues who have stayed by us right through, of helping to maintain a place of refuge for the sick and wounded."[13]

On Christmas Day, a Japanese plane hovered low over the main hospital building, weaving back and forth over its whole length – but did not drop any bombs. The missionaries believed that the large flags painted on the hospital roof deterred the Japanese and were somewhat reassured of their safety as British subjects. Their optimism did not last long. Within two months, the NCM stations were in the hands of the Japanese.

Japanese Occupation of North Henan

On the morning of 13 February 1938, missionaries at the Weihui compound were awakened by the sound of guns. Refugees started flooding into the compound, although it was already filled beyond its capacity: more than three thousand jammed into the neutral property, hoping for safety. Four shifts of twenty men were organized to patrol the overcrowded compound. Three days later, the Japanese entered the city of Weihui unopposed. It was devastating news, but it could have been worse – at least there were no new wounded for the harried hospital staff.[14]

Huaiqing's takeover was not as peaceful as Weihui's had been. On 18 February 1938, the North China missionaries at Huaiqing watched as the Chinese army retreated along the road close to their compound. To their horror, Japanese planes began dropping bombs on a column of soldiers just outside the compound wall. The seriously wounded near the gate were immediately brought into the mission compound. Rev. H. Stewart Forbes took the newly acquired ambulance into the village to collect other wounded. The medical staff worked until midnight as refugees poured into the compound. The next afternoon, shells began exploding right at the Huaiqing compound gate. Panic ensued, and while some of the staff rushed to the Forbes' cellar for protection, Mrs. (McNeely) Forbes grabbed her coat and "rushed to the hospital to join Miss Brydon in caring for the wounded."[15] Over the course of twenty-four hours, 102 seriously wounded victims were brought in. With the assistance of Brydon, Forbes, and the Chinese nurses, the two Chinese doctors operated on nearly all of them.

Dr. Bob McClure was impressed by the work done by Janet Brydon and Mr. and Mrs. Forbes in his absence. In a letter to Dr. McCullough on 20 April 1938, McClure wrote: "The Japanese bombed them, shelled them and machine-gunned them from the air. Our folks wheeled out the ambulance that we had the forsight [sic] to buy last Spring and took in 110 wounded in 24 hours. They filled our little hospital and all the branch ones and when the Japanese came they listed 29 of them as wounded soldiers and the rest as wounded civilians ... Really the stuff that those people in Huaiqing have learnt to put up with and still carry on would make history in most countries."[16]

Within days, the Huaiqing compound had 2,500 refugees. Soon the whole Huaiqing area was involved in hostilities. The crisis demanded the full attention of medical personnel, and anyone who was able lent a hand – even if it was traditionally unacceptable for them to do so. For example, at the Wenhsien Branch Hospital (one of the Huaiqing rural system hospitals), Dr. Chou's two young female assistants got around conventional Chinese mores by shaving their heads and dressing as boys in order to help care for the wounded men.[17]

As the danger mounted in North Henan, foreign consuls warned the missionaries to evacuate. Surprisingly, most chose to stay. According to Margaret Brown, "they were one with their Chinese brethren in distress. Mutual sharing of dangers prevailed over barriers of race and creed."[18] Unlike the events prompting the exodus of missionaries in 1900 and 1927, the 1938 crisis was not initiated by nationalism or anti-foreignism; Chinese aggression was not aimed at the British. Not only were Canadians and Chinese united in their condemnation of the Japanese, but the Canadians also had something very tangible to offer the Henanese: medical care and a safe haven. Their efforts did not go unnoticed. On 1 April 1938, Chiang Kai-shek paid tribute to the missionaries, stating that "thousands of people had escaped pain, suffering and death as a result of missionary effort, and girls and women have been saved from a fate worse than death."[19] Having their hard work recognized by Chiang was reassuring for the Canadian missionaries, especially after the desertion of their Chinese colleagues in 1937. Apparently, China still needed and wanted their help, after all.

Three Mishkids Appointed to Occupied China

By early 1939, nurses were badly needed at the NCM. Three of the missionary nurses had resigned to be married: Isabel Leslie to the recently widowed Rev. John T. Fleming of Weihui in 1937, Allegra Doyle to Douglas Smith of Canada in 1935, and Georgina Menzies to Dr. John Lewis of the Baptist

Missionary Society in 1939.[20] The Woman's Missionary Society (WMS) had appointed Miss Hargrave to the NCM in 1937, but the Sino-Japanese War delayed her arrival.[21] In May 1938, Miss Hargrave regretfully sent in her resignation "in view of the strong opposition of her family to Mission work of any kind."[22] The NCM missionaries were feeling desperate. The need for nurses was so great that the NCM was offering three-year contracts, rather than the usual five-year terms.[23] Interestingly, the three nurses appointed to replace those who had left were each Henan missionary kids: Mary and Dorothy Boyd, who were daughters of Rev. and Mrs. H.A. Boyd, and Elizabeth (Betty) Thomson, who was the daughter of Andrew and Margaret Thomson. Like the majority of the NCM nurses, Thomson and the Boyd sisters were all graduates of the Toronto General Hospital (TGH) nurses' training school. Indeed, all of the NCM nurses appointed after 1922 were TGH graduates (see Appendix 4: Missionary nurse education).

The prevalence of TGH graduates at the NCM is noteworthy, and raises some questions about the relationship between the two organizations. While the unavailability of TGH archives (in temporary storage during this study) hindered a thorough exploration of the relationship, it seems reasonable to assume that the "culture" of nursing school could influence a nursing student's decision to become a China missionary.[24] For example, Margaret Gay was supported by schoolmate Marion Fisher Faris and the nursing administration of the Vancouver General Hospital during the 1920s. Similarly, Margaret Straith Fuller was one of seven Winnipeg General Hospital graduates working in China in 1928.[25] Winnipeg General Hospital alumnae records from the 1920s and 1930s highlight the work of missionary nurses in general, and of China missionary nurses in particular. Students interested in mission work did not have to look far for mentors.

As with the Vancouver and Winnipeg hospitals, the culture of the TGH School of Nursing likely supported students' decisions to become China missionary nurses. Having missionary nurse alumnae was not new to Toronto: Jennie Graham and Margaret MacIntosh had both graduated from Toronto before 1889. Nursing students interested in mission work and mishkids interested in nursing could conveniently prepare for both in Toronto, since the TGH and the University of Toronto were within walking distance from the Presbyterian (later the United Church) headquarters. Nor did prospective missionaries have to go far to find mentors – there was always a number of missionaries on furlough close by. But did the TGH administration itself support prospective China missionary nurses? Dr. Robert McClure credited administrator Jean Gunn for supporting his efforts to recruit China nurses in 1938 since, after he met with her, there were "a number" of nurses who signed up.[26] McClure was probably referring to the Boyd sisters and Elizabeth Thomson, who all came out to China in 1938. Thomson's family, however, maintains that Gunn actually tried to dissuade her from going to China.[27] Gunn, it seems, wanted Thomson to stay in Toronto as an administrator. McClure may have underestimated his *own* persuasive abilities (in comparison to Gunn's), and may have overlooked the fact that the three new appointees had compelling reasons to go to China with or without the support of their school.

Elizabeth (Betty) Durie Thomson was born at Anyang in 1911 as the third of eight children. She attended grade school at Weihui, returning to Canada with her mother and siblings for high-school education. Thomson attended nursing school with her best friend and fellow mishkid Florence MacKenzie, graduating from the TGH School of Nursing in 1935 (see Figure 36).[28] After working for a year as a general duty nurse, Thomson went to the University

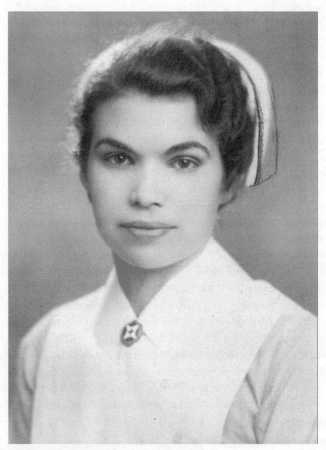

Figure 36   Elizabeth Thomson, TGH graduation, 1935.
Margaret Gale Wightman private collection

of Toronto, where she took a two-year course in hospital administration, finishing in 1938. Thomson was a bright student – having been awarded the gold medal of her graduating year at TGH – and a promising administrator. Thomson made a good impression on her supervisor, Jean Gunn. According to Thomson's family, Gunn had hoped Thomson would take over her supervisory role at TGH after Gunn retired; Gunn was not pleased to see Thomson give up a promising career in Toronto.[29]

Elizabeth Thomson had not always intended to return to China. Given the opportunities in Toronto, why did she choose to go to a country at war? According to Thomson's family, China offered personal attractions and professional challenges not available in Canada. To someone in her mid-twenties, life with the NCM looked like fun: Thomson had fond memories of family vacations at Beidaihe and of the tight social network among missionaries. Friendships begun at Henan often developed into deep, lifelong relationships. One could expect to find like-minded friends – and even spouses – within the missionary community in China. Indeed, Thomson met her future husband, London Missionary Society missionary physician Dr. Godfrey Gale, at Beidaihe. Moreover, Thomson already had personal connections in China: her father still lived there, and her friends Mary and Dorothy Boyd were planning to return. Besides the social opportunities, there was an even more compelling reason to go to China: there was an urgent need for medical workers.[30] Janet Brydon had written to *Canadian Nurse* in 1937 of the "wonderful opportunities [in China] for people with initiative and perseverance," and in 1938, Dr. Bob McClure was in Toronto seeking to enlist more nurses for China.[31] Thomson took notice. When she later read a newspaper article depicting a Chinese orphan sitting by a railroad, her mind was made up to put her skills to meaningful use in Japanese-occupied Henan.[32]

Nursing under Japanese Rule

Clara Preston returned to Anyang in the spring of 1939 after her furlough in Canada and found new challenges under Japanese rule. The Anyang women's hospital and training school for nurses had been carrying on with a limited staff and more patients – Chinese, Japanese, and Korean. Preston worried about the language barrier between Chinese nurses and "enemy" Japanese patients, believing that the consequences of miscommunication could be dire. After she discovered that the Japanese patients could make out Chinese written characters quite well, writing became the main means of communication between nurses and patients. The tension in the hospital could be overwhelming at times. The emotional and mental anguish experienced by the nursing staff is exemplified by the "breakdown" of one male student. Unable to cope with the stress, this student was admitted for "special" (that is, psychiatric) care at the Peking Union Medical College. Preston accompanied him on the trip to Beijing. Some of the other staff had already left the Anyang hospital because of the difficulties posed by Japanese occupation.

The Japanese authorities were making it difficult for patients to come to the Anyang hospital, sometimes fining patients if they were caught trying to sneak in. Although the mission hospital admitted Japanese patients, there was also a Japanese hospital in Anyang. Like the NCM hospitals, the Japanese hospital was short-staffed. The Japanese authorities asked the NCM for Chinese nurses and, much to Preston's dismay, Miss Jen, the head nurse, volunteered to go. This was a self-sacrificial act: by working for the enemy, Jen faced being persecuted by the Chinese. Yet Jen hoped that her going might prevent the need for others to do so. She also hoped that she might be able to care for Chinese patients. After praying together, the hospital staff agreed to let her go. Although Jen's fate is unknown, she did visit Preston later that summer when Preston was under house arrest.[33]

The hospital staff at Weihui was also experiencing difficulties with the arrival of Korean and Japanese patients. To Mrs. Ratcliffe, the ensuing "Tower of Babel" led to difficulties as the patients and nurses sought to understand each other. On one occasion, a young Korean woman was carried into the hospital, very ill, very frightened. Her response to offers of food, medicine, or treatment was simply to yell. One of the Chinese nurses found an innovative way to respond:

> The oldesr [sic] nurse prepared a tray, put a flower on it, carried it in herself, prepared to feed the sullen and suffering girl. (Youth does not expect to be so served by age in the Orient) ... the nurse put down the bowl and chopsticks, covered her face with her hands, and burst into what she hoped would sound like loud weeping. Startled attention from the patient. Then by pantomine [sic] [the nurse] explained her grief and how it might be comforted. The Korean girl looked astonished, then amused, then laughed outright. The food [and medicine] was taken.[34]

At Huaiqing, work carried on much the same as usual – that is, short-staffed. Janet Brydon worked alongside her colleague Miss Chiu, and continued to rely on the part-time assistance of Mrs. Maisie (McNeely) Forbes. Despite the wartime conditions, Brydon, Chiu, and Forbes managed to graduate their first "official" class of four nursing students, in 1938. According to Brydon, this was the first class at Huaiqing to go through a regular, systematic course of required lectures. Although it is not clear whether the school was actually registered in 1938, Brydon's goal was for the Huaiqing students to meet governmental standards and earn government diplomas. While Miss

Chiu managed the nursing school, Brydon oversaw patient care. War-related injuries were common and complicated by various forms of infection:

> Have a leg amputation on a child today. They nearly made it an emergency to relieve its pain but it was already of two days standing, so we got it put off. One man died today and one the day before yesterday and we have two others with dreadful temperatures and we do not feel at all sure of the diagnosis ... We had one who ran a temperature for weeks on end up to 106 [degrees Fahrenheit] once. He was a shrapnel or bomb case but he [also had gangrenous] toes, ascaris, syphilis and I think hookworm but I am not sure of the last.[35]

The Japanese invasion heightened rather than diminished the Canadian nurses' desire to work in China. There was more risk, but also more need. The nurses sought to create corners of order among the chaos, putting up with personal inconvenience (for example, the lack of proper footwear and the lack of radio communication) and threat to their well-being in order to respond to the physical needs of those who sought medical and nursing care.

Qilu Moves to Free China
After the outbreak of the Sino-Japanese War in 1937, the Nationalist government urged all educational institutions to move to Free China (that is, parts of South and West China not occupied by the Japanese). The West China Union University at Sichuan invited the Shandong Christian University faculty and students to come to West China. Like Qilu, the West China Union University was an inter-denominational institution supported in part by the United Church of Canada. In response to the invitation, the three upper classes of the medical college and four staff members started on the thousand-mile overland journey to West China in the fall of 1937. The Qilu hospital at Jinan remained open, but it was seriously understaffed. As in Weihui, patriotic Chinese doctors and graduate nurses in Jinan left Qilu to work with Chinese (as opposed to foreign) organizations. Some joined the Red Cross. The staff shortage was further intensified with the departure of Dr. E.B. Struthers, who was on furlough in Toronto.[36] Coral Brodie stayed at Qilu, and found herself in charge of heavy hospital work with a very limited staff (see Figure 37). By the end of 1937, however, the Japanese took over Jinan without a fight, and as the immediate threat of fighting abated, student nurses began to slowly return to Qilu.

By June 1939, forty-seven institutions had moved to Free China, and twenty-one to the foreign concessions of Shanghai. This mass emigration involved thousands of students and hundreds of professors travelling by boat, bus, and/or foot over hundreds of miles of dangerous territory – something C.H.

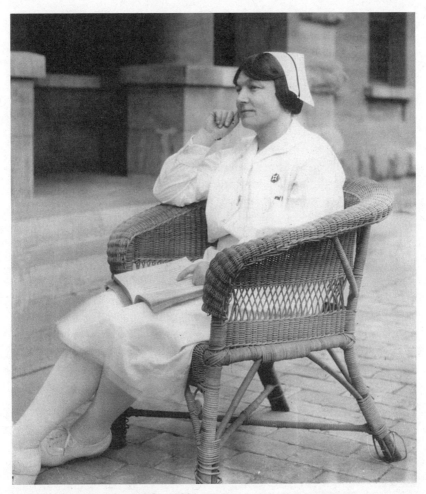

Figure 37 Coral Brodie at Qilu, 1930s.
Karen James, Brodie Family private collection

Corbett called, "one of the most astonishing phenomena in the struggle against Japan."[37] Brodie, however, stayed at Qilu, teaching and working in the wards. As the war escalated, the relationship between the NCM and the West China Mission would become increasingly important to missionaries from both sites.

The Anti-British Movement
In July 1939, summer rains came earlier than usual, and once again the Yellow River flooded its banks. At Huaiqing, walls and buildings collapsed, cellars filled with water, and gardens were destroyed. At Weihui, it was again

necessary for residents to travel by boat within the city. In the midst of these conditions, the Anti-British Movement took hold at Henan. According to Henan missionary Margaret Brown, it was the Japanese who instigated the movement. For example, at Kaifeng, south of the Yellow River, the Japanese forced the Chinese to boycott the British.[38] The nickname for foreigners had been "foreign devils" for as long as anyone could remember, but in recent years the term had been used more lightheartedly. Now foreigners were being depicted as fiends again. At Anyang, Japanese authorities commanded that the mission close. They increased restrictions against the hospital, threatened the Chinese staff, and prohibited Chinese patients from attending clinics. An anti-British demonstration was staged on 9 July by a mob of two hundred Chinese, accompanied by armed Japanese. According to Clara Preston, "[Chinese demonstrators] went to the east compound first, then marched onto our [West] compound. One of the leaders had been one of [the] medical assistants some time before, then had been with the Chinese army ... He had been put in prison and beaten, and was to have been shot, but was granted his life if he would work for the Japanese."[39]

On 30 August 1939, the Japanese gathered the Anyang hospital staff together in the chapel. The Chinese were told of supposed Canadian offenses and warned that those Chinese who did not leave by noon the next day would have arms or legs cut off. Everyone at the Anyang mission took the threat seriously. Within hours, Clara Preston and the others distributed equipment and supplies to the departing staff. Students received their class records and extra books, graduate nurses received instruments and an obstetrical bundle, sewing women received a sewing machine, cooks received the kitchen equipment, and goatherds were given the goats. At 9 p.m. everyone celebrated the Lord's Supper together and said farewell.

By noon the next day, Clara Preston, Rev. Don Faris, and Dr. Isabelle McTavish were the only ones left at the West Compound. Bill Mitchell, Grace Sykes, and Rev J.C. Mathieson were ten minutes away at the East Compound (later Faris and Mitchell traded places). The six missionaries stayed at their respective compounds for three weeks and kept in contact with each other by telephone. By refusing to leave, the Canadians held out hope that the Japanese would allow them to remain in China. A Japanese guard stayed at the compound gate to ensure that Chinese staff members did not return. The missionaries became virtual prisoners.

With no staff to help them, the missionaries were kept busy cooking meals, cleaning house, taking inventories of supplies, and sending some of their belongings to Beijing. At the East Compound, Rev. Faris milked the goats. At the West Compound, Preston, McTavish, and Mitchell pulled the belt each night to start the electric power plant – not so much for lighting as for their radio connection with the outside world. Every night, Preston sent a basket and rope over the compound wall; one of the Chinese hospital staff living on the other side would fill the basket with milk and other needed supplies. For some inexplicable reason, the postman was allowed onto the compound. He would ask Preston if there was anything he could bring in or buy to help out. Preston was overwhelmed by his generosity, realizing the risk he was taking. According to Preston, "he realized we had come to this country to help the sick and needy and now when we needed a friend, he was willing to do what he could even if he paid dearly for it."[40]

The situation was difficult, but the missionaries were still somewhat in control of their destiny: it was their choice to barricade themselves within the protective compound walls. Before long, however, it became clear that the walls would not protect them indefinitely. One night, the gate of the West Compound was set on fire – presumably by anti-foreign mobs. Preston, McTavish, and Mitchell formed a makeshift fire brigade to fight it: "We had water in our large water tank so we attached a heavy rubber tube to the tap which helped to fill the fire pails, and then got our operating room stretchers and carried the pails on them. Dr. McTavish and I kept the pails full while Bill Mitchell threw them on the fire. The beams were dropping ... Mr. Mitchell stepped on a nail, so we had to give him tetanus toxin."[41] The three missionaries at the West Compound saved their gate. The gate of the East Compound was similarly set on fire, but there was no running water at that compound. The gate burned down, leaving those missionaries exposed to a greater threat of danger. In the midst of this crisis, Preston experienced what would become one of the highlights of her career at Anyang. One day, two of the Anyang nurses came to the compound. They had walked for two days through Japanese lines to visit the Canadians, and to invite them to stay with them at their home until the situation settled. As Preston wrote, "hearing of our plight ... these two nurses walked back two days in the heat ... although it meant real danger to them. We only had time for a few hurried words as we were being watched by the guard, and it was with tears in our eyes that we thanked them but told them it would not be wise. We can never forget that offer, and it wasn't the only one."[42] Tired and anxious, the missionaries' resolve began to falter; it broke on the night of 16 September 1939. That night, nine grenades were thrown over the East Compound wall, of which four exploded. A poster pasted to the compound gate showed a prostrate foreigner with blood running from his neck. It read, "Englishmen, within three days if you are not away from this place, there will certainly be danger on your lives."[43] This was the end: staying any longer would mean danger to themselves and to their Chinese friends. Within days the missionaries left Anyang. Preston and Sykes took a train to Beijing, where Preston went to the Peking Union Medical College for a month's work and observation of the wards.[44]

At Weihui, things remained relatively quiet until 4 September 1939. On that day, staff members were called to the hospital where Mr. Chang, head of the local anti-British committee, ordered the missionaries to leave at once and not return. Margaret Gay later recalled "a white-faced frightened look-ing little Chinese man" telling the staff that the hospital was to be closed without delay, and patients, employees, and foreigners had to leave on threat of death.[45] Dr. Duan Mei-Qing pointed out that this would cause great per-sonal loss since the workers' homes were in the compound and forty pa-tients were still in the hospital.[46] So the missionaries were given a day's grace. Dr. Duan consulted with the missionaries, and it was agreed that he would take over responsibility for the hospital. Despite the orders to leave, some of the missionaries stayed on. Margaret Gay later wrote, "I had ten minutes in which to leave the place where for ten years I had worked amongst nurses and patients. Opening a drawer I gathered up a handful of vials of narcot-ics, and put them in my pocket. Then I went up to the storeroom on the third floor, where there were thousands of dollars worth of new goods ... [and gathered] as many new hot water bottles as I could [carry]."[47]

Gay took the supplies home, then proceeded to move into Isabel (Leslie) Fleming's house. The Flemings had left for Canada the previous month due to illness.[48] There Gay waited, terrified, for three days before someone came along and helped her light the Chinese stove for warmth and cooking. Much to Gay's surprise, Dr. Li from Huaiqing summoned her in person a few days later. Huaiqing missionary Violet Stewart was ill with typhoid, and Dr. Li requested Gay's help to nurse her. Gay left for Huaiqing on the afternoon train, leaving the other missionaries at Weihui.

On 5 October 1939, the missionaries at Weihui received word that they must leave by 12 October or "drastic action" would be taken on 13 October. They planned to leave in small parties and reunite in Beijing. Mrs. Ratcliffe was the only Canadian nurse at Weihui. She left on 12 October 1939, with Helen McDougall. Two months later, Ratcliffe described her final days at Weihui in her annual report. Although Ratcliffe did not know that subse-quent events would have her back in Canada within a year, she may have suspected that her three decades of missionary service at Weihui were com-ing to an end. Ratcliffe started her report by recalling Dr. Grant's words to the missionaries evacuated in 1927: "Our work here has been in vain unless we have succeeded in leaving behind a body of men and women with a deep love for their Lord and a willingness to sacrifice for the building up of His church."[49]

To Jeanette Ratcliffe, the missionary nursing work would have similarly been in vain if no Chinese nurses were in place to take up the task after the Canadians departed. When Ratcliffe left Weihui in 1939, her dream of pass-ing the work over to the Chinese became a reality – albeit more abruptly and under more trying circumstances than she could have imagined. It is interesting to note that, while little pre-1947 documentation related to Can-adian missionaries exists at Weihui, Jeanette Ratcliffe's parting actions are recorded in China thus: "Before returning to homeland [Jeanette Ratcliffe] looked into the distance from a high place in the hospital ward building to the west, saying 'I have been in China for 28 years. How beautiful the Chinese [scenery] is! Who [would not want] to come to China?'"[50] While it is impossible to verify Ratcliffe's words, it is significant that almost seventy years later, Ratcliffe is remembered in Weihui for her commitment to – and love for – China. In 1939, Ratcliffe's protégée Li Shuying became the superintendent of nurses. The Weihui Hospital and training school for nurses was poised to continue without the Canadians. Among the Chinese nurses (male and female) at Weihui during this period were Li Shuying, Lang Zicheng, Fan Wenhua, Zhang Fengzhi, Li Xiuzhen, Liu Quanxi, Liu Qingyin, and Liu Ze. There were twenty-four nursing students, including Zhao Liqing, Li Suping, Zhou Baoshan, Zhang Weihan, and Fan Mingyi.[51] It would be six years before a Canadian nurse would return to Henan.

The Last NCM Station Closed

At Huaiqing, the missionaries heard of evacuations at Anyang and Weihui and suspected they would be next. Young people had been slowly filtering out of Huaiqing over the previous two years, making the long trip to Free China by foot. Many were students determined to continue their education. Huaiqing missionaries estimated that at least a thousand children aged seven to fourteen escaped from Henan to Free China during that period.[52] The Japanese authorities had been treating the missionaries with increased suspicion and active opposition, "insinuating that we were supporting Communistic influences in our schools and church and hospitals."[53] Japanese authorities also suspected patients in the wards of being Chinese spies.

On 6 October 1939, the Japanese started to occupy the Huaiqing compound. Eighty soldiers entered the compound requesting "tea and a rest." That evening, the Japanese Propaganda Department asked for billets for six hundred Japanese soldiers, who remained for three days. On 19 October, the Japanese asked Dr. Chang to co-operate with them in "taking over the hospital after the foreigners had been driven out."[54] Dr. Chang told the Canadians of the Japanese plans to take over. It was decided that everyone must evacuate. Dr. Chang was the first to leave, escaping with his family in wheelbarrows at midnight on 24 October.[55] They arrived safely in Xian, having "gone across the country in several kinds of conveyances, walking a good part of the way."[56] On 26 October, the first Canadian party made their escape from Huaiqing. Margaret Gay – who had gone to Huaiqing from Weihui to nurse Miss Stewart through a bout of typhoid – was among this group of exiles.

Margaret Gay's party included four single women and an English doctor, who had been helping out in the absence of Dr. Bob McClure. This group had enough time to pack "the things we cared for the most," which for Gay meant her best bedding, books from Dr. McClure's medical library, and books from Dr. Bruce Copland's theological library.[57] The group was harboured for a while at the Catholic Mission at Xinxiang. Much had changed in the relationship between Catholic and Protestant missionaries since the 1800s. Unlike earlier times when Jonathan Goforth viewed the "Romanists" as deceptive and deluded rivals,[58] North China missionaries now viewed Catholic missionaries as having a common, faith-inspired goal – to provide humanitarian aid to the poor and oppressed in China. In turn for the kindness shown them by the Catholic missionaries at Xinxiang, Margaret Gay's group left behind "Red Cross money for famine relief and other necessities" plus "drugs for use in their clinics."[59] Despite the impending crisis, the Catholic missionaries resolved to stay in China.[60]

When the North China missionaries left Huaiqing and Anyang in 1939, they did not know how, or whether, their work would be preserved. It is not clear if anyone was left in charge of medical work at these two stations. At Weihui, however, the missionaries formally placed the NCM hospital under the care of Dr. Duan Chia Pin *(Duan Mei Qing)* before they left. Although it had seemed obvious to the Canadian missionaries that the threats to them and their Chinese colleagues necessitated their evacuation from Henan, doubt plagued them once they reunited in Tianjin. NCM secretary Rev. G.K. King *(Jing Zuozhi)* asked in a report of the October events, "Were we right in leaving the property and work in this way?"[61] With the exception of Elizabeth Thomson's father Andrew, who stayed on for a few more months at Daokou, all the NCM missionaries were evacuated in 1939 – the third mass exodus in the mission's history.[62]

Scattered Dreams

As a result of the Anti-British Movement and the worsening war conditions in Japanese-occupied Henan, the North China missionaries were exiled from Henan and scattered around China and Canada. At the end of 1939, Clara Preston, Margaret Gay, Dorothy Boyd, and Mary Boyd were in Tianjin working among refugees. They lived in the home of Mr. Hugh MacKenzie, the NCM treasurer, and father of Canadian nurse Florence MacKenzie Liddell.[63] Jeanette Ratcliffe was in Beijing undergoing treatment at the Peking Union Medical College hospital for an undisclosed illness, Janet Brydon was on furlough in Canada, and Elizabeth Thomson and Coral Brodie were at the nurses' training school at Qilu. (See Figure 38.)

Over the course of the next few months, there was a flurry of letters back and forth between Tianjin, the temporary NCM headquarters, and Toronto as the mission tried to figure out how best to situate their nurses. With the NCM temporarily closed, the West China Mission naturally hoped to secure the services of some of the free NCM nurses. This was not easily accomplished, however. Of the eight NCM nurses, only two could realistically

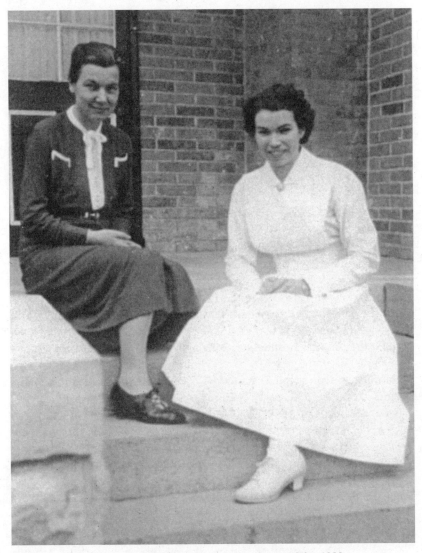

Figure 38   Coral Brodie and Elizabeth (Betty) Thomson at Qilu, 1939.
Mary Struthers McKim private collection and Margaret Gale Wightman private collection

leave their current assignments to go to West China: Dorothy Boyd and
Coral Brodie. Mary Boyd and Elizabeth Thomson were engaged to be married; Clara Preston, Margaret Gay, and Jeanette Ratcliffe had already accepted other assignments; and Janet Brydon was still on furlough. Even the
five married nurses who occasionally helped out were unavailable: Mrs.
Roulston and Isabel (Leslie) Fleming were on furlough in Canada; Georgina

(Menzies) Lewis was with her husband in Shandong; Maisie (McNeeley) Forbes was in Kobe, Japan; and Marion (Fisher) Faris was with her husband at Qilu.[64]

Dorothy Boyd was the first to go to West China. She had just recovered from a bout of diphtheria contracted in the Tianjin refugee camps and was interested in joining her parents in Sichuan. Her sister Mary Boyd preferred to stay close to Beijing since her fiancé, John Stanley, was studying at Beijing's Yenching University. Elizabeth Thomson was at Qilu with her fiancé, Dr. Godfrey Livingston Gale of the London Missionary Society. Thomson originally intended to complete her three-year commitment to the United Church of Canada WMS but resigned a month before her marriage.[65] Jeanette Ratcliffe planned to stay in Tianjin to finish revisions for an updated version of her nursing textbook *Communicable Disease*.[66] Once finished, Ratcliffe expected to either work at the University Hospital at Nanjing or return to Canada to retire.[67] Ratcliffe's health was fragile, however, and she had been losing weight since the late summer. Although Ratcliffe "bore up wonderfully all summer in Weihui [and] was a tower of strength" through the armed conflict, she had been hospitalized in Beijing for two weeks.[68] Realistically, her future with the NCM was tenuous. Clara Preston was doing relief work connected with the Yenching University at Beijing, and Margaret Gay had just been appointed to head up a hospital for contagious disease for the British Municipal Council at Tianjin.[69]

Tianjin had five hospitals staffed by Canadian and Chinese nurses and doctors. A medical clinic was open seven days per week. Gay's "hospital" was the basement of the British Municipal Hall. There, with Dr. Hoyt, an English doctor from the China Inland Mission, Gay turned the basement into a general ward, setting up a partition and arranging beds in rows, one side for men, the other for women and children. The International Red Cross provided funds for the bedding, food, and medicine. To Gay, not having to ask patients for money was "one of the happiest bits of hospital work we had done in China."[70] Gay worked with six Chinese graduate nurses – two men and four women – each trained at a mission hospital. After a morning in the wards, Gay would go out among the huts, looking for sick people needing care. Two stretcher bearers transported patients to a waiting ambulance. When the ambulance was filled, Gay went along to "distribute the sick ones to whatever Hospital they needed to be in."[71] She recalled caring for a ninety-year-old refugee: "We took her in, bathed her and put on clean new clothes, and put her comfortably in bed, with one of the English afghans [from the Red Cross] wrapped around her. On her pillow was a pillow slip with fine hand crocheted lace, and some holes had been expertly mended. The old lady was delighted beyond words to find herself so well looked after ... How she appreciated her bowls of hot food, and all the comforts of our makeshift ward."[72]

To Margaret Gay, working among Chinese refugees in Tianjin was the epitome of missionary nursing, giving her an opportunity not only to use nursing skills to care for the ill and injured, but also to showcase "the kindness of the Western world,"[73] by providing material and human resources to those who could least afford it. With Gay and the other Canadian nurses thus occupied, the only possible candidate to join Dorothy Boyd at West China was Coral Brodie.

Paralyzed Plans

After twelve years at Qilu, Coral Brodie was ready for a change, and in June 1939, she requested to be transferred to work in Henan. Although the records are vague, they do suggest that Brodie had been experiencing a difficult time at Qilu related to an inadequate housing arrangement of some sort. In August, Brodie changed her mind, requesting to remain at Qilu after all since a transfer to Henan would not "solve her problem."[74] Brodie expected to "meet with somewhat the same difficulties in Henan that she was experiencing in Jinan." Brodie asked to be moved into the hospital compound at Qilu, indicating that a change of residence would remove "her former difficulties." By December, Brodie changed her mind again, this time requesting a transfer to West China. The United Church of Canada WMS field secretary wrote a letter to the WMS secretary in Canada supporting the transfer, writing: "Although Miss Brodie's past difficulties in Tsinan [Jinan] have been removed, she is feeling the effects of the strain of last winter and early spring of this year, and feels that a change would be helpful and that she could do better work in a different environment."[75] Brodie had been ill during the summer and was tired. In December 1939, while she waited to be transferred to West China, Brodie was reportedly "in a reasonable state of mind ... [a] dependable [and] congenial worker."[76]

Two months later, forty-three-year-old Coral Brodie suffered a stroke. This came as a shock to everyone. Rev G.K. King reported on her condition on 14 February 1940: "Coral M.B. is suffering from a partial paraletic [sic] stroke which affected her right side. We are glad to report a very marked improvement. She is now able to stand and walk and move quite freely, and some movement has returned to the fingers of her right hand. Speech has not yet returned, but there is still room for hope. She seems bright and happy, and can communicate by writing."[77]

As King understood it, Brodie's stroke was triggered by a combination of prolonged stress and illness. He reported that she had been under a "terrible strain" of some sort, after which she contracted malaria – which she did not take seriously, despite being troubled with it "for some time."[78] King's implication was that the stroke could have been prevented, had Brodie's stress and malaria been attended to earlier. As it was, Coral Brodie's remarkable seventeen-year career in China had come to an end.

Since the time of her designation service with her friend Jean Menzies and Dr. Robert McClure at Bloor Street Church in 1923, Brodie had gained a reputation as a trustworthy, kind, patient, and – not least of all – determined woman: according to G.K. King, Brodie had both "grit and good humour."[79] Eighty years later, her descendants would use similar words to describe the woman they came to know and admire during her post-China years.[80] During her tenure in China, Brodie faced struggles similar to those of other NCM nurses, but there were some distinct differences. For example, Brodie bore witness to Japanese atrocities in 1928 – an experience that haunted her decades later. Also, although Brodie went to China as the "chum" of mishkid Jean Menzies, she spent most of her career as the only nurse among the NCM cohort at Qilu.[81]

If true nature is revealed through one's response to crises, Brodie's stroke revealed something of the nature of the NCM and the individuals it comprised. Jeanette Ratcliffe "hastened to Jinan" from Tianjin to assist Brodie and to escort her back to Canada.[82] This sealed Ratcliffe's future: she would take a year of furlough and then retire. Ratcliffe's offer was not unusual; Canadian nurses had often gone to the aid of fellow missionaries in need of medical attention. Yet this was the first time that an NCM nurse had to be accompanied all the way back to Canada because of a severe medical condition. Even though Brodie had worked in Shandong for fifteen years, she remained part of the Henan sisterhood.

For her part, Brodie faced her life-altering personal crisis matter-of-factly and without complaint. She was hospitalized in Jinan, but was clear-minded enough to make sure her hospital bill (Mex$413.00) was paid before she left China.[83] Brodie and Ratcliffe were given a farewell party, and then travelled by boat through Kobe, Japan (see Figure 39). At Kobe, Brodie visited mishkid Mary Struthers, who was attending boarding school there. Struthers later recalled that Brodie was able to walk, but communication was difficult.[84] Brodie and Ratcliffe reached Toronto by train on 17 April 1940, where Brodie's family anxiously received them.[85]

Brodie was placed under the care of a neurologist and speech therapist. Her sister Jessie Brodie – a nutritionist at the University of Toronto – worked closely with Coral, having her try the "latest theories" for rehabilitation.[86] A neatly handwritten letter dated seven months after her stroke exemplifies Coral's determination and clear-mindedness. In it she wrote: "I cannot use my right hand for writing yet. I cannot get much of a grip that you need for writing, but I can eat with a fork and spoon certain kinds of foods and I make a clumsy mess of it though. My speech is improving a lot faster than my arm, [but] that is not saying a great deal. I can carry on a very simple conversation with my family and Miss Lewis. I talk so painfully slowly that I pity those that have to listen to me."[87]

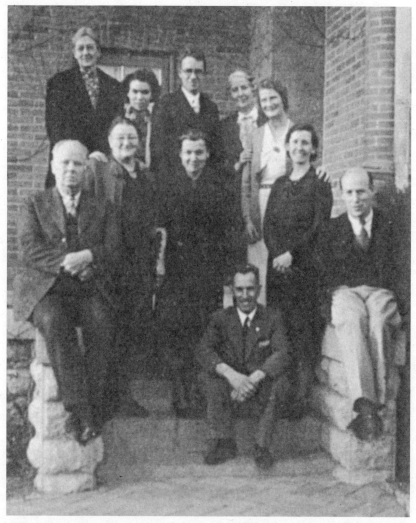

Figure 39   Farewell party for Coral Brodie at Qilu, 1940. *Last row, left to right:*
Jeanette Ratcliffe, Elizabeth and Godfrey Gale, Margaret Struthers, Carrie Scott;
middle row: George Ross (seated), Mrs. Ross, Coral Brodie, Marion Faris, Don Faris
(seated); *centre, seated:* Jimmy Scott.
Margaret Gale Wightman private collection

In September 1940, the mission's medical board recommended that Coral
Brodie be invalided out of service to the United Church of Canada WMS.
The board did not believe that it would ever be possible for her to be physically able to undertake missionary service again. Thus, the WMS moved
that Brodie be granted six months' furlough from the date of her arrival in

Canada, then one year's sick leave – until September 1941 – after which "she will retire."[88] Much to everyone's surprise, Brodie improved sufficiently enough to undertake part-time nursing in Canada in 1942. Although she never returned to China, Brodie did not retire from the NCM until 1 November 1943.[89]

West China Calling

The loss of Jeanette Ratcliffe and Coral Brodie brought United Church missions in China to a crossroads during the spring of 1940. With the NCM staff in exile, the WMS in Toronto was pressuring the NCM secretary G.K. King to send nurses to West China, but King was reluctant to do so. Dorothy Boyd was already in West China at Chengdu, and Margaret Gay had indicated her willingness to follow after an extended rest in Hong Kong over the summer. Gay had been under a "rather exhausting physical strain" in Tianjin.[90] According to Rev. G.K. King, Gay's exhaustion was "not due to overwork so much as to a dearth in fuel and table nicetles resulting from the barbed wire and the imposed control of traffic and supplies." A change of scenery in West China, he thought, would do Gay good.

The WMS had been criticizing King for sending NCM nurses to help neighbouring missions (in Jinan, Beijing, and Tianjin, for example) rather than "help[ing] to relieve the difficult situation created by shortage of staff in West China ... where our Woman's Missionary Society has accepted responsibility."[91] Yet what the WMS did not realize was how limited the options were. Three of the eight NCM nurses were in Canada (Ratcliffe, Brodie, and Brydon), and two were preparing to resign (Thomson and Mary Boyd). Since Gay and Dorothy Boyd were already committed to West China, this left only Clara Preston. G.K. King recognized that Preston was the only NCM nurse qualified to take on responsibilities at North Henan, should the field open up again:

> [The] most urgent nursing need [at the West China Mission] is someone to head up the training schools for our Chinese nurses ... Miss M. Boyd does not desire to go to West China. Miss Brydon [in Canada] is interested in the nurse's training but, we understand, does not feel particularly attracted to that aspect of the work. Miss Preston, on the other hand, is keenly interested in the nurses training work and in the individual nurses ... But, were you fully acquainted with the full situation [here] would you urge us to send Miss Preston west and so shatter our hopes of continuing [Henan] nursing schools?[92]

Preston's ability to manage a nursing school in Henan was not the only reason that King was reluctant to send her to West China. Preston was also involved in some type of clandestine activity in Japanese-occupied China. Of this activity King cautiously wrote, "she has a fairly intimate contact with her former pupils ... We hesitate to enlarge." Although the records are vague about what Preston was doing, it was something prohibited by the Japanese but valued by the NCM. It was something dangerous. According to her family, Preston thought of the Chinese as her own children, and was not averse to putting herself at risk in order to protect them. King's 1940 letter was intentionally cryptic and protective of Preston.

King's letter from Beijing to Mrs. Taylor, the WMS Secretary at Toronto, exemplifies the difficulty posed by long-distance communication between China and Canada during the early war years. The hierarchical structure of the WMS and the Foreign Mission Board gave decision-making power to those farthest removed from the ever-changing local situation – that is, those in Toronto had the ultimate authority over their missionaries in China. The missionaries had to accept the recommendations of the mission boards in Canada, even when the latter had incomplete or outdated knowledge of the situation. Because areas of China were increasingly cut off from communications and supplies, it was difficult to get messages to and from China. And, because of Japanese censorship, messages that did get through from China were often intentionally vague. King hoped the mission boards would recognize the difficulties, and alerted Mrs. Taylor to the censorship by writing, "we deeply regret the necessity laid upon us of being somewhat reticent and cryptic in our communication."[93] The WMS decided to send Preston to the West China Mission at Chongqing despite King's recommendation otherwise. King was obligated to accept their decision. A few weeks later he reluctantly consented, with one caveat: "However, we put after [Preston's name] 'temporary' as indicating that, should the work open up in Henan, we will expect that upon due notice, she will be available, speedily, to return and head up our Nurses Training [back in North Henan]."[94]

The fall of 1940 was pivotal for the NCM. Elizabeth Thomson and her friend Mary Boyd both married China missionaries, thus resigning from the NCM. Clara Preston and Margaret Gay joined Dorothy Boyd at the West China Mission in Sichuan, at Chongqing and Chengdu, respectively. Janet Brydon was in Canada making preparations to return to China. Her sailing date was set for 2 November 1940. Brydon was, however, having second thoughts about returning – due not to the escalating war, but to her progressive hearing loss. In September 1940, Brydon was prescribed a hearing aid. Although Brydon had struggled with hearing loss for a while, she had managed to work around it at Huaiqing. For example, in the operating room Brydon would repeat Dr. Bob McClure's instructions to be sure she understood ("Scalpel?" "Scalpel").[95] Yet now she would be unable to manage without a hearing aid, and would need a constant supply of fresh batteries.[96] While

Brydon wrestled with her decision, the Canadian government issued an advisory that ultimately decided for her. Due to the escalating war, the Department of External Affairs in Ottawa advised all women and children to leave Japan and the occupied territories. Brydon's passage to China was cancelled. Brydon was "loaned" to the United Church Home Mission department and was appointed to the United Church WMS hospital at Smeaton, Saskatchewan, with the hope that she would be able to return to China the following spring.[97] Shortly after Brydon left for Smeaton, an invitation came for her to work at the University Hospital at Nanjing. The NCM decided, however, that all sailings to China should remain cancelled for the time being.[98] This turned out to be Brydon's last opportunity to return.

At the close of 1940, three Canadian nurses remained in China under the auspices of the NCM but seconded temporarily to the West China Mission: Dorothy Boyd, Margaret Gay, and Clara Preston. Three other Canadian nurses associated with (but not presently employed by) the NCM were in China: mishkids Elizabeth (Thomson) Gale and Mary (Boyd) Stanley decided to stay with their husbands in northern China, and Florence (MacKenzie) Liddell had recently returned to Tianjin with her husband Eric Liddell and two daughters after a year's furlough.[99] Another Henan mishkid would return to China in 1943: Dorothy Lochead, daughter of NCM missionaries Rev. and Mrs. Arthur William Lochead, was at the TGH school for nurses at the end of 1940. She returned to China in 1943 as the wife of fellow mishkid Norman Hall MacKenzie – and sister-in-law to Florence MacKenzie Liddell.[100] All of these nurses were about to enter the most trying years of the missionary era.

Summary
During the "golden decade" before the Sino-Japanese War, Canadian nurses had measured success in terms of organization, coordination, and standardization of nursing services. Using the Canadian system as a guide, missionary nurses attempted to develop a program of nursing that emphasized student labour and a hierarchical staffing structure. Experience and education were rewarded through promotion to a higher level in the nursing hierarchy. That is, students would move through four annual levels, each represented by a different nursing uniform. Graduate nurses, in turn, could move up the ranks from ward nurse, to head nurse, to nursing supervisor. Those with postgraduate education (usually at Qilu or Peking Union Medical College) could work in nursing education or public health. Although the early Canadian nurses initially occupied the upper ranks of the nursing hierarchy, those who arrived in China after 1931 followed a career trajectory similar to that of graduate Chinese nurses. Starting as ward nurses, they were given increased responsibility (and status) according to experience,

education, and need. By 1937, Chinese nurses were replacing Canadians in the highest organizational positions.

The clash between Japanese and Chinese soldiers at the Marco Polo Bridge in 1937 set China on a turbulent course. The chaotic reality of 1937 to 1940 gradually stripped the Canadian nurses of the organizational and physical structures they strove so hard to establish. By 1940, they had lost many of the features of modern nursing they had attentively imported and devised, including modern medical equipment and supplies, access to state-of-the-art hospital buildings, and carefully designed curricula. Instead, they were nursing "on the fly" – untethered and unprotected. Nursing success was no longer measured in terms of organizational achievements, but rather by sheer survival – that of themselves and their patients. Through this period, they found that nursing could be successfully practised in the most primitive of settings and under the most tenuous of circumstances; alleviating suffering of humankind was still possible.

Between 1937 and 1940, the nurses' lives had become increasingly constrained as the Japanese occupiers encircled northern China and squeezed in toward Henan. As the Japanese surrounded Weihui, Anyang, and Huaiqing, the missionaries retreated behind the brick compound walls. For a while, the missionaries counted on the British flag to protect both them and the hordes of Chinese refugees wedged into the compounds with them. Ironically but inevitably, the compound walls came to represent imprisonment rather than freedom, and the Canadians fled north to the relative safety of Tianjin and other large cities – and to a new, nomadic existence. There the nurses found alternative ways to fulfill their common calling to serve ill and injured "strangers" while waiting for their beloved mission field at Henan to reopen. They were scattered around China and Canada, homeless but surprisingly at ease, surprisingly fulfilled.

Despite their exile and subsequent homelessness, the nurses experienced a sense of deep-rootedness and purpose in China that followed them into Chinese refugee camps and makeshift wards in Tianjin, temporary classrooms in Beijing, and under-staffed mission hospitals around northern, eastern, and southern China. Perhaps their "homeless belonging" should not be surprising, given the nomadic nature of missionary nursing. To commit to missionary work in the first place involved severing geographic, familial, and cultural ties. Successful missionaries learned how to straddle cultural boundaries – moving easily between two cultures, but fully belonging to neither. Home was a fluid, portable concept – created rather than received. Moreover, life as perpetual foreigners was by no means a solitary experience; missionary nurses did not journey alone. Newly arriving Canadian nurses were received into established missionary communities, and became part of an informal, global network of Christian workers. In China, they were connected to the Chinese Christian community. In the vernacular of mission circles, it was not a matter of *who* you were but rather, *whose* you were: "We belong to Christ." Identifying oneself as a follower of Christ (a Christian) implied that one adhered to a particular set of values, of which service, hospitality, generosity, honesty, integrity, and compassion were central. Thus, when the Sino-Japanese War changed Canadian nurses into inadvertent nomads, they could – and did – rely on the hospitality and goodwill of other Christians whom they met in their wanderings. And even if other Christians were not immediately accessible, God was. They believed in a personal divinity who was concerned with the very minute details of their lives. God, they believed, was ever-present, all knowing, and all-powerful. Even if they were "scattered to the ends of the earth," they were never alone.

If it were not enough to belong to a personal God and a fellowship of Christians, the Canadian missionary nurses also belonged to the broader nursing community in China. They nurtured their relationship with their Chinese students and staff who, in turn, showed respect to the Canadians. A rift in the relationship between Canadians and their Chinese staff during the early war years came as a shock to the Canadians. Despite their own nationalism and allegiance to Britain, missionaries considered themselves to be politically neutral. They did not consider their presence a threat to Chinese self-determination, and were surprised when staff members' loyalty to China overrode their loyalty to the community of Christians. Yet to the Chinese, nursing under the British flag undermined their allegiance to China. When the Japanese first attacked in 1937, the Chinese staff abandoned the mission hospitals for those bearing the Chinese flag. Their actions baffled the Canadians, who felt deserted and affronted.

Ultimately, the strongest relational ties were between the missionary nurses themselves. These women were bound by similar worldviews, difficult circumstances, and a genuine need for each other. They had forsaken the relative comfort of their homeland, investing their intelligence and health for the opportunity to enter into the suffering of the Chinese people; some gave up material and marriage prospects to nurture a dream of their missionary forbears. Despite the geographic distance that typically separated them, their sisterhood expressed itself in tangible ways. For example, when Jeanette Ratcliffe made the hasty journey from Tianjin to Jinan after Coral Brodie's stroke, she was offering more than nursing skills – Brodie was, after all, in capable hands at the Shandong University Hospital. Ratcliffe acted as a surrogate sister, dropping everything to be at Brodie's side and to accompany her back to Canada.

If the North China missionary nurses as a whole had much in common, nurses who were children of missionaries (mishkids) had even more. Not only did mishkids share similar formative years in Henan – which bred in them a unique bicultural, bilingual understanding of the world – many of the women also shared formative nursing years at the TGH. Mary and Dorothy Boyd, Elizabeth Thomson, Dorothy Lochead, and Florence MacKenzie had been reared in northern China. As children, they had acquired an ability to live comfortably in the cultural no man's land of missionaries. Their ability to be at home anywhere would serve them well in the upcoming war years.

6
War Years, 1941-45

Peace is not the absence of trouble, but the presence of God.

– J. Oswald Sanders, China Inland Mission

Behind Enemy Lines

By early 1941, there were no more United Church of Canada missionaries behind the enemy lines in Japanese-occupied Henan. Instead, the Canadian missionaries were spread around various "safer" areas of China, including the northern cities of Tianjin, Jinan, and Beijing, and in the western province of Sichuan. In North Henan, only one hospital remained open after the Canadians left. The Weihui Hospital had been left under the care of the Chinese Church, with Dr. Duan Mei-Qing as acting hospital superintendent and Li Shuying as nursing superintendent and principal of the Weihui training school for nurses. Dr. Duan, Miss Li, and five other Chinese nurses were determined to keep the hospital running – no easy task under wartime conditions. Dr. Duan sent a report to the North China Mission (NCM) temporary headquarters in Tianjin, summarizing the hospital work of 1940. He wrote, "Of course we have many difficulties in the war time. We are very weak both in personal and financial standpoint as you may think. All our friends left us especially [Canadian] doctors and nurses whom [are] very important in the hospital. [We] carry on so heavy work, as ninety in-patients for several monthes [sic]. Again our income is so limited, we cannot do the things what we like. The beddings, sheets and clothes are wear [sic] off but we have no [sic] enough money to buy the news [sic]."[1] Dr. Duan was optimistic, however, and "very proud" that he and his staff were able to care for as many people as they did. Indeed, the Weihui Hospital staff cared for an astonishing number of new and returning patients during 1940. In total, 9,043 patients were treated (1,063 of whom were in-patients), 745 operations were performed, and 58 babies were delivered. The operations included twelve appendectomies, fourteen "amputations of the breast," nine hernia repairs, eight intestinal obstructions and six removals of "blad-der stone[s]." In addition to providing medical statistics, Dr. Duan described the Chinese Church's religious involvement with the hospital. For exam-ple, Miss Yang Chin Hwa led prayer meetings and Bible class for the nurses once each week, nursing students led morning services in the wards each morning, and Mr. Chang Tin Siu and his daughter preached in the hospital every day. Duan measured evangelistic success in terms of how much Chris-tian literature was sold in the hospital: in 1940, the hospital sold one hun-dred hymnbooks, fifty "pieces of single Bible," and three hundred small gospel books, and distributed three hundred sheets of "Christian lecture." Under the direction of Dr. Duan, the training of Chinese nurses continued to be a priority at Weihui. According to Duan's report, four students com-pleted their Nursing Association of China exams in 1940, and two others were seeking postgraduate education: Miss Li Kwang Ling planned to at-tend the Peking Union Medical College for four months of operating room training, and Miss Liu Chi'ing Lin (*Liu Qing Yin*) was currently studying at Qilu (after which she planned to return to Weihui as the new head nurse). In addition, Weihui's Miss Fan Wen Hwa (*Fan Wen Hua*) was joining Miss Jen Hwiu Ying at Anyang to open a dispensary together there.

Dr. Duan's report gives some indication of the daily routine, struggles, and priorities at the Weihui Hospital. It also marks where the Chinese Church was at in terms of meeting the oft-cited goal of becoming self-governing, self-propagating, and self-supporting.[2] That is, it was the Chinese Church in North Henan that supported the development of medical services as well as other missionary activities. When the Canadians departed, Chinese Chris-tians stepped into the gap at the Weihui Hospital. If there was ever an op-portunity for the Chinese Church to exercise more autonomy, it was in 1940. The relationship between the hospital staff and their absentee Canad-ian "landlords" was, in some ways, a microcosm of the relationship between the Chinese Church and the United Church of Canada mission organiza-tion as a whole. On the surface, the Weihui Hospital appeared to be self-governing – at least insofar as Dr. Duan was in charge and the administrative staff were entirely Chinese. It also was reportedly self-supporting. Yet, on closer inspection, it is apparent that, of the so-called "three selfs," it was only in the area of propagation that the Chinese Church was self-sufficient.

In terms of self-governance, not only was Dr. Duan directly accountable to the absentee Canadians but his letter also underscores the tacit expecta-tion that Weihui would continue to use Canadian, Western structures. For example, despite the fact that the Weihui staff was entirely Chinese, and that North China missionaries were generally fluent in the local language, Dr. Duan wrote his report in English – the mother tongue of his Canadian overseers. In addition, most of Duan's report centred on descriptions of medi-cal and evangelistic achievements – proof, perhaps, of his mission-minded intentions and abilities as a superintendent. If his objective was to reassure the exiled North China missionaries of his ability to maintain the status quo, Duan met it. Duan's report provided a sense of relief to the missionaries, some of whom had been experiencing misgivings about leaving the field. After all, the better the reports out of Weihui, the more the missionaries could reassure themselves that they had made a good decision by leaving their colleagues behind in a war zone. And if the Weihui Hospital blossomed under the circumstances into a self-governing, self-supporting organization that was all the better.

Dr. Duan's positive report gave the Canadian missionaries the chance to recast their sudden departure as an unanticipated opportunity for the Chinese Church mission to fulfill her three-self mandate. In 1940, the NCM reported back to the home board that Dr. Duan was a "capable leader."[3] The NCM reassured the homeland supporters that, while the hospital staff faced difficulties, they "know how to endure and overcome" because they were, after all, Christians. Finally, ignoring Dr. Duan's indirect appeal for finances, the NCM report of 1940 indicated that the Weihui Hospital was "caring for itself financially." Although the NCM advocated for Chinese success in independently maintaining mission-initiated programs, in reality the Canadians' abrupt departure actually undermined the Chinese ability to continue the programs. For his part, Dr. Duan stood awkwardly in a cultural no-man's land, trying to meet the demands of his overextended Chinese staff and of his absent Canadian supervisors and financiers. The Weihui Hospital was a Western institution, minus the Westerners. The survival of the Weihui Hospital would be the ultimate litmus test of the missionary enterprise in Henan.

If the Chinese Church at Weihui was not exactly self-governing or self-supporting in medical work, it *was* self-propagating in terms of the Christian Gospel. Duan's emphasis on evangelistic statistics reveals his belief that the mission hospital was to be used as a centre for dissemination of Christian values and beliefs in general, and of the Christian message of salvation in particular. Duan's report is strikingly different from those by Canadian hospital administrators; the latter are characterized by a decided lack of evangelical emphasis. Since it is improbable that the evangelistic strategies noted by Duan were new to Weihui, the relative silence regarding evangelistic activities in the Canadian reports suggests that Canadian missionary physicians and nurses either did not directly participate in evangelistic strategies or that evangelism was implicit. The former is more likely. That is, most Canadian nurses emphasized the professional nursing aspects of their missionary work. Although Margaret Gay used evangelistic metaphors to describe her Chinese experience ("Who needed Him more than that city full of Chinese people, most of whom had never heard His Name?"), Canadian nurses more commonly used nursing images to describe their experiences (such as Clara Preston's "We wondered if Florence Nightingale found things much worse than we did?").[4] For the most part, missionary nurses viewed their wartime practice as a practical expression of, and opportunity to deepen, their own Christian faith. Propagation of the Christian Gospel was generally the responsibility of the self-propagating Chinese Church.

From Henan to the West China Mission (WCM)

After the Canadian NCM nurses were evacuated from North Henan, there was still one Canadian nurse remaining in the province. Susie Kelsey was a 1923 graduate of the Winnipeg General Hospital. She had been working at the Church of England in Canada (Anglican) St. Paul's mission hospital at Sanqui for seventeen years when Canadians were advised to evacuate Henan. Other Anglican missionaries left Henan, but Kelsey decided to stay, at her own risk.[5] From "time to time," those from within the Anglican Church urged her to leave, but the bishop had given Kelsey "full authority to leave at [her] own discretion," and she kept opting to stay.[6] Kelsey's reluctance to leave stemmed from the belief that her "local contacts are good and the work of the hospital is held in high esteem by the [Japanese] authorities and, of course, is greatly appreciated by the local community." Kelsey hoped that the Japanese would simply ignore her presence: whereas there "might be trouble" if a number of foreigners stayed, the Japanese might overlook the presence of a single woman.[7]

Susie Kelsey was well known to the NCM nurses. Not only did she work in the same province but she also served on the same District Auxiliary of the Nurses Association of China. In 1940, shortly after the North China missionaries had been evacuated from North Henan, Kelsey worked closely with both Mary Boyd and Clara Preston at Sanqui. At that time, Dr. Joseph Hsu was the only doctor at St. Paul's hospital, and had been attending to an average of 150 outpatients per day, in addition to 120 in-patients. Efforts to secure an American doctor and nurse and more Chinese doctors had met with no success. Thus, when the NCM agreed to send Dr. Isabelle McTavish and nurse Mary Boyd to help out at Sanqui in May 1940, the Anglican missionaries were delighted.[8] Mary Boyd took over teaching new students so that Kelsey could spend the requisite time with her advanced students. Mary Boyd viewed Susie Kelsey as the embodiment of an ideal missionary nurse, "bravely and successfully [carrying] the load of the busy little hospital there in Sanqui through a year and more of very critical events."[9] Kelsey's Canadian classmates also thought highly of her. Kelsey, like a number of the NCM nurses, had acquired a reputation as a brilliant student during her nurses' training, as exemplified in a poem written about Kelsey in the Winnipeg General Hospital 1923 nursing yearbook:

Susie, oh! please won't you tell us
For we have wondered in vain,
Just where, in that small anatomy,
You store up that bountiful brain?[10]

Susie Kelsey worked with Mary Boyd at Sanqui for five months. Clara Preston joined them for some of that time; she was called over to help nurse Boyd back to health after Boyd became ill with "typhus, relapsing fever or malaria" shortly after her arrival at Sanqui.[11] In October 1940, the Canadian Department of External Affairs in Ottawa advised women and children to be evacuated from occupied China. In response to the advisory, Rev. G.K. King sent a letter to Dr. McTavish at Sanqui suggesting that Boyd and McTavish head to safer regions, such as Tianjin, Beijing, or Jinan.[12] Boyd left Sanqui for Beijing, where she met up with her fiancé, Charles Johnson Stanley, who was studying and lecturing at Yenching University.[13] There, Boyd and Stanley decided that this was "no time in the world's history to become widely separated and lead separate lives."[14] Mary Boyd tendered her resignation from the WMS on 17 November 1940 and married Mr. Stanley. When the Japanese attacked Pearl Harbor thirteen months later, Susie Kelsey was the only Canadian nurse remaining in Henan, at Sanqui. Here the Japanese placed her under house arrest.[15]

After responding to the "S.O.S call to go down to Kweiteh [Sanqui]" to care for Mary Boyd, Clara Preston agreed to help out at the West China Mission.[16] Mary Boyd's sister Dorothy had been at the WCM station at Chongqing since January 1940, and Preston planned to join her there.[17] The WCM was established by the Methodist Church of Canada in 1892. After Church Union in 1925, the WCM and the NCM became sister organizations under the umbrella of the new United Church of Canada. There were remarkable similarities between these two missions. That is, both valued educational and medical work in addition to evangelism, opened a number of main stations and outstations at cities and villages around the province, established hospitals and nursing programs, employed female nurses through women's missionary societies, emphasized educational preparation for their missionaries, and had their mission offices in Toronto. The WCM, however, was a larger organization. While the NCM had three central mission stations in Henan (at Weihui, Anyang, and Huaiqing), the WCM had ten central stations in Sichuan, seven of which had hospitals (for example, Chongqing, Rongxian, and Chengdu). And while the NCM was only peripherally involved in university education in another province (Qilu), the WCM played a major role in the establishment and operation of the West China Union University, right within their mission.

The West China Union University was established in co-operation with other foreign missions at Chengdu in 1910. It boasted a school for physicians, dentists, and pharmacists, as well as a baccalaureate program for nurses. The WCM took great pride in the medical and nursing work around Sichuan. Between 1892 and 1937, forty-six male and female medical missionaries, including six dentists and two pharmacists, had served at the WCM.[18] In total, fifty-two Canadian nurses served at the WCM between 1894 and 1951, twenty-four of whom worked under the auspices of the Woman's Missionary Society (WMS).[19] During this period, Canadian WMS missionary nurses established the first health care services for women and children in southwestern China, and were instrumental in developing both hospital-based (diploma) and university-based (baccalaureate-level) nursing education programs.[20] In comparison, the NCM developed four-year diploma nursing education at Weihui, Anyang, and Huaiqing, but not a baccalaureate nursing program.

Preston headed to Sichuan in July 1940, where she was to act as superintendent of nurses at the WCM Chongqing hospital during the furlough of Canadian nurse Irene Harris. Preston left Tianjin for Shanghai, arriving in Hong Kong as residents were making preparations for the inevitable war. Hong Kong was considered to be a natural target for Japanese bombers, so foreign women and children were being evacuated from the island. Chinese women and children, of course, had no choice but to stay. Inflation was rampant in Hong Kong. Preston was astonished to find that the cost of her flight to Chongqing had gone up one hundred and forty dollars from the time she booked her ticket ("I thought it would be more reasonable to *lessen* the rate when we were going into a bombed area!").[21] Not knowing what to expect on the mainland, Preston focused on the excitement of her first plane ride, a four-hour trip on a "beautiful moonlit night." Once in Chongqing, Preston took a rickshaw ride through the streets to the river, and ferried across to the south bank of the Yangtze to the WCM compound.

The WCM hospital was at the top of a steep embankment – there were exactly 532 stone steps from the river to the hospital compound, then another sixty from the gate to some of the missionary houses.[22] The hospital, built eight years earlier, was a four-story building "with electric lights but no running water and, owing to the shortage and high cost of coal, our wards were not heated in the winter."[23] There were usually 180 to 220 patients in the hospital.[24] Dr. Stewart Allen was the hospital administrator. There was usually a "ward full" of typhoid and dysentery cases, a large children's ward, and a "good sized obstetrical service," but the chief work was surgery. Preston described the nurses' residence as "unusually good," but actually roomed in the nearby "Medical House" where she and Dorothy Boyd were set up with furniture, dishes, and stoves.[25] Preston felt fortunate to have such a good home to live in; on the other side of the river, Chongqing was very crowded with refugees. When she arrived, the WCM hospital had eleven doctors, twenty-four graduate nurses, and about eighty nurses in training.

Some of these nurses, she was thrilled to discover, were from Henan. In fact, one of them was Preston's "first graduate nurse," with whom Preston had developed a strong friendship over the years.[26] The presence of Henan nurses helped alleviate any sense of loneliness Preston may have otherwise felt. Even so, Preston soon discovered that nursing in North China could "hardly be compared to a war-conditioned program in the West."[27] The West, she discovered, had problems all its own.

"Hell Let Loose": Japanese Air Raids

An air raid alarm sounded the day Preston arrived. For the next fourteen months, alarms continued off and on. Clara Preston found the air raid sirens nerve-racking, later recalling: "Often a scouter plane would be seen in the morning and a warning would go up. When the planes had left Hankow [Hankou], a red ball would go up ... and the whole atmosphere told you that an air raid was expected. Then we would hear the first alarm, and everyone was hurrying to get the most essential things done, treatments completed, medicine secured, or food sent to the wards before the raid started."[28] Frightened as she was by the air raids, Preston was also impressed by how the staff and patients learned to cope with them. When the siren sounded, the hospital staff jumped into action, cancelling or hurriedly performing operations, evacuating patients from the wards, bringing laundry in off the line (where planes might spot it), and scrambling to dugouts under the hospital or up the hill. Patients from the third and fourth floors of the hospital were carried down to the main floor, from where coolies would take them on stretchers down the front ramp. Although most patients were evacuated during the air raids, some found the evacuation too strenuous: the tuberculosis patients, who were accommodated on the hospital verandah, usually preferred to stay quietly in their beds and take their chances with the bombings. Similarly, if the sirens caught nurses and doctors in the middle of a delivery or complex surgery, the staff would stay in the case room or operating room during the bombings. To Preston, crouching in a dugout during the bombing was "as if heaven was ripped open and hell let loose."[29] West China missionary Rev. James Endicott later called Clara Preston "the unsung heroine of the war" because of her "constant heroism during raid after raid of Jap bombers, when she would sit by the side of patients, too ill to be moved to the shelters, to assure them that all was well."[30]

The nurses had one additional, peculiar task during air raids: changing from white to blue nursing uniforms. It was considered dangerous to wear white during air raids. The Japanese were reportedly employing Chinese men to join a crowd when a raid was on, and to be dressed in a white suit covered by a dark cloak. When the planes came, the designated man would throw off his cloak and run into the open waving a white piece of cloth to attract the plane to the spot for bombing.[31] The nurses at Chongqing solved the problem of white nursing attire by "quickly changing into blue uniforms which we had specially for air raids."[32] It is curious that nurses did not wear blue uniforms *all* the time, thus avoiding the need to change. Preston apparently did not even entertain the idea; since she did not elaborate on this, her reasons for insisting on white uniforms are not entirely clear. One can surmise that the symbolism of white uniforms, caps, and pins was extremely important to the nurses – not only identifying the wearers as nursing staff (as opposed to medical or support staff), but also indicating their relative achievement and rank, since nursing students wore different styles of uniforms based on their year in the school.

After an air raid, patients were carried back to their beds and made comfortable. According to Preston, the evacuations took a toll on everyone – emotionally, physically, and materially. For example, meal preparation was interrupted since all fires were supposed to be extinguished during an air raid so no smoke could be seen, and the constant moving of patients caused much wear and tear on the mattresses and bed linen. It was a very poor atmosphere for patients to recover in. Yet Preston marvelled at the way the nurses held up. She had come to Chongqing expecting nurses to be "breaking down mentally and physically under these conditions."[33] Instead, she found that, despite the extreme heat, routinely interrupted sleep, and unrelenting air raids, nurses focused on the task of caring for patients – both existing and new. The WCM hospital was designated the Fifth Red Cross Emergency Hospital in Chongqing. As such, it received cases from bombing in their own area – as many as seventy-two at a time: "We had our staff organized into teams so everyone knew their own responsibility. As soon as possible morphia was given [to the newly arrived casualties], emergency treatment rendered, accommodation found in the hospital and then the operating rooms made ready for the cases which needed it."[34]

Like Clara Preston, Margaret Gay found the air raids to be the most distressing aspect of working in West China. According to her memoirs, Gay encountered the air raids en route to Chongqing, and the bombing of southwestern China postponed her arrival in Sichuan. Indeed, it took Gay four months to travel to Sichuan, via Beidaihe, Shanghai, Haiphong (Indo-China), and Kunming. When Margaret Gay arrived in Kunming, Yunnan, all that was left of her long journey to Chongqing, Sichuan, was a one-hour airplane flight. Yet she was delayed in Kunming for weeks, where she relied on the hospitality of two English Methodist missionary families, the Harrisons and the Evans. Gay got her first taste of Japanese air raids the day after she arrived in Kunming. The air raid warnings came while Gay was at the British Consulate with Isabel Harrison arranging for letters of permission to travel on to Chongqing. Harrison and Gay hurried out along the

road and, spotting an open field with grave mounds, decided to hide themselves among the graves. To their surprise, Chinese soldiers were also hiding
there. As Gay later recalled, the women were placed under the guard of two
bayonetted soldiers, who "made us lie down in a muddy gully, not allowing
us to raise our heads" when the planes flew over.[35] Gay and Harrison returned to the Harrisons' home later that evening, only to discover that bombs
had demolished the neighbourhood. Ted Harrison met them at the street
corner and together, by the light of his flashlight, the threesome "stepped
along over piles of rubble, passing dead bodies here and there" before arriving at the Harrison house. There they found "walls were smashed in,
windows all broken, plaster and glass lying everywhere." Many of the surrounding buildings had been destroyed, including a home for English Methodist nurses nearby. After a restless night's sleep "in any corner that seemed
safe" the cook's little boy awakened them at six o'clock in the morning. The
first air raid alarm of the day had sounded: "The Japs," recalled Gay, "were
coming again."

The air raids were relentless. According to her memoirs, Gay spent her
days "dodging air raids" and shopping for flashlight batteries – the only
means of lighting – and food.[36] One night, there was nothing to eat but
soda crackers and clear tea. Gay grew somewhat accustomed to the air raids:
running from the city after the siren sounded, hiding in rice fields and under bean stalks, covering her head with a steamer rug when a pistol shot
indicated the planes were almost overhead, and then returning to Kunming
to "see and hear of the terrible things" that had happened. Finally, Gay was
able to arrange for a flight to Chongqing. She got as far as waiting on the
airfield to board her plane, but at the last minute was turned away; the
plane was overloaded. Although she was disappointed, Gay would later report that her delay was divinely inspired: God orchestrated her delay so
that she would be available to nurse Mr. Albertson, the only other United
Church of Canada missionary in the province of Yunnan. Albertson had
become ill while in Haiphong, Vietnam, where he had been arranging for
the transport of missionary luggage and large pieces of furniture to the WCM.
When Gay returned to the Evans' home after being refused passage on the
airplane, she found Mr. Anderson lying on their living-room couch, "not
being able to walk up to the bedroom he was meant to occupy upstairs."[37]
Albertson had developed an infection from sunburn on his ankle, and was
running a fever of 105 degrees Fahrenheit. Gay decided on the spot to post-
pone her plans another two weeks in order to nurse him. That same evening,
a visiting physician diagnosed Albertson with "malignant malaria," from
which he was not expected to survive. Margaret Gay and two Chinese nurses
stayed by his side through the night. At 5 a.m., Albertson passed away. To
Gay, this experience proved that God was in control of her destiny and

that, regardless of how frustrating and unpredictable her circumstances might be, she could rest assured that God would steer her to situations where she could best fulfill His plan for her and for others. It seems that Gay perceived herself as a tiny thread in an immense divine tapestry – not clear on the whole design, but confident in the Designer. It would give great comfort to Albertson's family, Gay believed, to know that a fellow Canadian was by his side when he died. Gay stayed at Kunming for a couple more weeks under constant threat of bombing, until finally she was able to board a plane for the one-hour flight to Sichuan.

Reunion at the WCM

After her gruelling journey from north China, Margaret Gay was reunited for a few days with her NCM colleagues Dorothy Boyd and Clara Preston at Chongqing. Soon afterward, Gay made the four-day journey (by bus, truck, and coal cart) to the WCM station at Rongxian, where she was to take charge of the WCM hospital. For the next few months, Gay worked at WCM hospitals at both Rongxian and Chengdu – rooming with veteran WCM nurse Caroline Wellwood when at Chengdu. As isolated as Sichuan was from the rest of China, it was not peaceful. Besides dealing with air raids, the nurses discovered that both human and material resources were expensive and in short supply. Of immediate concern to the missionaries was the high cost of fuel, used for heating and cooking. WCM missionary Winifred Harris wrote to the church offices in Toronto in November 1940 with her concerns: "With fuel the price it is to-day one wonders what one ought to do. I tried to cut down here by buying less than half the amount we usually buy, and by doing without fire in the office. I bought a Chinese fire basket and determined I was going to make that do for the winter, but the very first day I used it I got a chill that sent me to bed for a few days, so I decided it didn't pay."[38]

Although Margaret Gay later recounted that "we had a very happy time" at Chengdu and that her period at Rongxian was "one of the happiest times I had ever spent in China," she did have difficulty adjusting to the rigours of wartime work in Sichuan.[39] According to a letter sent by WCM field secretary Adelaide Harrison to the WMS headquarters in Toronto in February 1941, both Margaret Gay and Clara Preston struggled with wartime conditions: "Misses Preston and Gay are finding conditions in our hospitals vastly different from Henan where they had ample supplies of all kinds to work with. Here after three and a half years of war, transportation difficulties, [and] soaring prices, our hospital supplies are almost down to rock bottom which makes effective medical work, particularly in the nursing department, very difficult. Also, we do not have modern conveniences like running water and central heating."[40]

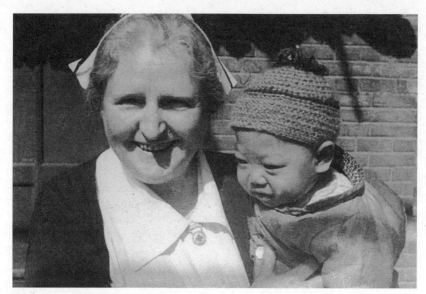

Figure 40   Margaret Gay with refugee at Tianjin, 1940.
UCCVUA 76.001P-2114

Reports that Gay and Preston were struggling must have been surprising, considering that they had experienced their share of challenges over their decades in China, and had successfully adjusted to primitive and chaotic working conditions in northern China in the past. On the other hand, although experience and tenacity were valuable missionary attributes, so was the physical vigour commonly associated with youth; compared with the other NCM nurses, neither Preston nor Gay was young. Preston was now fifty years old, and Gay was fifty-five (see Figure 40). In addition, Margaret Gay did not receive her promised four-month furlough in Hong Kong, and West China certainly did not offer relief from the "dearth in fuel and table niceties" that had reportedly "exhausted" her in Tianjin.[41] While it is difficult to imagine that Preston and Gay expected wartime Sichuan to offer any luxuries, they evidently were not expecting the situation to be as dire as it was. Neither, it seems, was Dorothy Boyd. By June 1941, both Boyd and Gay made plans to return to Canada.

Departure of Dorothy Boyd and Margaret Gay

On 6 May 1941, Dorothy Boyd wrote a letter of resignation to Adelaide Harrison, the WMS field secretary for the WCM. It read: "For personal and family reasons I find that I shall have to put in my resignation to the WMS and go home in June when my parents sail. My father has already fixed [a] sailing date for me on the *Pres. Coolidge* leaving Hongkong on the 14th of

June, and I have booked a seat on the CNAC plane leaving Chungking [Chongqing] on June 6."[42] Dorothy Boyd's resignation came as a complete surprise to the United Church WMS – if not to Boyd herself, who wrote: "I am sorry that I have to spring this thing so suddenly, but I did not know myself until yesterday." While Boyd did not articulate her specific reasons for resigning, the wartime conditions and imminent departure of her parents to Canada for furlough undoubtedly influenced her decision. In addition, the Canadian government had again issued an order for women and children to leave occupied China. Although the Boyds were in Free China, the war was escalating elsewhere; Canada was safer. There may have been an additional compelling reason for Dorothy Boyd to return home. According to North China missionary Margaret Brown, Dorothy Boyd returned to Canada to be married to Phillip Johnston.[43] Although Boyd did not mention marriage in her resignation letter, she did marry Johnston within four months of her return to Canada.[44] Whatever her reasons for resigning, Boyd was still a year away from the end of her three-year contract – a matter that irritated field secretary Adelaide Harrison. Since Boyd had already made travel arrangements, Harrison felt forced to "accept the inevitable," leaving it up to the mission office in Canada to deal with Boyd's broken contract.[45]

At about the same time as Boyd's resignation, Margaret Gay made the sudden decision to return to Canada "at once" to help care for her sisters.[46] According to WMS executive secretary Mrs. Ruth Taylor, one of Gay's sisters "is finding it impossible to carry on at home without [Gay] because of the continued illness of her other sister."[47] In the past, Gay had taken seriously her obligations to ill family members (for example, nursing her father through an illness before returning to China after her nurses' training in Vancouver); this was no exception. Gay left Rongxian by sedan chair, travelling four days over the mountains to Chengdu; she then travelled with a mail truck driver for two more days to Chongqing, before flying to Hong Kong ("I had not the slightest sense of fear; I had made so many strange journeys throughout the years)."[48] Whereas Gay's trip to Chongqing had taken four months, the return trip from Chongqing to Hong Kong took only four days. She sailed for Canada on 14 May 1941.

The WMS was sympathetic toward Margaret Gay. It tried to find ways to bend the rules to accommodate her needs. Since Margaret Gay recognized that she could be "detained at home for a matter of possibly three years," the NCM secretary G.K. King directed her to request a leave of absence from the WMS "on account of home conditions" rather than resigning; this way the board would agree to pay her full travel home.[49] Margaret Gay reached Toronto in July 1941, after having spent some time with her brother and father on the coast of British Columbia. According to Gay's niece, Margaret moved to Toronto to help her older sister Elizabeth care for another sister, Jessie, who had epilepsy – a stigmatized condition that was not discussed, even with other family members.[50] None of the four sisters in Margaret's family ever married (one died young); Elizabeth, a teacher, cared for Jessie. Elizabeth's appeal for help from Margaret came at an auspicious time; conditions in West China were unbearable. Responding to a genuine need at home legitimized Gay's abrupt departure from China, and the WMS honoured her request for a three-year leave. Gay's thirty years of service to the NCM did not go unrewarded. In September 1941, the WMS generously granted Gay a four-month furlough and a three-year leave of absence, and also agreed to bear the expenses of her travel home.[51] Despite the generosity of the WMS, however, Gay was now without an income. In Toronto, she moved into the nurses' residences at the Toronto General Hospital, and put her name in at the Registry of Nurses for work in Ontario. Later, she moved with her sisters to Victoria, where they lived together until Jessie's death, in 1946.[52] Gay's leave of absence was later extended indefinitely, and lasted until her retirement from the United Church WMS on 12 August 1951.[53]

The WMS was not as generous with – or as sympathetic toward – Dorothy Boyd. After Boyd's abrupt departure, there was some confusion over the length of her appointment; had she fulfilled the terms of her three-year contract? When she resigned, Boyd had been on Chinese soil for only two years. Yet since she had been appointed by the WMS in 1938, Boyd was actually closer to the end of her contract than the WMS field secretary in West China may have realized.[54] Unfortunately, Dorothy Boyd was the third of three new recruits to quit early. Mary Boyd, Dorothy Boyd, and Elizabeth Thomson had each been given reduced contracts as a way to attract them to China. Instead of the usual five- to seven-year commitment, these women were given three-year contracts. Both Mary Boyd and Elizabeth Thomson had broken their already shortened contracts to marry. Dorothy's unexpected resignation compounded the disappointment felt by the WMS secretaries. Since the WMS was responsible for a missionary's travel and outfitting costs only if contract terms were met, Dorothy Boyd was required to reimburse the WMS $195.00. Her sister Mary, however, had her incurred expenses waived, since Mary's husband was a student.[55] It seems that the WMS was not beyond bending the rules, but held steadfast in the case of Dorothy Boyd. Finding replacements for Dorothy Boyd and Margaret Gay proved to be an impossible task.

With the departure of Dorothy Boyd, the WMS in Toronto hoped Janet Brydon would be able to go to West China. Brydon was agreeable to this; she was not enjoying her time as a home missionary at the WMS hospital at Smeaton, Saskatchewan (see Figure 41). According to Brydon's nephew, the working conditions at Smeaton were "very bad; primitive."[56] All through 1941, Brydon made it clear to the WMS that she was anxious to return to China. Sending Brydon seemed the perfect solution to the shortage created

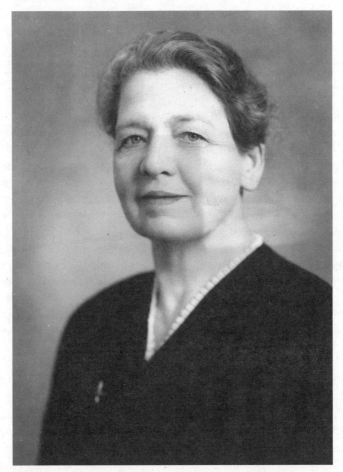

Figure 41 Janet Brydon, home mission's portrait, c. 1941.
UCCVUA 76.001P-705

by Boyd's departure, and to Brydon's dissatisfaction with her home mission assignment. Much to everyone's surprise, however, the WCM gave an "unfavourable recommendation" to Brydon in June 1941 because of her hearing problem.[57] Their concern was not so much her disability as the fact that hearing aid batteries would be unavailable in Sichuan. The batteries were available through the Sonotone Company (a hearing aid company) in Shanghai, but supplies from Shanghai were not easily obtainable for those living up the Yangtze River in Sichuan. Undeterred, the NCM field secretary began looking into other openings in China for Brydon. Rev. G.K. King requested that the NCM interim committee consider sending Brydon to Nanjing, where the need for nurses was deemed urgent.[58]

By September 1941, an interim committee determined that prospects for Brydon did not look promising at either Nanjing or Qilu. "Perhaps in 1942," the committee ventured.[59] Having had enough of the heavy work and "different conditions" at Smeaton, Brydon requested a one-year leave of absence.[60] She preferred to wait for an opening "in her own line of work in China" rather than "trying to adjust herself to the very difficult situation in our Home Mission hospitals." On 3 December 1941, the NCM secretary wrote that he would be "be glad to welcome Miss Brydon back; there is an abundance of work awaiting her," but that "general conditions [in China] now are so uncertain and menacing that we cannot assume the responsibility for asking her to come now."[61] Brydon was disappointed. Not one to shy away from hard work, Brydon's heart was nonetheless not in just *any* kind of nursing practice; it was to be China or nothing. While Brydon waited, news of the extreme need for nurses in China kept coming. For example, the Student Christian Movement of Canada had recently advertised a need for missionary nurses to China in *Canadian Nurse*.[62] Not only was there a need in Sichuan, Nanjing, and Qilu (in exile), but also at the Canadian Anglican Mission hospital at Sanqui, Henan, where Susie Kelsey was still working. Perhaps Brydon could work there?[63] Any hopes that Brydon might have held of returning to China were dashed when Japanese planes attacked Pearl Harbor on 7 December 1941.

Reverberations from Pearl Harbor
On 3 December 1941, Rev. George K. King wrote a letter to Mrs. Ruth Taylor describing, among other things, the location of some of the Canadian nurses.[64] As secretary of the NCM, King wrote most of the mission reports. He kept in close contact with Mrs. Taylor, the WMS executive secretary, who was in turn responsible for overseeing and coordinating all WMS missionaries in the various mission fields, including Korea, Japan, and China. It was not unusual for King to write two or three letters in one week to Taylor. His letter of 3 December 1941, however, would be his last from China. He would not write Taylor again until two years later, from aboard the repatriation ship *MS Gripsholm*.[65]

In this 1941 letter, King took stock of the location of various missionaries, including three mishkids who were former NCM nurses: Mrs. Georgina (Menzies) Lewis was en route to visit her mother, Mrs. D.G. Menzies, in Jinan, and Georgina's sister Mrs. Jean (Menzies) Stockley had been in Xian, where she and her husband occasionally took in refugees, but was now in England. It is not clear when Jean Menzies Stockley left China. According to a *Globe and Mail* article in August 1942, one of Mrs. D. Menzies' daughters was living in England. According to two letters written by G.K. King, Georgina was in China in December 1941 and in November 1943. Thus, it must have been Jean who was in England. Jean's husband, however, must have remained in China, since the NCM later credited Dr. Handley Stockley for "what they [?] did for refugee students from North Henan." Apparently, Dr. Stockley left Xian in April 1943 with other English Baptist missionaries, after receiving evacuation orders.[66]

Mrs. Elizabeth (Thomson) Gale was with her husband at Qilu, where she "[continued] to carry nursing responsibility in the hospital [and was] in charge of the private patient ward."[67] Elizabeth Gale had given birth to a daughter the previous July and had recently returned to work part-time. "Dr. and Mrs. Gale and family," wrote King, were "looking hale and hearty and healthy." Four days after Rev. King wrote this letter, Japanese planes dropped bombs on Pearl Harbor, Hawaii. The United States declared war on the Japanese on 8 December 1941, and foreigners in Japanese-occupied China immediately became "enemy aliens."[68] All correspondence between China and Canada stopped.

News of the Japanese attack on Pearl Harbor reverberated through the United Church offices in Toronto, giving "the [mission] board secretaries some of the most anxious days of their years of service."[69] Twenty-five United Church missionaries, including nine from the NCM, were in Japan, Korea, and occupied China, and an additional eleven single women, including Dr. Margaret Forster, were on the ocean en route to or from their respective fields. It was not until February that the mission learned through the International Red Cross that all the North China missionaries were safe and well. Dr. Forster, having unwittingly observed the attack on Pearl Harbor, made it safely home from Honolulu. Nine remained in occupied China: Rev. and Mrs. G.K. King (Beijing), Miss Bertha Hodge (Tianjin), Miss Winifred Warren (Shanghai), and Dr. G. Struthers, Rev. A. Thomson, Mrs. D.G. Menzies, Dr. McTavish, and Rev. D.K. Faris (all in Jinan).[70] Dr. Godfrey and Elizabeth Gale were also at Jinan, with the London Missionary Society. Clara Preston was the only North China missionary nurse who remained in China after Pearl Harbor.

Few documents exist from the North China Mission from the period between December 1941 and April 1946. In the months leading to Pearl Harbor, there was the usual flurry of correspondence between Rev. G.K. King and Mrs. Ruth Taylor. Then, silence. Reasons for the dearth of documents are likely related to the extremely dangerous situation in China. For example, Dr. R. Gordon Struthers reported to the *Globe and Mail* in 1942 that the missionaries "dared not keep diaries and were nervous about writing anything at all, since Japanese police are apt to walk into their homes at any time."[71] Other missionaries were reluctant to talk about their life under Japanese dominion "for fear of reprisals against those left behind." Some, like Peter and Helen (Turner) Nelson, were advised to destroy all personal letters before they left China.[72] Even Margaret Brown's *History of the North China Mission* – a meticulous, 1,500-page unpublished opus – contains fewer than thirty pages on the period between 1941 and 1945.[73] One "brief confidential message" written by Rev. G.K. King on 19 May 1942 was smuggled out of China by an American being "repatriated" (that is, released by the Japanese, and returned to America via ship). In it, King gave an update of the situation at NCM sites after Pearl Harbor: "At 8.15 Dec. 8th received news state of war existed. Pastor Liu C.C. [Chinese Church] and Messrs. Hu and Kuo [Daokou] were in compound. They departed forthwith. At 10 a.m. were courteously informed of new conditions and confined to compound one week, since when have enjoyed normal life within limits of city walls ... [Qilu] University disbanded Dec. 8 the hospital closed three weeks later, radium etc. commandeered."[74] In the same letter, King also gave an update on Weihui. "Weihwei Hospital," he wrote, "continues to serve the whole area, self supporting and helps provide maintenance of pastors and evangelists who continue labour with unabated zeal." After 8 December, the Japanese required that all missionaries register with them their personal and mission property. "Great pressure" was placed on them to sign all property away to the Chinese Church. Rev. G.K. King reluctantly signed over the Canadian property under his care in Tianjin, including two motorcars, "drugs, radium, portable x-rays and the bloodless knife" the missionaries had brought with them from the Huaiqing hospital – albeit with a clause stating that his decision would have to be endorsed by the Canadian church. This was the last record pertaining to NCM hospitals until after the war. [75]

Left Behind

The sole NCM nurse in China during the post–Pearl Harbor period was Clara Preston, in Sichuan. There *were,* however, a number of Canadians directly associated with the NCM who were in northern China after Pearl Harbor, including Elizabeth (Thomson) Gale, Mary (Boyd) Stanley, Georgina (Menzies) Lewis, and Susie Kelsey. At the time of Pearl Harbor, Mary Stanley was with her husband at Yenching University at Beijing, where she was working as a secretary while he was studying for a master's degree in Chinese; they planned to be in Beijing for two more years.[76] These nurses became "internees" in civilian internment camps.[77] A full examination of these nurses' experiences during the war is the subject of a new study, currently in progress.[78] Their experiences deserve mention here, however, since each had a close association with the NCM: Susie Kelsey worked with the NCM in Henan; the other four Canadian nurses were NCM mishkids, born and reared in North Henan. The husband of Henan mishkid and nurse Florence MacKenzie Liddell was also interned. In 1941, Florence Liddell, who was expecting their third child, had returned to Toronto with her two daughters because of the increasingly dangerous situation in China.

Immediately after Pearl Harbor, foreigners were placed under house arrest. At Qilu University in Shandong, Betty Gale went to work at the hospital "as usual" at 7:30 a.m. on 8 December 1941 to examine student nurses for their registration exams. After a couple of hours, Gale headed home in order to nurse her daughter, Margaret. According to her diary entry that day, when Gale arrived at the university campus gates en route to her house, "a lorry [was] unloading dozens of [Japanese] soldiers – all armed to the teeth. Then, following a shouted command they proceed to march into the Campus. I have a moment of wild panic – war must have been declared."[79] The campus gates clanged shut behind her, temporarily separating Betty from her husband Godfrey, who was also working at the hospital. The Japanese immediately informed the campus personnel of their plans. Betty was told that "the university is to close immediately. No new patients may be admitted into the hospital – and as soon as the patients now there are better – the hospital will also be closed. Doctors and nurses will be 'convoyed under guard' between the Campus and the hospital. Our servants may not leave the Campus – and *we* will do the necessary shopping, always with a guard. We must carry a 'pass' at all times." The Japanese authorities had immediately closed down clinics at Qilu, where Dr. R. Gordon Struthers had been caring for fifty outpatients per day. Dr. Struthers later reported that guards armed with bayonets marched behind him whenever he moved between his home and the 180-bed hospital.[80] The last in-patient was discharged by mid-January, at which time the Qilu University hospital was closed, although Dr. Godfrey Gale managed to smuggle out some instruments and medicine afterward.[81]

The seventy foreigners at Qilu were initially allowed to remain in their own homes. Among these were the five NCM missionaries, Dr. Isabelle McTavish, Mrs. D.G. Menzies (mother of nurses Jean Stockley and Georgina Lewis), Rev. Andrew Thomson (father of Betty Gale), Dr. R.G. Struthers, and Rev. D.K. Faris (husband of Marion Fisher Faris).[82] Dr. McTavish wrote a letter to Clara Preston on 2 February 1942 from Jinan, noting that Georgina (Menzies) Lewis had just given birth to a baby girl via a caesarian section – her second – at Chow Ts'un, a community two and a half hours by train from Jinan.[83] The missionaries were anxious to get news of each other, and passed along any snippets they received. Yet since mail service was frequently interrupted, the information was not always accurate. For example, on 26 February 1942, Clara Preston wrote to Annie Waddell (Dr. McTavish's sister in Manitoba) that Mrs. D.G. Menzies and her daughter Georgina were living with Dr. McTavish in Jinan. Concerned about how Dr. Isabelle McTavish was coping since the Qilu hospital had been closed, Preston remarked: "She will have Georgie Menzies' two children to help look after [at Jinan] and that she will enjoy."[84] In actuality, Georgina Menzies was not in Jinan, but at Chow Ts'un.

Situated in unoccupied China, Clara Preston had more access to international mail services than some of the other missionaries. In early 1942, Eric Liddell sent two letters to Preston from Tianjin, where he was under house arrest at the British Concession. Because of his connection with the NCM through his wife Florence, Eric had developed relationships among Florence's China friends and nursing colleagues, and relied on their help during the war. He hoped Preston would be able to send along news to Florence via Ruth Taylor at the United Church office in Toronto; Preston had more access to international mail services than he did. In the first letter, on 23 January 1942, Liddell described the conditions at the British Concession, where he lived with the other foreigners except hospital staff. According to the letter, food was not restricted, but all work stopped except that of the mission hospital.[85] A week later, on 1 February 1942, Liddell wrote again to Preston. This time, he had a specific message of encouragement to pass along to his wife:

> [Let Flo know] how fortunate I am ... There are some simple thoughts that I
> thought Flo might like just to get a right attitude to all that happens so that
> we can in all circumstances live on "top of the world": "All things work
> together for good to them that love God" ... "My grace is sufficient for thee,
> for my strength is made perfect in weakness" ... Everything I ought to do,
> I have strength given to me to do. I know it isn't easy for Flo not to be
> anxious; perhaps these will give a way to overcome anxiety.[86]

On 6 April 1942, Godfrey and Betty Gale and the group at Jinan were required to vacate their private homes and move in together in two rows of houses on the campus. The group filled their days with ordinary tasks, such as buying food (accompanied by a Japanese guard) and tending to a garden. Although no longer allowed to practice medicine, according to Betty Gale's diary, a few doctors and nurses would meet together "for an experimental prayer-circle for spiritual healing of sickness among our own community, and such Chinese as we are able to contact outside the Campus."[87] The group planned to keep track of the illnesses, and make an attempt "to discover the conditions necessary for the spiritual healing of sickness – its scope and limitations." While no conclusions were drawn, their experiment gives insight into the philosophy of medicine that guided the Gales and their medical compatriots, as well as their desire to somehow assist the ill – even when there were no facilities or resources available to do so: "Rather than pray for direct physical healing, [Godfrey] would prefer to pray that each sufferer should find God's Will for himself – or herself – in the particular circumstances in which they are placed – for this is ultimately a higher objective than to seek simply for relief from physical disability."[88]

After a few months of living under house arrest, word came that "Americans" (those living in North and South America) were to be repatriated home. On 12 June 1942, Betty Gale attended a farewell party for all those who were leaving, including her father, Rev. Andrew Thomson, and the four other North China missionaries. It was one of a number of farewell parties around the campus gardens that week, where members of the group sang songs, put on skits, and shared in the sacrament of the Lord's Supper. After the group left, Betty felt "glad for them – but very sad for ourselves – and left behind."[89] Betty Gale was the only Canadian left at Qilu.[90] Although Betty did not explain in her diary why she opted out of leaving with the other Canadians, her daughter Margaret has suggested it was because, as English citizens, neither Godfrey nor Margaret would have been allowed to leave China.[91] Even had Margaret been allowed to leave with her, Betty refused to leave her husband. As Godfrey later wrote, "Betty put her foot down and refused to return to Canada."[92] It was a decision Betty later questioned – if only temporarily – writing on 20 August 1942: "Oh, should I have taken [Margaret] home when the Canadians left?"[93] A family friend heard a different account:

> We were talking about the need for prayer and how God does answer prayer if we are open to His response. Betty said that her father definitely wanted her to go back to Canada where she would be safe and he had arranged for her travel. She started to pack her trunk but felt uneasy about leaving Godfrey. She unpacked and then started packing again etc. She was really confused and torn. Then that night, she decided to hand it over to God in prayer. She told Him that she could no longer see clearly what to do and left it in His hands. Betty said that when she woke up the next morning she was no longer confused and just knew that she should stay ... so she unpacked her trunk. She also added that when Godfrey got so sick, she [felt] that he would not have lived if she hadn't been there to care for him. She knew that was why God had led her to stay in China.[94]

On 25 August 1942, the five repatriated NCM missionaries arrived safely in Montreal. Rev. Andrew Thomson, Mrs. Davina Menzies, Rev. D.K. Faris, Dr. Isabelle McTavish, and Dr. R. Gordon Struthers had been taken to Shanghai, where they boarded the Italian liner *Conte Verde*. On arrival at Lorenco Marques (Maputo, Mozambique), they were exchanged for Japanese prisoners from Europe and placed on the Swedish diplomatic ship the *MS Gripsholm*.[95] United Church foreign mission secretaries Dr. J.H. Arnup and Mrs. Ruth Taylor met the group and brought them to the United Church office in Toronto, where they were met by some one hundred church leaders and friends.[96]

On 13 July 1942, Betty Gale wrote in her diary of her excitement to find out that the remaining missionaries at Qilu were to be repatriated back to their homelands. Most of the foreigners at Jinan were "wildly happy" – although some were "mildly depressed" at the thought of leaving their adopted country.[97] Three days before their departure, the group was told to sell all their furniture to the Chinese. The Gales set their belongings out on their front lawn for a yard sale. Although they made little money, they were not terribly concerned ("Who cares? In three days we will be *on our way home!*"). On 10 August, the Jinan group boarded a train for Shanghai. There they were taken by bus to the Columbia Country Club – formerly an exclusive club for wealthy British residents. Trainloads of foreign refugees arrived at the club, 90 percent of whom were missionaries. In Shanghai, the Gales' excitement turned to despair after receiving the news that only seven of those from the Jinan area were included on the list of those to be repatriated; the Gales were not among them. Betty wrote, "So here we are – for the duration, whatever that may be." A total of 350 people lived together at the "country club" internment camp for the next seven months, under cramped and difficult conditions.

Civilian Internees

By March 1943, the Japanese had decided to move "enemy aliens," kept under house arrest to that point, into large internment camps. From the Japanese point of view, the idea of internment made sense. Keeping thousands of people under house arrest in the major cities of North China required too much time, money, and effort.[98] On 13 March 1943, Godfrey and Betty Gale and their daughter Margaret were moved from the Columbia Country Club to a concentration camp at Yangzhou (by the Grand Canal) and then, the following October, to a camp at Pudong, across the Huangpu River from the famous Shanghai Bund. They remained at Pudong until the end of the war – finally being released on 1 September 1945.

In March 1943, Canadians in other parts of northern China were also transported to internment camps. Susie Kelsey (Anglican – Henan), Rev. and Mrs. G.K. King (NCM – Beijing), and Bertha Hodge (NCM – Tianjin) were among those transported from various locations for internment at the Weixian Camp in Shandong province.[99] Georgina (Menzies) Lewis and Mary (Boyd) Stanley also became civilian internees, although it is not clear where.[100] Weixian Camp comprised a large compound surrounded by a tall gray wall, whose corner turrets served as guard towers, with searchlights and machine guns. Over the course of ten days in March 1943, six groups of "enemy nationals" from three different cities were transported to Weixian.[101] The total camp population was 1,800, including Canadians, British, Dutch, Americans, and Belgians.

Susie Kelsey was among those who had been kept under house arrest prior to being imprisoned at Weixian. After Pearl Harbor, the Japanese allowed the Anglican hospital to continue to function, but Kelsey was confined in her own home for more than a year. She became lonely and isolated. The move to Weixian Camp in March 1943 was, therefore, paradoxically exciting for Kelsey. She later explained in a letter to the *Canadian Nurse* journal that "the busy, complex society [at Weixian] was a great contrast to my loneliness and isolation in the interior and, in spite of various discomforts, I quite enjoyed the change."[102]

The Weixian Camp was in the former Civil Assembly Centre at Weixian (now Weifang) in Shandong province. The centre was itself a former American Presbyterian compound established in 1883. Inside an area of about one city block were school buildings, a church, some four hundred individual rooms, and a hospital. Japanese officers and guards now occupied the five large Western-style missionary houses.[103] According to the letter written by Kelsey to *Canadian Nurse*, the Japanese provided food and accommodation, but the internees themselves undertook all the internal organization and work of the camp. Before long, the internees had organized three kitchens, schools for the children, adult classes, religious services (half of the camp were missionaries), baseball matches, and concerts. The health of the camp was important to the doctors and nurses interned there. Kelsey reportedly found her niche in this area. The hospital had been "one of the finest in North China" before the war. Now, the heating system and water pipes had been ripped out, all the surgical furniture and equipment had been removed, and dirt and plaster covered the floors. Kelsey and the others were given the use of the first floor, but the upper two stories were to be used as dormitories ("and were occupied by Dutch priests").[104] The hospital was cleaned and stocked with supplies brought into camp by nurses and doctors from Beijing and Tianjin who had been able to rescue them from their own hospitals. According to Kelsey's letter, sufficient beds were available, but patients had to bring their own mattresses and bedding, which meant "friendly neighbours had to rally around to carry the patient, on a stretcher or chair, with his roll of bedding from his dormitory to his hospital bed." The hospital, she wrote, was staffed by a number of doctors and nurses "who had ignored consular advice to leave China before the war broke out." The hospital superintendent and nursing superintendent were both from the Peking Union Medical College. Almost all the nurses had held executive positions in Chinese hospitals, and "we now enjoyed the chance to do humble nursing," including visiting the less seriously ill in the dormitories and working in outpatient clinics, the laboratory, the pharmacy, or the hospital wards. The hardest worked were the nurses in charge of the combined operating and labour room, who not only had to prepare and sterilize supplies, but also had to wash all the linen afterward. Eight babies were born in the camp during the six months that Kelsey lived there, including a "fine set of twins."[105]

Susie Kelsey was released from the Weixian Camp in September 1943. She was with Rev. G.K. and Mrs. King on the second repatriation ship to North America (the *MS Gripsholm*). They spent ten weeks at sea before arriving in New York on 1 December 1943. In a letter written from the *Gripsholm* on 2 November 1943, Rev. G.K. King clarified why he had included Kelsey in his original cable to Canada notifying the NCM of their release, indicating the relationship between Kelsey and the NCM: "I think you would recall – or someone from Honan [Henan] could remind you – that Miss Kelsey was a nurse of the Ch. of Eng. in Canada resident at Kweiteh [Sanqui], and that it was with her that Dr. McTavish worked for a year. Miss Kelsey desired to be included in our cable."[106]

Kelsey felt a certain kinship with the NCM. She was, after all, the last Canadian nurse to leave the province of Henan and had forged relationships with the other Canadian nurses in the province. Kelsey's affinity for the United Church missionaries would come to the fore in 1945. That year, Kelsey, eager to return to China, expressed a desire to join those Canadians returning to the WCM. In response, the Missionary Society of the Church of England in Canada (the Anglican Church) gave permission for Kelsey to be seconded to the United Church WMS for work as a nurse in West China. The WMS began to make arrangements for Kelsey's travel and inoculation.[107] Apparently Kelsey changed her mind after VJ day in 1945, however, when Sanqui again opened up.[108] Rather than heading to West China, Kelsey returned to St. Paul's Hospital in Henan, where she worked alone for almost two years before being joined by her former colleague Mary Peters.[109] Kelsey remained at Sanqui until the Communist takeover in 1949.[110]

When Susie Kelsey and the Kings left Weixian Camp on the second repatriation ship in October 1943, they left behind Bertha Hodge and Eric Liddell. Miss Hodge was reportedly well when the Kings left ("a little thinner – as we all are – but as cheerful, self-denying and full of good works as ever").[111] Diplomats continued to work toward further prisoner exchanges via the *Gripsholm,* and the hope of leaving Weixian sustained those remaining. Eventually winter set in, and imprisonment stretched on for another sixteen months. By February 1945, Eric Liddell was exhausted, and Annie Buchan, a nurse from Siaochang, insisted that he be hospitalized at the camp. On 11 February 1945, Liddell suffered a small stroke that left him with a slight limp and a strange reflection in one eye. He was diagnosed with a possible brain tumour.[112] On 21 February, he typed a letter to his wife Florence, back in Canada, "Slight nervous breakdown. Am much better after a month's rest in hospital. Doctor suggests changing my work ... Special love to yourself and children."[113] That same evening, Eric Liddell died at the Weixian Camp hospital. Because of war-related communication disruption, Florence did not actually hear of her husband's death until two months later, when Rev. G.K. King and Rev. Armstrong of the NCM delivered the news in person, on 2 May 1945. All of the North China missionaries remaining in China after Pearl Harbor survived the war. But since Eric Liddell was like a member of the NCM family, the missionaries mourned his loss.[114]

Clara Preston: The Last NCM Missionary Nurse in China

By the summer of 1941, when the North China missionaries in occupied China were interned, Clara Preston was in Chongqing, Sichuan. One of Preston's responsibilities at the WCM hospital at Chongqing was teaching in the nursing school. The Chongqing nursing school was composed primarily of female students who had started their studies in other parts of China – which complicated their training. For example, only four of the twenty students in one class were from Sichuan. The newcomers from Hong Kong found it difficult to adjust to Chongqing because they were used to a higher standard of living and more up-to-date hospitals. In addition, some of the new nurses lacked knowledge of Mandarin, making it harder to fit in with the work at Chongqing.[115] Furthermore, food was expensive – the price had risen from $6 per month to $60 per month for nurses during Preston's first six months – and malnutrition had resulted in anemia among the students.[116] Finally, it was difficult to obtain supplies. Books, formerly bought in Shanghai, were no longer obtainable. Neither were drugs or equipment. In response, the pharmacy department at West China University in Chengdu was producing "useful drugs made from native products."[117] As a result of the difficult conditions at the school, only five out of the class of twenty-eight finished their program in 1942.

Preston did not like the school principal. When he left in April 1941, Preston wrote to Mrs. Ruth Taylor: "We have lost our principal of our Training School – for which we are *thankful*."[118] Dr. Stewart Allen became the acting principal of the nursing school, which pleased Preston because "he has a marvelous disposition, unbounded energy and [is] very good in surgery."[119] Besides, Preston and Allen had both graduated from McGill University in Montreal; "it is a bond between us." When a new (unidentified) principal for the nursing school arrived in March 1942, Preston was impressed. He was a graduate "from one of the Hankow [Hankou] mission hospitals" and had been the first vice president of the Nurses Association of China for many years.[120] As such, he had a "wide acquaintance among the government officials so is a big help with linking us with the Educational and Public Health Departments of the Government." According to Preston, he was strict with pupils, but was also good to them and "always seeks their best interests."[121] Upon graduation, the Chinese government conscripted nurses into a year of public health service, military service, or Red Cross work. The hospital was allowed to keep only 15 percent of its graduates, which worsened staff shortages at Chongqing. Preston had overseen two groups of nursing graduates, thus sending out twenty-five nurses to "serve their country in this needed time."[122] There was constant staff turnover. Within two years of Preston's arrival, the number of graduate nurses on staff had dwindled from twenty-one to seven, and the number of doctors from seven to two.[123]

The conditions at Chongqing wore on Preston. Lack of heating in the hospital wards made bathing the patients difficult. Lights often went out and kerosene was expensive, so night nurses had only a small lamp to carry. There were mice and rats, flies and mosquitoes, bedbugs and cockroaches – for which netting and screens were placed around patient beds and baby bassinettes. Supplies were so difficult to get, and cost so much, that Preston would debate whether she could afford an article or not. For example, "when we wanted [rubbing] alcohol there was so much red tape in getting it that it took hours of the coolie's time."[124] Items cost thirty times more than they did when Preston first arrived, and predictions were that this amount would double by the following year. Preston's new policy was: "Eat it up, Wear it out, Make it do, and Do without."[125]

After the fall of Hong Kong and Singapore to the Japanese, Chongqing received a number of foreigners as patients – many of whom could not speak Chinese.[126] This meant more work for Preston since few of the Chinese nurses spoke English. Furthermore, the foreign patients required foreign food – which would be sent over from Preston's house. "We marvel at our houseboy," Preston wrote, "who can carry 2 of those heavy trays over at once and has many trips to make in a day and never seems to mind."[127] Eternally optimistic, Preston claimed in a letter to friends that she was "glad to be able to help in this way, and it makes our lives so much more interesting as we often have 4 different nationalities in at one time." She ended the letter with the line, "Just two more years 'til I will be home again to see you all." As it was, illness would send Preston home just six months later.

By the summer of 1942, Clara Preston was feeling unwell. The WCM had agreed to an extended summer holiday for her, hoping that would help her condition. But within a few months, Preston was diagnosed with active tuberculosis. On 18 January 1943, the WCM field secretary wrote to the WMS secretary in Canada that Preston had been given permission to leave on a furlough as soon as the necessary arrangements could be made.[128] Preston was, simply, exhausted. The hot and humid weather, overcrowded surroundings, poor nutrition, and constant bombing had contributed to her ill health.[129] According to Preston's memoirs, doctors had told her that it would likely be two years before she could work again or take much responsibility.[130] She was urged to leave the unfavourable climate of Sichuan, even if it meant she had to find a hospital or sanatorium en route to Canada. Preston began packing immediately, and flew out of Chongqing on 17 January 1943, accompanied by Dr. Gordon Agnew.[131] She travelled as far as India, where she convalesced for a month – mostly at a United Church hospital in Indore – before beginning the four-month journey to North America via South Africa and South America.[132]

After arriving in Canada on 15 June 1943, Preston spent another eighteen months recuperating in Ontario. By 1945, she was well enough to take up nursing work again, and in January of that year, Preston was appointed as the acting superintendent of nursing at the WMS Hospital at Hearst, Ontario. Although Preston worked diligently in Ontario, her heart was not in it. Like Janet Brydon, Preston preferred work in China to "home mission" work in Canada. She was determined to return. Preston kept in regular contact with the United Church office, hounding WMS secretary Mrs. Taylor with letters of inquiry as the end of the war seemed imminent. One letter in particular sounds almost breathless, as Preston fires one question after another:

> What are your plans for the return of the Honan [Henan] workers? ... Will this civil war [between the Communists and Nationalists] have any bearing on the subject? Are you planning on sending as many as can go back? What about my physical? Where would I have it done? ... Has there been any word at all from the Christians of Honan? ... Would it be too much to ask for you to let us know what the plans are and when you would expect me to go and if you think I could go Physically?[133]

To Preston, a return to Henan could not come soon enough. When the NCM field reopened after the war, Preston was among the first to return.[134]

Summary
China held a certain "power" over the Canadian nurses in China during the height of the war against Japan. For single North China missionaries such as Clara Preston, Margaret Gay, and Janet Brydon, nursing in China was their destiny. Despite the dangerous and tenuous conditions, they could not imagine themselves doing anything else – including nursing at home mission hospitals in Canada. As long as Canadians were allowed to stay in China, the only legitimate reason to leave would be physical illness or disability – theirs or their family's. For the married missionaries reared in North Henan, like Elizabeth (Thomson) Gale, Mary (Boyd) Stanley, Dorothy (Boyd) Johnson, Georgina (Menzies) Lewis, Jean (Menzies) Stockley and Florence (MacKenzie) Liddell, China was the glue that connected their past with

their future. Training as nurses opened up the door to return to China, but nursing was more a means to an end rather than an end in itself. China was the attraction; China was their home.

After Pearl Harbor, the Japanese army became the wedge that separated Canadian nurses from what they valued most in life. Most of the single and married Canadian nurses were locked *out* of their China homes. Betty Gale, Mary Stanley, Georgina Lewis, and Susie Kelsey were locked *in* it, in civilian internment camps. NCM nurses waiting to return to North Henan felt locked out of their place of belonging and purpose, and felt a keen sense of loss being separated from their Chinese colleagues and friends. To Preston, West China was a fine temporary refuge, but the geography, the people, and the living conditions were so different from North China that it did not feel like home. By 1945, all the NCM nurses had departed China. Although attempts would be made to resuscitate missionary medical services in the upcoming two years, missionary nursing was already becoming unsustainable between 1941 and 1945. The mishkids, for the most part, had already officially left missionary nursing for commitments to their children and husbands. Those career missionaries who had committed decades to China were getting older and were distracted by illness and obligations at home. With the exception of Clara Preston, they had neither the energy nor the opportunity to start over.

7
The Last Days, 1946-47

> It is not the crisis that builds something within us –
> it simply reveals what we are made of already.
>
> > – Oswald Chambers, message to prospective
> > missionaries[1]

Postwar Planning

The Sino-Japanese War came to an abrupt end after atomic bombs were dropped on the Japanese cities of Hiroshima and Nagasaki by the American military. Japan surrendered on 14 August 1945. After eight years of war, some missionaries were incredulous; the end of the war had seemed a distant dream. Other missionaries, however, had already begun contemplating their return to China the previous spring, when the war in Europe was drawing to a close. In April 1945, a group of North China Mission (NCM) missionaries in Toronto ("Honan Toronto Committee") named fourteen missionaries to go to China before the end of the year. Among these were D.K. Faris, Norman MacKenzie, and Clara Preston.[2] Dr. Bob McClure, who had spent much of the war working in China with the Friends Ambulance Unit (FAU) and the International Red Cross, was also returning to China, after recovering in Canada from a bout of typhus. McClure's wartime experience had equipped him as an excellent resource for the returning missionaries. McClure knew more than most about what kinds of conditions the missionaries were likely to find in Henan, and believed that medical relief work would have high priority in postwar China. McClure anticipated that returning missionaries would work closely with the newly formed United Nations Relief and Rehabilitation Administration (UNRRA), which was planning to build new hospitals in China and possibly re-establish some mission hospitals.[3] As the commander of the FAU China Convoy, McClure had an idea – about which Doug Crawford, one of the FAU members, composed a ditty:

Old McCurdle has a plan
Based upon Chengchow [Zhengzhou],
To save the people of Honan,
Starting with Chengchow.[4]

The FAU was a wartime organization associated with the Quakers. Composed of approximately forty conscientious objectors from the United Kingdom, the United States, New Zealand, Canada, and China, the FAU had a mandate to assist in wartime suffering. The China Convoy had spent the war hauling approximately 95 percent of the medical supplies being distributed to civilian hospitals in "Free China," as well as providing ambulance services.[5] Upon hearing of Japan's surrender, Dr. McClure immediately began plans to get rehabilitation work underway in Henan. Since the convoy was committed to rehabilitation work, McClure worked to convince members of his idea to rehabilitate medical work in Henan, using the Baptist hospital in Zhengzhou as a starting point. Once the FAU re-established the hospitals, the UNRRA would take over. The FAU endorsed McClure's plan.

McClure wrote to the United Church offices in Canada, urging medical and nursing missionaries to return to China immediately. He was concerned that, even if the FAU could reclaim the hospitals, there would not be enough Chinese personnel to staff them since many Chinese doctors and nurses were temporarily under the employ of the US Army. If enough foreign personnel could come out at once to re-establish the hospitals, the mission would be able to attract Chinese doctors and nurses when their army terms were complete. Time was of the essence. If the mission board procrastinated, it might lose the opportunity to secure Chinese staff since Chinese medical personnel would soon be in high demand everywhere. McClure was certain that "CNRRA," the Chinese government section working with the UNRRA, would be willing to re-establish mission hospitals if missions worked closely with the National Health Association.[6] Indeed, the International Relief Committee promised two million Chinese dollars each for Anyang and Huaiqing hospitals and one million for Weihui, which, when converted into Canadian currency, totalled approximately five thousand Canadian dollars.[7] In addition, if Weihui could promise to provide forty beds for refugees for three months, the CNRRA would provide a thousand pounds of drugs. Only hospitals on refugee-returning routes could get these grants.[8] According to McClure, the missions had to act quickly or lose a golden opportunity to rehabilitate the mission hospitals. There was one caveat: the UNRRA money could not be used for staff salaries. McClure quickly consulted with fellow missionaries Mr. Mitchell and Mr. J.B. MacHattie *(He Yage)* in Chongqing, and sent a cable to Toronto requesting Cdn$40,000 from the United Church mission boards. Of this, $20,000 would be used for reconstruction, the rest for travel and other emergency costs.[9] The mission boards were "stunned" by the large amount requested and offered $10,000 instead.[10] McClure moved forward on his plans without a clear idea of how, or if, appropriate funds would arrive.

Reoccupation of the Mission Hospitals: An Expensive Prospect

Dr. Bob McClure travelled to the Baptist hospital south of the Yellow River at Zhengzhou, Henan, with the hope of reclaiming the former NCM hospitals in nearby Anyang, Weihui, and Huaiqing as soon as the Japanese moved out. McClure wanted to be physically close by the mission hospitals so that the FAU could move in and reclaim mission hospitals before the Chinese military could move in and use them as barracks.[11] He was already in Zhengzhou in October 1945 when NCM missionaries Grace Sykes, J.B. MacHattie, and Norman MacKenzie passed through, on their way back to Weihui. Sykes, MacHattie, and MacKenzie received a warm welcome at Weihui and a house was hastily prepared for the three of them to move into. The house was in rough shape; MacHattie fell through the floor of an upper verandah and landed on a concrete floor ten feet below, cracking some ribs.[12] In fact, most of the mission buildings were badly damaged. MacHattie estimated the cost of repairs, excluding the hospital, at $13,385.00.[13] Re-establishing the NCM was an expensive prospect.

It is difficult to obtain a comprehensive picture of the NCM's financial situation in the postwar years. The records are fragmented, currencies are used interchangeably (Chinese or Canadian "dollars"), and the rate of exchange fluctuated on an almost daily basis. Sources of funding for the NCM were varied, and included grants from the United Church itself, plus a myriad of sometimes-indistinguishable relief committees, including the International Relief Committee, the International Red Cross, "HIRC," the UNRRA, the CNRRA, Canadian Aid to China, and the China War Emergency Relief Committee. Furthermore, there was sometimes a discrepancy between the amount of the grant promised and that received at any given time, since funds were not usually paid out in one lump sum. Add to this soaring inflation rates, estimated at anywhere between 1,000 percent and 100,000 percent per year, and the figures become almost indecipherable.[14] One thing is clear, though: by 1947 the NCM was facing a severe and seemingly unresolvable financial crisis.

At Weihui, a 1946 financial report estimated the 1939 replacement cost for hospital land, walls, buildings, and supplies at a total of Cdn$115,000.[15] While the report estimates wartime destruction of the hospital buildings by percentage, it does not translate any of these numbers into replacement costs for 1946. One way to estimate the 1946 costs would be to add up the percentages: if 50 percent of a building worth $20,000 was deemed to be

Table

Weihui reconstruction costs in 1946

Buildings	Est. Cdn replacement cost, 1939	Est. destruction	Replacement cost, 1946*
Foreign residences	22,000	25%	5,500
School classrooms	14,350	35%	5,022
Chinese buildings	11,800	25%	2,950
Subtotal			**$13,472**
Hospital land, buildings, walls	60,000	15%	9,000
Hospital equipment	25,000	?	?
Hospital supplies	25,000	40%	10,000
Hospital bedding	4,500	60%	2,700
Hospital library	500	80%	400
Subtotal (minus equipment)			**$22,100**
Total (Cdn)			**$35,572**

* Estimated by author.

damaged, the replacement cost might be $10,000. Using this formula, an estimated replacement cost of the non-hospital buildings would be $13,492, which is close to MacHattie's figure of $13,385 (see the table above). Using the same calculation method, the 1946 estimated replacement cost would have been $22,100, plus equipment – yet a report in 1946 placed the estimate closer to $50,000.[16] Either way, Dr. McClure's request for $20,000 was, in fact, rather low. As it was, Weihui would have to rely on its portion of the United Church mission grant (approximately $3,000), the IRC (likely the International Relief Committee) grant for hospital reconstruction ($1,000), and a promised UNRRA grant ($2,000).[17] Thus, while the costs would be somewhere between $22,100 and $50,000, the NCM had secured only $6,000. The grants, while generous, were grossly insufficient. Debt was piling up before reconstruction and refurbishing had even started, and this was without taking into account salaries, travel expenses, and operating costs.

By July 1946, the actual cost of running the Weihui Hospital was becoming clearer. For one month, expenditures such as salaries, food, and heat added up to Ch$2,289,585 (approximately Cdn$2,289).[18] Because the various grants could not be used for salaries or operating costs, the hospital was reliant on income from patients themselves. In July 1946, in-patients and outpatients paid the hospital a total of Ch$784,270. While this income helped to offset the costs, it still left a deficit of Ch$1,505,312 (approximately Cdn$1,505) at the end of just one month.[19] Although the records do not indicate whether or not the NCM requested operating funds from the United Church mission boards, it seems it would not have gotten far even if it had. The United Church in Canada was also suffering from a deficit. In fact, missionary travel from Canada to China was delayed because the money simply was not available. Clara Preston, who had been ready to return to China in the fall of 1945, had to wait until the question of funds could be addressed.[20] She would not return until October 1946.[21]

Disappointment at Weihui

Finances were a problem at Weihui, but North China missionaries were focused on a different matter: low staff morale. McClure facetiously expressed regret that the Weihui Hospital had not been destroyed during the war: damaged bricks and mortar could be repaired, but what of the spirit of the place?[22] The Canadians had been away from Henan since the Anti-British Movement of 1939. For the first few years after their departure, the renamed "Hwei Min" (Huimin) Hospital reportedly thrived under the leadership of Dr. Duan Mei-Qing, who was hailed as a "capable leader" in 1940.[23] The evacuated missionaries had reason to believe that the hospital would continue to reflect mission standards and values under Duan, based on his report in 1940, where he stated: "We are very proud that this hospital still can going on [sic] so we can continue work here not only for ourselves but for so many people whom got the propper [sic] treatment. Again the learning something about our Jesus Christ and believe Him."[24]

After Pearl Harbor in 1941, communication between the Weihui staff and the departed missionaries was difficult, if not impossible. The dearth of mission records suggests that the NCM had little idea of what was going on at the hospital. According to postwar reports, the Japanese occupied the mission compound after Pearl Harbor, and the hospital was constantly under suspicion. Wartime difficulties were aggravated by a three-year famine. Standards gradually deteriorated and "order and discipline broke down."[25] When the missionaries returned to find the hospital in a deplorable state, all fingers pointed to the acting hospital director, Dr. Duan. Although the postwar mission records are vague about the situation, three allegations emerge from the documents. First, Dr. Duan was fraudulent. Second, he allowed hospital service to devolve into disarray. Third, and perhaps most significantly, he was unwilling to work under the leadership of the Chinese church. In terms of the first allegation, although the North China missionaries never directly charged Duan himself with fraud, they suggested that he, along with other members of the Chinese staff, had been pilfering hospital funds for personal profit. Always circumspect, the missionaries wrote comments such as "the lust for gain entered and got control of the souls of some,"[26] or "the problems [at Weihui] are also plentiful and of a serious nature."[27]

Although missionaries avoided the use of names, thirty years later Dr. McClure identified Dr. Duan as the source of trouble. According to McClure, Duan had capitulated to the Japanese during the Sino-Japanese War, hastening to make his staff sing the Japanese national anthem and quickly denouncing anyone who objected. McClure also blamed Duan for selling drugs and instruments and using hospital income to buy copious quantities of land in his own name, while employees were paid only food for their services.[28]

Contemporaneous mission documents neither confirm nor deny McClure's later charges against Duan of fraudulence and collaboration with the Japanese. Records do, however, suggest that Duan was considered a troublemaker and affirm the second allegation – that is, that the hospital under Duan's care had fallen into disarray. The FAU arrived at Weihui in July 1946 to assist with the rehabilitation of the hospital. Whereas the FAU had expected to find a running hospital where only minor changes, re-equipment, and gradual improvement of staff standards were required, what they found was a hospital requiring complete renovation – a six-month prospect – plus complete re-equipment of the wards and operating theatre. Walter Alexander, the FAU business manager, wrote: "We do not wish to be critical of those who carried on during the war years here, but there is no use covering up unpleasantness in vague words ... The hospital [has] fallen gradually though steadily into a deplorable state."[29] He continued,

> When we arrived about July 5th we found the medical superintendent, Dr. Tuan [Duan], laid up with a bruised shoulder; a graduate nurse, "Dr." Liu, was seeing 90 patients in the OPD [Outpatient Department] each day (though no examining table was being used); 190 persons were attending a daily Kala Azar clinic and [were] receiving one half or less of the usual dosage so that treatment was taking 25 to 35 days; all the post-operative cases in the wards were septic; and since three nurses were required for the Kala Azar clinic, only two were working in the wards most of the time; and of the 40 or more patients in the hospital ... [it was] possible and necessary to discharge over one half immediately.[30]

There was little evidence of the core ideals (such as patient-centredness, cleanliness, and efficiency) that physicians and nurses had emphasized previously at Weihui. According to the third allegation, Dr. Duan did not consider himself accountable to the Chinese church. Although the missionaries placed Duan in charge after they left, they still considered the church to be the ultimate authority when it came to mission-sponsored programs. Yet according to McClure's later account, Dr. Duan felt no such obligation to the Chinese church – nor, by extension, to the NCM missionaries: "[The missionaries] were trying to get the Weihui Hospital back under the full control of the Chinese presbytery, but Dr. Tuan [Duan] did not wish to let go. He was demanding payment for having saved the buildings and, in McClure's estimation, had gone quite money-mad."[31]

McClure's allegation of Duan's unwillingness to work co-operatively with the Chinese Church is more direct than anything found in the NCM documents. Yet subsequent events confirm that, for whatever reason, missionaries considered Duan a liability: they had him fired. To the FAU, and to the North China missionaries, the best way to get the hospital back into good running order would be to dismiss those staff members who seemed to be working counter to prewar goals and ideals. This was a delicate prospect – one that the missionaries, not surprisingly, seemed loath to undertake. According to Walter Alexander, the missionaries invited the FAU to "replace some of the senior members, and to do all they could to raise the standards of work in the hospital generally."[32] The FAU team agreed that the only way to solve the problem of "staff who have gotten into very bad habits" was to replace them rather than "try to retrain staff who have worked under bad conditions for many years." As a result, Dr. Duan, two nurses, and the hospital business staff were "invited" to resign. They and any others who wished to resign were offered three months' salary.[33] The nurse called "Dr." Liu was not asked to resign, but did so anyway, "and on the whole we feel he is the loser, [but] the situation will be made considerably easier by his leaving."[34] By the end of July, there were ten FAU members on staff at the Weihui Hospital, including Walter Alexander's wife Harriet, who became the temporary superintendent of nurses. She oversaw the remaining three Chinese nurses, as well as nine nursing students. One of the graduate nurses was reassigned to the operating theatre, one to the nursing school as a full-time teacher, and one – who had little recent nursing experience – as a full-time housekeeper. Hospital servants, many of whom had been employed since the hospital first opened twenty-four years earlier, had become accustomed to providing nursing care such as dressing changes and were retained as ward orderlies. The FAU was satisfied and hopeful about the new staff; Walter Alexander playfully remarked: "All are doing very good work ... [including] a very good male nurse whom even Harriet praises highly (though it is against her policy to admit that male nurses can be useful)."[35]

It is not clear what became of Dr. Duan Mei-Qing and the nurses after their dismissal. Although Dr. Duan recognized his role as temporary, even signing his 1940 report as "Acting Hospital Superintendent," over time he and others may have come to see his position as permanent and his leadership as unconditional. Indeed, according to the official history of the First Affiliated Hospital of the Xinxiang Medical University at Weihui (originally the Weihui/Huimin Hospital), "[the Canadians] handed over the hospital to

Chinese management *unconditionally* and represented both sides respectively for the signing on the handing-over book. After the Chinese take-over of the Huimin hospital, [a] seven-people management committee was formed. [Dr.] Duan Mei [Qing] was appointed by all as chief."[36] It is probable that some disagreed with the dismissal of Dr. Duan and the others. Although there is no record that anyone tried to defend Duan's wartime actions or that Duan or the others resisted their "invitation" to resign, Margaret Brown later commented: "These were men who through the long years of war had carried heavy burdens and who, at times, risked their lives to prevent the Japanese from gaining control of the Hospital."[37] The North China missionaries may have felt sombre about the personnel changes, but the FAU forged blissfully ahead, with the missionaries' consent. In the conclusion of his July 1946 report, Walter Alexander enthused: "Really, we are just one big happy family, all loving each other to death."[38]

Weihui Hospital: Open for Business

Within one month, much had improved at Weihui. According to the FAU Team Report for August 1946, "everyone is going full blast [which] gives very much the feeling that the hospital is 'open for business.'"[39] Carpenters, tinsmiths, and "med machs" (medical mechanics) refurbished the hospital, restored electricity, hooked up the X-ray machine, and painted ("many gallons of paint have been slapped on, and the resulting brightness almost dazzles the eyes of those accustomed to the former gloom"). Two wards were reopened, allowing for a potential of fifty beds. Due to the shortage of graduate nurses, however, only thirty to thirty-five beds were being used. It was difficult to attract new nurses to Weihui – possibly because the hospital offered only half the salary paid to nurses by organizations such as the UNRRA.[40] There were two additions to the nursing staff, but one was temporary: June Straite was "on loan" for three months from the Mennonite Central Committee. Miss Chu came to Weihui as the fiancée of the FAU chief surgeon Philip Hsiung, and was helping out in the operating theatre. After their marriage, the Hsiungs continued working at Weihui until days before the final crisis in 1947.

By the time Clara Preston and Dr. Isabelle McTavish finally arrived in October 1946, the hospital was in good running order.[41] There were eight graduate nurses on staff, plus three different classes of nursing students. Under the principal, Miss Li Shuying, the nursing school had opened on 15 September 1946 with approximately ten new students.[42] Miss Li had been the principal of the training school for nurses after the Canadians left in 1939 and was no stranger to the NCM. She was the daughter of a Huaiqing biblewoman, and was among the first NCM nursing school graduates.[43] Although it is not clear whether Miss Li continued as principal of the school

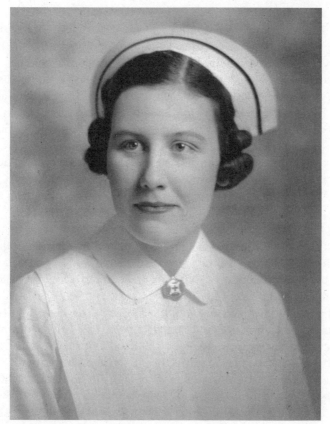

Figure 42 New recruit Helen Turner, c. 1941.
UCCVUA 76-001P-6765

during the war years, there is evidence that nursing education continued during the absence of the Canadians. The 1941 graduating class included five graduates: Zhou Bao Shin, Fan Ming Yi, Zhang Wen Fan, O Yang Bin, and Zhang Shu Ai. Among the 1942 graduates are Li Shu Ming, Guo Rui Wu, and Suixiulian – each of whom worked for the Huimin hospital after graduation.[44] There is no record of nursing education at Weihui between 1942 and 1946, when the missionaries returned.

In addition to Clara Preston and Dr. Isabelle McTavish, the United Church of Canada Woman's Missionary Society (WMS) had secured two new Canadian nurses for three-year terms in China: Margaret Hossie and Helen Turner.[45] (See Figure 42.) Matters seemed to be falling into place. The FAU made plans to turn direction of the Weihui Hospital back over to the NCM in November 1946.[46]

Losing Huaiqing

At the end of the Sino-Japanese War, control of China was not well defined. The departure of the Japanese created a vacuum of power that both Communists and Nationalists hoped to fill. Having suspended their own hostilities as they fought together against the Japanese, the Nationalists and Communists now turned against each other. There was fighting in every county held by the Communists. Although the Nationalists had control of most regions in China, the Communists controlled 80 percent of North Henan, including Huaiqing.[47] Huaiqing was inaccessible to the North China missionaries, and they were anxious to find out how the mission site fared during the war. One of the earliest reports came from a Roman Catholic bishop, Megan, who had managed to secure a pass to visit Huaiqing. He reported that the NCM compound was a "total loss," describing his experience as "like [that of] Jeremiah amid the ruins."[48] Dr. Bob McClure, who escorted Dr. Stewart Allen to Huaiqing in 1946, confirmed Megan's findings.

Dr. Stewart Allen, the McGill graduate who had worked with Clara Preston at the West China Mission during the war, arrived unexpectedly in Henan during the spring of 1946. He had been on furlough in Canada when the Canadian Aid Committee and Canadian Red Cross approached him to visit the hospitals in China ordinarily supported by Canadian funds. His purpose was to investigate and report firsthand knowledge to his sponsors as to the conditions, needs, and prospects of these institutions, "with a view to securing for them assistance in equipment and funds."[49] Escorted by Dr. Bob McClure, Dr. Allen travelled between Communist and Nationalist military lines to Huaiqing. In separate accounts, McClure and Allen described the devastation they found. Huaiqing was in ruins. The compound walls were jagged remnants. Missionary residences built years earlier by Dr. James Menzies were mere fragments: no roofs, no chimneys, and no people. There was no bell tower and no bell tower gate. The hospital was an empty shell. According to McClure and Allen, the Japanese had stripped the mission of everything, and then the Chinese Communists had destroyed whatever was left.[50]

The tour of Huaiqing clarified the state of affairs there. It also brought disastrous consequences.[51] For McClure, the bright spot in an otherwise depressing visit was the opportunity to reconnect with Chinese friends – particularly Li Hung Chang, an elderly evangelist and one-time principal of the mission boarding school. After meeting with the two doctors in Huaiqing, Li Hung Chang, Li's son, and twenty-six others were arrested and taken to the hills, purportedly by Communists. Some managed to escape, but Li, his son, and sixteen others were "liquidated."[52] As far as the NCM missionaries understood, the men were killed because of their contact with Allen and McClure during their visit to Huaiqing. The tragedy did not end there. That is, while in Shanghai after his hospital tour, Dr. Allen had been urged to submit a written report to a Communist committee on his findings in Huaiqing. In it, Allen was critical of the Communists. He was subsequently "blacklisted" and, three years later, was arrested by the Communists in Chongqing. After a "public trial," Allen was placed in solitary confinement for a year. His arrest in Chongqing reportedly resulted from his visit to Henan and his subsequent written criticism of the Communists.[53] After Allen was released, he was heavily fined and expelled from China. According to Bob McClure, Allen became permanently deaf due to vitamin deficiency during his confinement.[54] The NCM mission at Huaiqing was never reopened.

Rehabilitating Anyang

When the North China missionaries returned to Anyang, they found that many of the buildings had been destroyed. Buildings in the east compound were stripped to the walls – not a chair, table, or utensil of any kind could be found. The Japanese had used the girls' school dormitory as stables. In the west (hospital) compound, the men's hospital and doctors' residence were in ruins.[55] As the Canadian missionaries set out to reconstruct the houses and schools, the FAU moved in to rehabilitate the men's and women's hospitals into one functioning unit called the "Kwang Sheng" hospital. At Anyang, the FAU staff included a doctor, an operating theatre nurse, a business manager, and three mechanics. Assisting them were eight Chinese graduate nurses, a laboratory technician, and a pharmaceutical dispenser. By March, twenty beds had been opened.

Within a few months, the hospital had more than sixty in-patients (and were treating an average of sixty-four outpatients per day), and the hospital facilities were strained to their limits. Yet financially it was doing quite well. The Canadian Aid to China Committee donated an operating theatre worth Cdn$12,500. It also promised Cdn$20,000 for heating, lighting, and plumbing.[56] Funds available from outside sources were used to pay off "old cloth debts" and meeting the costs of rehabilitation materials and labour. The major portion of money was raised directly by the hospital through services rendered. In August 1946, a total of 144 patients were admitted, 158 operations were performed, 315 physiotherapy treatments were given, 68 X-rays were taken, and 1,892 laboratory tests were conducted. Unlike Weihui, Anyang actually had a surplus.[57]

Apart from the natural increase of work as the Chinese became more "hospital-conscious," two other factors were responsible for the great increase of work in all departments of the hospital: increased military activity and an outbreak of cholera – the scourge of war. Although many deaths from cholera were reported in the Anyang area, not many victims came to the hospital for treatment. The role of the staff was to provide mass immunizations with CNRRA-supplied cholera vaccine. For staff treating in-patients, the conditions were numerous and varied. The FAU kept meticulous records of the type and number of conditions treated, providing a rare glimpse into medical care in North Henan. The hospital treated patients with conditions as varied as carcinoma of the cervix, tuberculosis of the rib, strangulated inguinal hernia, carbuncle of the neck, "poisoning from Chinese drugs," tapeworm, hysteria, amoebic dysentery, ruptured ectopic pregnancy, and carcinoma of the left eyelid. Some of the more unusual diagnoses included conditions such as acute salpingitis, rodent ulcer, phimosis, and pemphigus. Yet one diagnosis stands apart from the rest: gunshot wounds. Thirty-nine of the forty-seven traumatic surgical cases listed were for gunshot wounds; almost half of the sixty-four in-patients at the end of August were admitted with gunshot wounds. The civil war was taking a toll.

By September, it appeared that the Anyang hospital was running well. The FAU reported "a competent staff of nurses and servants" and two interns in training. A nursing school was about to open under "competent Chinese supervision."[58] The FAU successfully helped both Anyang and Weihui to resume hospital work, completing its mandate at Henan in a surprisingly short period of time. Its plan was to depart Anyang by 1 January 1947, and then disband altogether by March.[59]

The relative swiftness with which Anyang was rehabilitated, as compared with the less-damaged Weihui Hospital, was striking. Anyang, it seems, was able to channel energy into rehabilitation, while Weihui was reeling over the breakdown of relationships between the missionaries and Chinese staff, and the low staff morale. Some missionaries undoubtedly recognized staff despondency as a natural outcome of wartime trauma, but others expected the Christian staff to have stoically endured their ordeal and to now move forward toward renewed mission goals with enthusiasm. Despondency reflected the state of the soul; it was a sign of weakness. Weihui missionary Jean Sommerville expressed it this way in a letter to the WMS secretary Mrs. Ruth Taylor in 1946: "They [in Anyang] have achieved better cooperation than we [in Weihui] have in church and hospital work. There is no doubt whatsoever about the reality of the postwar moral slump of which we hear so much. In those without any real Christian faith it shows itself in self-centredness, in getting all I can for me and mine; in those with the love of Christ in their hearts it shows in hopelessness and dependence on outside help."[60] Hope through suffering was a hallmark of the Christian faith, yet hopelessness was to remain a pervading feature of the NCM at North Henan until the mission closed in 1947.

Clara Preston: Restoring Nursing Relationships

War and political turmoil had been part of NCM history as long as anyone could remember. Summing up the postwar situation in China, Dr. Bob McClure remarked: "There are risks, but missionaries have to take these risks. It is a part of the modern job. I feel it is fatal to any mission work to wait for more quiet times."[61] Clara Preston was no stranger to the risks involved with missions in China, and she had eagerly anticipated her return to China for almost a year. While in Canada, Clara Preston had tried to prepare for the unique problems in postwar China. She planned to take more items from Canada than she had done previously, partly because she knew her former possessions in China were gone, but also because she understood the postwar difficulty of obtaining goods in China. Preston secured a professional shopper at Eaton's department store to assist her with shopping and shipping the goods to China. She had been advised to bring to China a folding organ, a bicycle, a Singer sewing machine, and anatomical charts for the nurses' classroom, as well as a steamer trunk of items for one of the West China missionaries who had lost a trunk in Shanghai. She also packed up a new afghan and typewriter, gramophone and records, kitchen utensils, a kitchen table with chairs, dry ink, and enough eyeglasses to last for the duration of her upcoming tenure in China.[62]

After a long journey across the Pacific from Seattle to Shanghai aboard the *Marine Lynx*, Preston and her companion Dr. Isabelle McTavish took the train through Nanjing to Kaifeng, then boarded a jeep for the final, dusty leg of the trip to Weihui, arriving in late October 1946. Before settling into her new role as nursing superintendent at Weihui, Preston visited Anyang, her former home. There she found the hospital and homes looking quite different from before. Only half the hospital buildings were being used; refugees were living in the others. Yet she was delighted to find "our first graduate nurse in charge of the nursing work and [our] students doing so well."[63]

Preston was also optimistic about the situation at Weihui. After her arrival, the two FAU nurses left, but Preston was pleased with the prospect of working with two Chinese nurses who had trained under Mrs. Ratcliffe and had been at Weihui for many years (probably Miss Li Shuying and Miss Liu Qing Yin). Having arrived at Weihui after the departure of Dr. Duan, Preston missed the early, anxious days of the postwar reconstruction. In a circular letter to friends back home in December 1946, Preston mentioned "a Chinese doctor" who ran the hospital during the Japanese occupation, but her focus was on how the situation had improved for nursing since she arrived in China twenty years prior: "How different from when we first started when there were no Graduate nurses, now we have 8 here. I feel better able to cope with the problems, and having the language makes such a difference ... Good co-operation among the nurses and an interesting group of students, 4 male and 18 female, all help to make the work more worthwhile."[64]

At about the same time that Clara Preston wrote the circular letter, she wrote what would be her last letter to *Canadian Nurse*. The letter was both nostalgic and hopeful. In it, Preston reflected on what she described as "the evolution of nursing work in China," including the changes she had witnessed over the previous twenty-four years.[65] Preston recalled the original hospital, comprising a chapel, a dispensary, an operating room, and private and public patients' rooms built around courtyards, "in true Chinese fashion." She remembered the woman who came twice each day – and paid the hospital a monthly sum – for the privilege of carrying away the human excrement ("night soil") to use in her gardens. Building the modern hospitals was complex; wood was cut by hand, bricks were brought by wheelbarrow, and paint was rubbed on by hand, using scraps of silk. Chinese workmen built hospital equipment such as bedside tables, bassinettes, mattresses, and "electrical bakers"[66] based on designs provided by the Canadians, who made rough patterns from memory. The central nursing school at Weihui was established with the idea that those trained there would be the future leaders of nursing in China. Canadian doctors and nurses created the curriculum, secured textbooks, and taught in Chinese. Although the first students worked without electricity or running water, eventually the hospital had both – which meant the hospital could use X-rays and electrical laundry equipment.

Preston remembered the years from 1931 to 1937 as progressing "like a story book." During this period, three nurses at Anyang graduated: "They were the first graduate nurses to pioneer the way in our city of Anyang, three thousand years old. What a thrill!" As many as twenty-five nurses would regularly attend meetings of the newly organized District Nurses Association in Henan, and the Nurses Association of China supplied structure to the neophyte profession, providing for graded salaries for nurses with experience or with postgraduate certificates. Postgraduate work was available in public health, obstetrics, dietetics, and hospital administration, and fellowships were available through the Peking Union Medical College. Some of the larger universities offered degrees in nursing. Then, the Sino-Japanese War began in 1937.

Preston told the *Canadian Nurse* readership that, during the Japanese occupation (1937-45), hospitals were closed, buildings and equipment were destroyed, training schools were abandoned, pupils fled, and nurses focused on providing emergency care. Despite the chaos, work continued in West China, where schools took in refugee students from other regions. Eighty-five percent of graduated nurses were sent to Red Cross hospitals, to public-health centres, and into military work, wherever there was the greatest need. "Our nurses just accepted this," wrote Preston, "and [drew] lots where they would go." Preston seemed to be drawing strength from the successes of the past; the future seemed less promising: "Now that the war is over, the difficulties seem insurmountable – rehabilitating hospitals, reorganizing competent staffs, getting equipment, inflation, civil war, famine, thousands suffering from tuberculosis and malnutrition. In addition there are outbreaks of epidemics occurring all over the country, besides the ordinary illnesses. There are some of the problems that face the doctors and nurses."[67] To Preston, the postwar period was a time of starting over. Just as the nursing program had to be built from the ground up after Preston first arrived in 1922, the postwar nursing program needed to be rebuilt in 1946.

Weihui nursing services and education may have been further ahead in 1946 than in 1922, but there were some problems particular to the postwar years. One recurring theme in Clara Preston's letters and memoirs was her distress over the lack of heating. The price of coal had skyrocketed during the postwar years, and heating the hospital became a major concern. Arriving in China just as winter was setting in, Preston sent letters home describing unique problems brought by the cold. Not only was it difficult to bathe patients and keep them warm, but nurses were also perplexed by what to do about water freezing in the sinks and toilets, and urine samples freezing in bottles.[68] Newborn babies were kept in the ward kitchen, where heat from the cooking warmed them.[69] Clara bundled up with layers of clothing – including a padded Chinese dress – but rarely felt warm. Even in bed Clara felt "too cold to read."[70] Weihui had an advantage over Anyang, however; it had glass rather than rice-paper windows.[71]

Preston was an avid letter writer. Besides publishing four letters from China in *Canadian Nurse* between 1935 and 1947, she sent numerous letters to friends and family, usually typed on her portable typewriter. From her letters home, it is clear that Preston drew considerable pleasure from her relationships with Chinese colleagues. At Weihui, the boundaries between work and home were blurred, and Preston frequently visited with Chinese nurses and students at her residence. For example, in one letter, Preston recounted a weekend visit with Miss Yang Ch'un Jung, who travelled from Anyang to visit, as well as an evening visit with some of the Chinese nurses from Weihui.[72] In another letter, Preston described her regular Saturday evening games with her nursing students, playing pin the tail on the donkey, Chinese checkers, and pick-up sticks.[73] When one staff member came down with tuberculosis and was hospitalized, Preston offered to pay for his food.[74] One evening, some of the nurses shared with Preston their stories of struggle during the famine and the Japanese occupation. Miss Li Shuying described the deaths of her husband, brother-in-law, and niece at the hands of the Japanese.[75] Preston depicted her relationship with nurses and nursing students as one of mutual trust, based on a shared history and common goals.

As prolific a writer as she was, Preston rarely wrote about her dreams and plans apart from missionary nursing. In a letter written in January 1947,

Preston provided a rare glimpse into her unfulfilled desire to be a mother, writing with characteristic good humour: "[Our house Amah] came with my hot water bottle and said here is your baby. I said I hadn't any baby and would like one so she said she would give her oldest daughter to me. I said I would love that but what plan would I have for her. She said, you wouldn't have to nurse her just give her [bottled] milk."[76] If Preston regretted her single life, she rarely made mention of it. Those she worked among became like her children; with colleagues, students, and patients, Preston found a place to invest her energy, skill, love, and hope for the future.

A Thief in the Night

In January 1947, Clara Preston wrote a letter reflecting on the difficulties associated with postwar work, including inflation and the high cost of living. "Perhaps," she wrote, "[it is] better that we can't see ahead, but we wonder what the next few months will bring us.[77] In a letter to family dated 16 March 1947, Clara Preston wrote of looking forward to the arrival of Margaret Hossie, one of the new WMS nurses. Although Margaret Hossie and Helen Turner travelled together to China, Turner had not yet arrived in Henan, for reasons that are not clear.[78] Miss Hossie would join Clara Preston and Dr. Greta Singer (a Jewish refugee from Vienna whose family had taken exile in Shanghai) in their Weihui residence (Dr. McTavish was now at Anyang). The letter was optimistic, with references to budding flowers, improved exchange rates and the arrival of some "luxury groceries" such as tinned milk, butter, chocolate, and flour with "only a few dead bugs" in it.[79] Almost immediately after Hossie arrived, everything changed.

On 26 March 1947, Communist soldiers tore up the railway between Weihui and Anyang. Days and nights of severe fighting ensued; approximately sixty thousand to eighty thousand Communist troops had joined together to attack Weihui.[80] Preston wrote a letter on 16 April 1947, describing her experiences: "The enemy came upon us like a thief in the night and before we realized our situation was serious some of the staff were [leaving the mission compound to go into the walled city proper] where they felt it was safer."[81] On the evening of 30 March, "most of the nurses were on duty" when Preston went to her residence to sleep. She heard bombs and shooting "all night long [so] I was regretting that I wasn't at the hospital but then it was impossible to go at least it wasn't very safe." The next morning, she discovered that most of the nursing staff had left for the city without telephoning Preston – their superintendent – about their plans. Dr. Philip Hsiung, now surgeon and chief of medical service at Weihui, and his wife were among those who left – an action that Rev. G.K. King would later harshly criticize.[82] This left Dr. Singer, Clara Preston, and the newly arrived Margaret Hossie in charge of seventy patients. The tone of Preston's letter is one of frustration and anger. She felt abandoned and in danger of being hurt or captured by the Communist army since "foreigners, Doctors, Nurses and Christians are the people most wanted by the enemy [Communists]." Preston and Hossie went to the hospital where they made rounds and kept watch with two ward aides and a junior student nurse. They spent the night listening to machine gunfire and bombing; one bomb hit the hospital roof. Preston returned home for two hours of sleep and then "word came that all the rest of the nurses were leaving." Authorities instructed the hospital staff to go to the city because the Nationalists wanted to use the hospital for their headquarters: "They already had guns up ... just behind us and all around."[83] The Nationalists would provide trucks to transfer patients to a hospital within the city walls. Hossie and Preston prepared patients for evacuation.

The Nationalists provided ten trucks to transport hospital personnel, equipment, and seventy patients.[84] None of the trucks actually reached the compound, however. Seven trucks retreated back into the city proper because of heavy gunfire. The remaining three trucks made it as far as Yen Tien village, approximately two hundred yards from the south gate of the NCM mission compound. Initially unaware of the "new development," the missionaries and other hospital personnel waited at the compound. Suddenly, they found the plans revised "without notification or coordination."[85] Confusion reigned as the group realized there were no stretchers to carry patients and that those who were able would now have to walk to the city – a thirty-minute trek under normal conditions. The most critically ill patients were left behind with a few servants and refugees who volunteered to look after them at the mission compound. The missionaries began escorting patients and their families through the north gate toward the city. Although the trucks were closer to the south gate, it was unsafe to exit there; the heaviest fighting was just outside that gate. Indeed, as the missionaries passed through the north gate with their patients, the Communist army was already positioned at the east end of the compound and was entering through the south gate.[86]

What happened over the next few hours is not completely clear from the records; there are slight discrepancies between the accounts. It seems that the group of about forty men, women, and children began walking down the main road toward the city at about 4:30 p.m. on 1 April 1947. Everyone carried a bundle of some sort. Some young children were carrying their little brothers or sisters. According to an account recorded in the United Church yearbook of 1948, Preston and Hossie took charge: "Our party had to break up into small groups and in the excitement families got separated. Our two Canadian nurses took charge of the patients and led them to safety. [Preston and Hossie] had the children under perfect control, led them by the hand as though off to a picnic. They certainly upheld the tradition of their noble profession!"[87] This last sentence ("their noble profession") typifies the way in which other Canadian missionaries perceived and portrayed missionary nurses – as virtuous, altruistic, and valiant. For her part, Preston did not mention taking charge of patients in her version of events. Instead, in a circular letter written two weeks after the incident, Preston wrote: "I got to the main street and met the truck ... A lot of the patients were let off in Ma Shih Chieh [Weihui city gate] and we wanted to get off with them but we were told to go on [into the city] and then we could come back and see them."[88] Although Preston's account suggests that she and Hossie accompanied patients by truck to Weihui, it is possible that they first led patients "to safety" – that is, to the trucks. Preston's omission may be due to modesty, or a desire not to recount all the details of what must have been a harrowing experience. In any event, the escaping group somehow met up with the trucks from Yen Tien. Preston and Hossie assisted "bed patients" onto the trucks, and then climbed aboard to accompany them to Weihui city, while those who could walk continued their trek on foot. That night, the normally thirty-minute walk took six hours, those who made the journey "being menaced the whole time by Communist bullets."[89]

Hossie and Preston accompanied the patients to the walled city. At Ma Shih Chieh gate, some of the patients were told to disembark. Apparently those guarding the gate were "on the alert against enemy infiltration" and refused entrance to the patients.[90] Hossie and Preston went on to the city, but Preston later returned to the gate at dusk to inquire about the patients, who were still waiting at the gate. They were still refused entrance and were left with their blankets to fend for themselves. Preston could do nothing to help them, and the patients later returned to Yen Tien and the mission compound. In Weihui city, Catholic missionaries received the Canadian missionaries and gave Hossie and Preston places to sleep in the dugout under the Catholic mission. "I wish you could have seen us settled for the night," Preston later wrote to friends, "Two catholic sisters, the mother superior, and the two of us. One bed had salted meat hanging from the roof, vegetables were stored there."[91] Preston and Hossie spent the next few days helping out at the Catholic mission hospital in Weihui city, taking care of more than three hundred wounded soldiers. Preston described it as a "grim" experience. There was little water and no coal for heating. Preston and Hossie went around the wards with two wash basins and a few pieces of cloth to wash the patients. They used the water until it got "too grim." They were disturbed by the lack of tetanus antitoxin; this alone accounted for more than 20 percent of the deaths. Preston wrote,

> They had no tetanus serum and already about 10 have died of tetanus ... there is nothing quite so terrible as to see soldiers die of tetanus and no serum to give them. You feel so helpless and so responsible and know it should not have been. There should be an international law against war

without tetanus serum ... We wondered if Florence Nightingale found things much worse [in Scutari during the Crimean War] than we did in the hospital, scarcity of water, no coal, they had to cut down the trees in the [Catholic] mission compound [for fuel].

The Communist soldiers spent two nights in the NCM compound, departing at daybreak on 3 April. On 4 April, all of the staff had permission to return to their residences, although Margaret Hossie, Dr. G. Singer, and Jean Sommerville remained at the Catholic mission to help care for the wounded there. The NCM hospital had not been greatly disturbed, but the compound was "a shambles" and many missionary belongings had been looted, including sugar, soap, bedding clothing, boots, watches, scissors, cutlery, and telephones. Some of the Chinese staff had lost their homes and possessions through the fighting but, incredibly, none of the hospital personnel were injured or killed. Although the records are vague, it seems that some patients may have been killed or injured on the trek to Weihui city, however, G.K. King wrote: "The failure of the trucks to arrive increased considerably our percentage of losses."[92] The hospital was now filled to overflowing with fifty of the most seriously wounded soldiers, who had been transferred back from the Catholic mission hospital, in addition to the previous patients. Tired, frustrated, and frightened, Preston found herself in charge of a "jittery" nursing staff and a distracted group of nursing students. The usually optimistic Preston was disheartened, writing: "It all seems such a discouraging and difficult world to work in."[93] She blamed the United Church organization for allowing the hospital to become so "poorly equipped with personnel." The Weihui missionaries had reached their limits of endurance. One report noted, "Whether we could stand another such storm is a matter to be seriously considered."[94]

Another Such Storm

Although the Canadian missionaries typically kept a neutral stance in mission records when it came to China politics, they had begun to voice their alarm about what they were witnessing and hearing about the Communists: "Reports from those who have been given permits to travel in Communist areas and who have had their way prepared for them are uniformly laudatory. [However, other reports] leave us convinced that Communism as carried out in these parts is for the people an enforced slavery, regimented and controlled by fear and cruel torture – torture unto death."[95] In terms of political conflicts in China, Clara Preston had always felt "we would work for either side and of course are neutral," and "if asked any opinion we do not say." After the Communist attack at Weihui, however, Preston cautiously but pointedly noted: "We do know that the people flee from one army [Communist] and not from the [Nationalist] government one, so that speaks for itself."[96] The Canadians feared Communist rule of China. More immediately, they feared another attack at Weihui.

At about 4:00 p.m. on 18 April 1947, the missionaries at Weihui received word that Communist forces were advancing. All military patients were to be immediately discharged from the hospital; the Nationalists were planning to transfer them to Xinxiang and south. A couple of hours later, Dr. Philip Hsiung telephoned the Canadian missionaries to urge them to leave immediately for Zhengzhou, south of the Yellow River. Dr. Hsiung was still in Weihui city, engaged as a private physician to one of the Nationalist generals. He promised that he would return to the mission hospital the next morning to discharge the remaining sixty patients before he and his wife headed with the Nationalist military south to Xinxiang.[97] Hsiung volunteered to assist the missionaries in trying to secure a truck to transport them to Xinxiang. The missionaries held a meeting at 8:00 p.m. to discuss the situation. While formally expressing gratitude to Hsiung for keeping them abreast of the military situation during the past couple of weeks, privately they expressed their mistrust of the former FAU surgeon. As far as the missionaries were concerned, Hsiung had deserted the mission, showing "no great interest in [the hospital] – and [taking] no practical measures to minister to the urgent needs of some five hundred seriously wounded soldiers."[98] Their belief that Hsiung had little loyalty to the mission was confirmed the next day (19 April), when, instead of returning to the Weihui Hospital to discharge patients, Dr. and Mrs. Hsiung fled on the first available southbound military truck to Xinxiang. The missionaries took stock of their situation. With the loss of Dr. Hsiung and the impending departure of Dr. Singer (whose contract was ending in May), the NCM was left with a modern hospital but no qualified doctor, and no prospect of securing one. The missionaries decided to close down the NCM (Huimin) hospital at Weihui. They planned to prepare refugee centres in Weihui city and Xinxiang, and then evacuate as a mission group to Zhengzhou.

The missionaries spent the day of 19 April arranging the details of discharging patients, preparing to leave, and directing those who would remain behind to take responsibility. At 11:30 that evening, they were aroused from sleep by torchlight in the central yard, and then a knock on the door. Retreating Nationalist soldiers had arrived from Hwa Hsien. According to a confidential report by G.K. King on 25 April 1946, "after two nights and one day of fighting they had walked 35 miles and now, supperless (nothing since breakfast – two meals a day) were ordered to rest in the 'Hospital.' They took the word 'Hospital' literally. It took us two hours to get them – an advance guard of some 200 men – moved into former school dormitories. The men were exhausted and for the most part slumped into slumber when allowed to rest."[99] The following morning, military trucks arrived; one was reserved for Canadian use. At 7:20 a.m. on 20 April, the Canadians departed the United Church NCM compound. Many of the remaining hospital staff were evacuated south by train. Although a few of the missionaries would return over the next few months to inspect the mission and assess the situation at Weihui, for all intents and purposes, Sunday, 20 April was the final day of Canadian missionary medicine and nursing at Weihui. The Nationalist army immediately took over the compound as a military fortress.[100] The group of Canadian exiles arrived in Zhengzhou on 21 April. Mrs. H.A. Boyd came down with pleurisy and was "on the thin edge of nothing," Mr. H.A. Boyd took to bed, Mr. Norman Knight had an attack of dysentery, and Mrs. Edna King was "badly frayed."[101] In contrast, the three single missionary women, the Misses Sommerville, Preston, and Hossie, were portrayed as extraordinarily hearty: "They have had a *tough* time [but] are out in front, and going strong."[102]

Evacuation of Anyang

The Communist army controlled the area surrounding Anyang, yet on 25 April 1947, hospital work was reportedly "uninterrupted and very busy."[103] Rev. G.K. King believed that Anyang would become the site of intense fighting between the Communists and Nationalists. He reported back to the United Church mission boards in Canada: "We feel it doubtful if our staff is in a fit physical condition to stand the strain of a protracted siege. We have asked the Canadian Embassy if evacuation by plane can be arranged."

After hearing about the evacuation of Weihui, the Anyang missionaries prepared themselves for the possibility of an emergency withdrawal. Still at Anyang were Dr. Isabelle McTavish, Rev. and Mrs. (Dorothy Lochead) MacKenzie, Rev. and Mrs. Newcombe, Rev. and Mrs. MacHattie, Miss Grace Sykes, and Miss Violet Stewart. The Canadians requested passage by military planes, and on 29 April 1947, they evacuated Mr. Newcombe and his wife (who was still recovering after the loss of a newborn baby), Miss Sykes, and Miss Tsoa, a Chinese student who had just been granted a scholarship to study in Canada.[104] The remaining missionaries worked with members of the Church of Christ in China to move the medical work into the city of Anyang. Plane passage for the remaining five missionaries was reserved for 6 May 1947. The day before the Canadians planned to depart, some of the Chinese leaders "expressed doubt as to the wisdom of our all leaving, although they had advised it previously."[105] As a result, Norman MacKenzie and Dr. Isabelle McTavish decided to stay. The very next day, however, the "situation again deteriorated," and MacKenzie and McTavish requested passage as well. It was too late: Communists had taken over the airfield. For the next five weeks, McTavish and MacKenzie helped to move the mission hospital into Anyang city and cared for refugees and casualties. Before leaving

Anyang, MacKenzie left the mission property in the charge of the "Assistant Superintendent," Pastor Liu Chang Djang, with Elder Wu Shao Hsien as a gateman.[106] When McTavish and MacKenzie were eventually evacuated to Zhengzhou, they were uneasy about their decision, feeling "unconvinced that they were following the path of duty and wisdom in remaining outside."[107] As a result of the NCM decision to pull out of North Henan, Clara Preston and Margaret Hossie were in abeyance from May until August 1947, moving between the Canadian Anglican Mission south of the Yellow River at Kaifeng and Chi Kung Shan with no clear sense of where they would be stationed next.[108]

The Confidential Report

Canadian nurses Louise Clara Preston and Margaret Hossie were among the twelve exiled missionaries who gathered with Dr. Stewart Allen at Zhengzhou, Henan, on the morning of 14 May 1947 to discuss the future of the United Church of Canada NCM.[109] Dr. Allen had come at the request of the Canadian Embassy to "clarify our diplomatic position." Allen believed that philanthropic work would be the only form of activity that might be permitted under Communist rule. The group discussed its options, including evacuation for a period of three to five years, and dissolving the mission altogether. The North China missionaries feared the Communists. In a letter to Dr. Armstrong written 15 May 1947, Rev. G.K. King made an oblique but pointed criticism of missionaries Dr. Stewart Allen and Rev. James Endicott of the West China Mission, who earlier had positive things to say about the Communists after having been invited to spend time among them at one point:

> We are especially sorry for the members of our Chinese church, particularly its leaders who are involved in the difficulties of these times and have no way of extricating themselves. They had a very difficult time during the past ten years, and I think there is no doubt but that they would all agree that the last few months have been worst of all. They have great fear for the future. They know, *as conducted tourists through Communist areas do not know,* that for the common man in the Communist area, divided loyalties will not be tolerated.[110]

A small committee was struck to prepare a strictly confidential report on conditions in Henan. Written on 1 June 1947 from Kaifeng, only three copies were made – one for the mission board, one for the Canadian embassy, and one for the NCM minutes. Its contents were not to be published. In Toronto, Dr. Armstrong read the report to a group of Henan missionaries there, but did not give them copies. Rev. G.K. King, who, according to NCM

missionary Margaret Brown, authored the report, was convinced that sharing the information indiscriminately, even among other missionaries, could
result in harm to Chinese Christians. King's comments in April 1948 underscored the intense fear Canadians had of the Communists, and highlight
how missionaries believed that even words carelessly spoken in Canada
could endanger lives in China: "Some repercussions are being felt by Chinese
Christians in Honan [Henan] because of unguarded criticisms of [Commu-
nist] activities made in Canada. You would hardly credit how sensitive Communist set-up is to adverse criticism and how diligently they trace
uncomplimentary remarks to sources within their sphere ... making individuals pay the penalty."[111] The confidential report contains gruesome details of
the torture and death of particular Henan Christians known to the NCM. In
her otherwise meticulously detailed history of the NCM, Margaret Brown
leaves out details of the confidential report, stating: "The accounts are too
many and too harrowing to relate in detail here."[112] Brown intimated that
the details of the reports should remain undisclosed, writing that the report
"was never published and still (1965) remains buried in the files in the [United
Church] archives." Although this is not the only mission record labelled "confidential" during the postwar period, the significance of this particular report
cannot be overemphasized. This report arguably shaped the future of missions in China by articulating the fear many missionaries felt, giving just
cause for dissolving the NCM altogether, and preventing returning NCM missionaries from voicing their China experiences in Canada. That is, the silence
surrounding Canadian missionary nursing in China after 1947 can be partially explained by the fear missionaries felt about possible repercussions.[113]

The confidential report of 1947 is a four-page, single-spaced, typed document with a nine-page appendix. Stapled to the front of the report is an
ominous note: "Failure to recognize the *confidential* nature of this report
may imperil the lives of Christian men and women, Canadian and Chinese."[114] The authors of the report criticized foreigners who supported the
Communist cause, such as "visiting newspaper correspondents, and others
capable of molding world opinion," who contributed to a "highly favour-
able impression of strength and virtues of Chinese Communism." Although
no names are listed, the report is likely referring to influential journalists
Edgar and Helen (Nym Wales) Snow and Agnes Smedley, who provided sympathetic portrayals of Mao Zedong and the Communists through the 1930s
and 1940s.[115] Their widely read articles and books contradicted the experiences described by Chinese refugees from Communist-controlled areas who
were given refuge at the Anyang and Weihui missions: "More and more we
were forced to realize the contrast between the ideal statements emanating
from Ya'nan [Fu-Shih, the headquarters for Mao Zedong's Eighth Route
Army] and the fearful conditions of life the common man must endure

under Communist rule in our nearby areas."[116] According to refugee accounts described in the report, Communist leaders banned all forms of Christian activity, prohibited worship, and eventually eradicated all leadership not under Communist control by arresting or otherwise "disposing of" Christian leaders through "cruel, brutal [and] inhuman means."

The nine-page appendix to the report is marked "very confidential" in red ink. It substantiates in clear, horrific detail otherwise vague claims by missionaries that Communists were threatening lives, torturing and killing Chinese Christians and any others who were thought to endanger the Communist cause (see Appendix 5: Summary of the 1947 confidential report). According to the appendix, the Chinese in Communist-controlled areas in Henan were subject to mob trials and punishment for "crimes" of wealth, association with the Nationalists, and association with foreigners. In the closing lines of the report, the authors ask: "Can we continue as a group to carry on effective mission work on a virtual battlefield or can effective mission work be carried on in a North Honan [Henan] that is Communist-controlled?" They concluded that, while some measure of work might be continued "if one is prepared to play hide and seek with contending armies," such a course of action would endanger Chinese Christian colleagues. Furthermore, Canadians themselves could become targets of attack since "contending parties may not be satisfied to leave unmolested a neutral observer, however innocuous he may feel his presence to be." Finally, since the Communists were demanding a "clean sweep of everything but Communism," sooner or later mission and church organizations "will be obliterated." In August 1947, the NCM Council convened and agreed that "the establishment of a Christian Church in North Henan will not be served by our attempting to re-enter North Henan for residence or work at the present time; therefore resolved that we now proceed with arrangements for the cessation of Mission activities in so far as they directly affect the North Henan area."[117] Six decades of Canadian missionary work at the United Church of Canada NCM in North Henan came to a reluctant end. Margaret Hossie was assigned to the United Church South China Mission in Jiangmen. Helen Turner was assigned to Qilu, where she stayed until 1951.[118] Clara Preston returned to Canada to do home mission work. In a letter to friends dated 3 September 1947, Preston informed her friends of her decision to leave China: "I think it is wisest, but very very hard to do."[119]

Canadian Missions in China between 1947 and 1951
After the closure of the NCM in Henan, missionaries came under considerable criticism, both in Canada and China, for having evacuated their field.[120] Reports of events in China were confusing to church members in Canada. As Margaret Brown expressed it, Canadians wondered: "Was the Gospel not

also for the Communists?"[121] Canadian missionaries such as Stewart Allen, Jim Endicott, Norman MacKenzie, and D.K. Faris publicly expressed a belief that mission work would be possible under the Communists. Others remained silent. According to Margaret Brown, "the real reasons for the Mission evacuation were withheld" from the Canadian public. She suggested that Norman MacKenzie's support of the Communists reflected the naïveté of someone fairly new to the mission field. Despite the mission's expressed intention to remain neutral about political matters in China, the decision whether or not to remain in China *was* a political one: If one believed Communist propaganda, continued mission work was possible. If one believed Nationalist propaganda, the impending Communist takeover would destroy both missions and the Chinese Church as a whole. The United Church missionaries were divided in their assessments of the feasibility and wisdom of staying.

Although United Church missionaries in other parts of China chose to remain, the North China missionaries were not the only ones to withdraw from northern China. For example, in a report to the Board of Overseas Missions (formerly the Foreign Mission Board) of a brief visit to Weihui on 10-12 September 1947, Rev. H.A. Boyd and Rev. G.K. King listed a number of missions that had either withdrawn personnel from outlying districts (deemed less safe than cities) or from North China altogether. These included Canadian, American, Scottish, and Irish Presbyterians; Assemblies of God; Mennonites; and the China Inland Mission. Furthermore, Roman Catholic missionaries – known for their policy of remaining on the mission field during national crises – were also considering withdrawal: "[Despite their] general directive that where formerly they expected their priests to remain with their people under persecution, now, for the well being of the people, Priests, Nuns etc., are expected to evacuate before Communist occupation."[122] The evacuation of other missions from North China lent strength to the NCM's decision to withdraw from North Henan. United Church missionaries now had the option of working in Shandong (Qilu), Sichuan, Hong Kong, Shanghai, or Jiangmen.

The civil war between Chiang Kai-shek's Nationalist army and Mao Zedong's Communist army continued until 1949, when Chiang fled with his army to the island of Taiwan. Mao established himself as the leader of the People's Republic of China on 1 October 1949. The number of missionaries remaining in China decreased, but those who remained in China did so with the hope that they would be allowed to continue philanthropic work. Canadian nurse Helen Turner was among those who continued to work under the auspices of the NCM at Qilu. After her marriage to missionary Peter Nelson in Jinan in June 1950, Turner moved under the auspices of the English Baptist Missionary Society. Between 1948 and 1949, the university functioned as separate units in Jinan, Fuzhou, and Hangzhou due to the war. Peter and Helen Nelson were among the last missionaries to leave Jinan, in June 1951.[123]

On 5 January 1951, the executive of the United Church Board of Overseas Missions and the WMS met to consider the future of the missionaries still in China, at Chengdu, Chongqing, and Jiangmen. Many had already evacuated, in part because of the mounting Korean War. One unnamed but "highly valued senior missionary, noted for his consistent optimism," had written: "We have had a couple of weeks of violent anti-American propaganda which has developed into general anti-foreign feeling with many slanderous remarks made upon almost every western member of the staff. Many of the leading Chinese here are of the opinion that the continued presence of westerners is only an embarrassment to them, and a cause of constant misunderstanding with government authorities. For this reason quite a few more [missionaries] have decided to leave. In addition, the very tense international situation [Korean war] has decided [sic] other westerners to leave."[124] It was unnecessary to "order" the missionaries to leave at once: almost all had already applied for exit visas or had signified their intention to do so. Jesse H. Arnup reported: "This action of the Executive records the failures of our effort to carry on the China missions under the Communist government. From the time of their approach to power I have consistently taken an optimistic view of the situation. In September 1949 I sent my own son to West China. Now he is home again, quite convinced that there is no future for a foreign missionary doctor in that field ... The remaining missionaries are advised to come home."[125]

Summary

Jesse H. Arnup's use of the word "failures" to describe the last days of the United Church of Canada missions in China in 1951 is telling; after the missionary era, the church would continue to ask itself how it failed in China. To missionaries returning to North Henan after 1945, failure was an inconceivable notion. They knew that mission work in postwar China was risky, but as McClure noted, China had always been a risky mission field. Since the Canadians first arrived in China in 1888, the NCM had survived innumerable difficulties, including violence, death, disease, war, revolutions, and imprisonment. Despite the ordeals, the missionaries had managed to establish and develop Christian institutions, including the Church of Christ in China, Christian schools, and church-run hospitals. Canadian missionary nurses had already met most of their goals by 1939. Veteran missionary nurse Clara Preston and her Canadian nursing forbears had established and developed a system of modern nursing service and education comparable to that found in hospital programs in Canada. Furthermore, the Chinese nursing students and graduates were acculturated and taught in a Christian milieu where nursing and Christianity were considered inextricable concepts. Their difficulty was not in establishing nursing services; it was in maintaining them under the chaotic conditions of war, and in a postcolonial nation that was in the process of reinventing itself as an exclusively Chinese Communist Republic. While Canadian missionaries enjoyed a certain measure of success in creating a supportive local environment for nursing in Henan before 1939, their ultimate success was dependent on a supportive national environment. Whereas being British subjects had once gained missionaries entrance into China, it now determined their exclusion.

Considering the circumstances under which the Canadians left – abruptly and under threat of attack – it is not surprising that missionaries felt a sense of failure. To observers, the missionaries had failed on many levels. They failed at their original intent to Christianize China. They failed to develop a *sustainable* system of modern medicine and nursing in North Henan. They failed to re-establish mission interests after the Second World War. They failed to stand by their Chinese colleagues at North Henan when other missionaries found ways to work under the Communist government. It would be easy, then, to dismiss the phenomenon of Canadian missionary nursing in China as one colossal failure. Yet to do so would be to undermine the accomplishments of Canadian missionary nurses, and to overlook particular ways in which missionary nursing shaped nursing and health care in both China and Canada. The sense of failure that pervaded the NCM after 1947, and that has persisted in discussions of Canadian missions in China since, is part of the story of Canadian missionary nursing – but only part.

The last five months of Canadian missionary nursing in North Henan were unlike any other period. The hospital infrastructure was destroyed, the staff was despondent, supplies were difficult to attain, finances were uncertain, and there was no escape from the cold. In addition, a loose expatriate network of returning missionaries, relief workers, and nurses on short-term assignments had replaced the cohesive familial community of NCM missionaries that historically supported missionary nurses. Finally, and most significantly, the relationship between the Chinese and the Canadians had eroded into one of mistrust. Although anti-foreignism had always been a feature of Canadian missions in China, this was the first time that Canadians had come to distrust members of their own staff; loyalty was not guaranteed, even among "brothers and sisters in Christ." This was also the first time that this generation of missionaries felt personally threatened by Chinese leaders. During the Sino-Japanese War, United Church missionaries banded together with the Chinese against a common enemy, the Japanese. Now, North China missionaries felt threatened not only as bystanders in the civil war, but also as targets of Communist aggression. To complicate matters further, United Church missionaries around China were divided on the issue of Communist governance. While some felt threatened by the Communists, others perceived Communist ideals of equality and socialism as common ground upon which Canadian missionaries could work. The Communist military attack of Weihui and Anyang was the final blow to a mission already fatally weakened by disinterest, distrust, disloyalty, and despair.

Conclusion
Creating a Cloistered Space

> God is our refuge and strength, a very present help in trouble.
> Therefore will not we fear.
>
> – Psalm 46, read at last NCM meeting at
> Zhengzhou, 14 May 1947

During the missionary era (1888-1952), China became a testing ground for Canadian nurses committed to a view of missionary nursing as a creditable, lifelong profession for well-educated Protestant women. Missionary nursing itself was not a new concept. As Sioban Nelson and Pauline Paul have documented, religious women had been spreading the gospel of nursing from Europe to the New World since the seventeenth century, and from eastern to western Canada since the mid-nineteenth century.[1] Yet the designation of Harriet Sutherland as "the first trained Canadian nurse to be sent to a foreign field" in 1888 represented a shift in Canadian missionary nursing from a predominantly Catholic phenomenon emanating across Canada from Quebec, to one that included Protestants, and emanated from Canada to sites abroad, including China, Japan, Korea, and India. While Canadian missionary nursing in North Henan is best understood as part of the larger Protestant missionary movement in China originally represented by the slogan "The Evangelism of the World in this Generation," it must also be recognized as an offshoot of nursing roots put down in Canada by religious women over the previous two centuries. Missionary nursing in North Henan provided an unprecedented opportunity for Protestant Canadian women to create communities of faith within which one's work identity could be fully integrated into one's personal identity. Being a "missionary" connected one's public and private lives.

A major, surprising theme emerging through the letters, diaries, and correspondence reviewed is the walled and, therefore, somewhat "cloistered" nature of missionary nursing that eventually and insidiously evolved in North Henan. Both physical and social constructs formed protective walls within which missionaries envisioned and developed a culture of health care. The system of modern nursing introduced by the Canadian missionaries was based on a combination of Canadian and Western ideals, which Canadian nurses and their Chinese protégés adapted and interpreted for Henan. The successful introduction of modern nursing in Henan (indeed, all over China) occurred within the small, protected enclaves called mission compounds and expanded from there. The centrality of the "wall" in China missionary nursing is most readily seen in its most tangible sense – the mission compound walls. Originally built to protect the missionaries from the threat of deadly, contagious disease, the walls also served to shield missionaries – and others who took refuge within their walls – from local bandits, Japanese soldiers, and Chinese militants. When waves of violence threatened to overcome the walls, especially during periods of national armed conflict, missionaries fled – and nursing came to a standstill. The image of Communist soldiers flooding into the Weihui compound in 1947 as Clara Preston and Margaret Hossie fled through a different gate with a harried group of patients exemplifies the vital role of "the wall" in Canadian missions during this chaotic period in North Henan. Missionary nursing would have been impossible without it.

Like the physically constructed walls, socially constructed boundaries served to define and protect a creative space for missionary nursing in North Henan. Nationality, religion, gender, and professionalism served as buffers to changing economic and political realities in China and Canada. The socially constructed meanings of these interrelated concepts shaped and connected nurses' private and public identities. They linked missionary nurses together in a core "sisterhood" of Canadian, white, married and unmarried, educated, Protestant women "set apart" at ceremonial designation services for a lifetime of Christian service.[2] Within socially and physically constructed walls, the missionary nurses created a unique, ambitious, complex nursing culture. As long as the walls offered protection, nursing flourished.

Generally, to be a Canadian nurse during the missionary era in North Henan meant to be of a particular race (Caucasian), language (English), and ethnicity (Scottish). It also meant embodying a paradox. Canadian missionary nurses were British subjects with colonial rights; they were inadvertent beneficiaries of unequal treaties between imperial powers and the Chinese. No matter how honourable their intentions, how politically neutral they perceived themselves to be, or how strong their relational ties with individual Chinese, they were ultimately part of a group of identifiable, uninvited occupiers of China – *yanggui* (foreign devils). Even if they donned Chinese clothing, ate Chinese food, studied Chinese history, and communicated in the Chinese language, they would never belong; even those born in China were not Chinese. Features such as white skin, light hair, blue eyes, and long noses proclaimed their status as part of a privileged élite, and as cultural outsiders. Thus the paradox: being Canadians granted political entrance to China, but hindered trusting relationships with the Chinese. Being easily identifiable foreigners marked Canadians as targets of anti-foreign sentiment, but foreign features also served as embodied pass-ports, enabling the missionaries' escape during the worst phases of anti-foreignism and armed conflict. They could hide under the protection of the British flag or flee from China altogether. Perhaps such contradictions are part of any expatriate experience; certainly the concept of straddling two worlds is not unique to Canadian missionaries. For example, Canadian jour-nalist Jan Wong writes of using her Chinese heritage to her advantage in Communist China during the late 1980s. She blended in with crowds of Chinese students at Tiananmen Square in order to glean information from them, but also used her Canadian nationality to her protective advantage by calling out in English when plainclothes police moved in to arrest her.[3] The interesting point, then, is not so much that Canadian missionary nurses used their nationality to their advantage, but that they were able to estab-lish a blended culture of Canadian and Chinese nursing within a milieu where race and ethnicity usually served as barriers to trusting relationships.

Like nationality, religion had particular meanings for missionary nurses during the missionary era in China. Religious identity defined boundaries of belonging and not-belonging by intersecting with constructs such as family and community. Missionary nurses were church kids, with family involvement in the Presbyterian Church often dating back two or more generations. They were the children and grandchildren of ministers, elders, mission board members, and missionaries. Significantly, many had family ties with the North China Mission (NCM) itself; Jennie Graham's sister Dr. Lucinda Graham and Jeanette Ratcliffe's sister Dr. Susan Grant worked in North Henan. Others were born and reared in North Henan themselves. The phenomenon of missionary kids as nurses is a fascinating exemplar of the interrelationship between family, religion, and missions. Mishkids played a major role in the development of medicine and nursing in the NCM after China-born Robert McClure and Jean Menzies returned to Henan in 1923. Mishkids comprised an influential group of second-generation missionaries, and were largely involved in the development of modern nursing care in Henan. They formed a new, influential community of cultural insiders, whose upbringing in China helped them to bridge the cultural divide be-tween Chinese and Canadians. Belonging neither to Canada nor to China, mishkids who became nurses were most at home in the distinct culture of the Chinese missionary community. Training as nurses in Canada provided mishkids with a means to return to China. Once in China, most of the mishkids married China missionaries; becoming missionary wives provided an opportunity to replicate the family nature of religion and to reproduce for their children something similar to their own Chinese childhood.

Being a member of the NCM community meant belonging to the larger family of missionaries in China as well, particularly after the Presbyterians were integrated into the larger United Church of Canada. Nurses felt a certain kinship with other United Church missionaries, particularly at Qilu and West China. For example, when Margaret Gay stayed by the side of Mr. Albertson in Kunming the night he died in 1940, she considered her presence to have extreme value, not because she was a friend with Albertson, but because she was the only other United Church missionary in the province of Yunnan. North China missionary nurses could be counted on – and could count on – the community of missionaries for hospitality, shelter, and emotional support, especially during the scattered years of the Sino-Japanese War. Their commitment to each other was underscored in times of illness, such as when Clara Preston travelled to Sanqui to nurse Mary Boyd, or when Jeanette Ratcliffe travelled to Qilu to care for the paralyzed Coral Brodie. In this way, the boundaries of religious community were flexible; wherever there were other Christian missionaries, there they belonged. Such fluid boundaries were not always part of the mission; turn-of-the-century missionaries such as Jonathan Goforth viewed with suspicion those with a different theology – especially French or Italian "Romanists" (Roman Catholics). After the formation of the United Church, denominational and national lines blurred – all Christians were "brothers and sisters in Christ" and could be depended upon during times of trouble or need. Being "Christian" became a more significant indicator of belonging than one's denomination.

Being Christian was also central to the nursing culture developed by Canadian missionary nurses at the NCM. Here was an unprecedented opportunity to test how well Christian faith fit together with nursing practice. Faith-based nursing was not new to Canadians. It was not unusual to see Christian themes threading through public nursing discourse (such as in *Canadian Nurse*) in Canada during the 1920s and 1930s. Nor, as Kathryn McPherson has noted, was it unusual to find Christian traditions such as prayer or Bible study incorporated into nursing education in Canada.[4] Christian discourse and traditions were part of the larger social fabric of Canada; one was not set apart simply by claiming Christian values. In contrast, to be a professing Christian in China meant being set apart from one's ancestral heritage. As members of the Church of Christ in China (CCC), Chinese nursing students and staff were part of a small Chinese subculture. The CCC, like the United Church of Canada, acted as a mediating agency, connecting nurses with practice opportunities.

To Canadian missionary nurses, nursing personified Christian service and was inextricably linked to Christian faith: Christian beliefs guided, motivated, and sustained them. They believed that Christianity, with its emphasis on moral responsibility toward the sick, the poor, and the dying, provided the foundation for successful nursing services. If nursing was suitable work for pious women, missionary nursing was the pinnacle of piety because it combined two New Testament directives: to heal the sick and to bring the message of Christ to the far ends of the earth. Chinese nursing in North Henan was meant to be a sinified offshoot of missionary nursing; missionary nurses sought their own reflections in their Chinese protégés.

To some of the earliest missionaries, such as Margaret MacIntosh and Margaret Gay, missionary nursing was a means to bring the Chinese to a "saving knowledge of Jesus Christ." To later missionary nurses, however, nursing was about providing state-of-the-art hospital care. It was not about soul saving. Indeed, Canadian nurse Clara Preston disparaged pioneer nurse Margaret MacIntosh for her emphasis on evangelism during the first quarter-century of the NCM. Sinologist Alvyn Austin described this shift in Canadian missions from evangelism to service in Canadian missions as a movement from "the saving gospel" to "the social gospel."[5] I suggest an alternate descriptor, based on what Sioban Nelson has described as "Martha's turn."[6] In her study of nursing, nuns, and hospitals in the nineteenth century, Nelson notes that the spiritual paths open to women over centuries of Christian practice were shaped by the New Testament story of Mary and Martha. Mary sat at the feet of Jesus, washing his feet in expensive oils. Her sister Martha fussed, preparing food for the apostles and followers and complaining about Mary's inactivity. Much to Martha's surprise, Jesus praised Mary's unworldly devotion while criticizing Martha's mundane and temporal preoccupations. As Nelson has described it, this story delineated two paths for pious women in Britain, America, and Australia: one of prayer and withdrawal from worldly concerns, and one of practical work. Prior to the nineteenth century, these religious women aimed to emulate Mary. Then they emulated Martha. Just as Nelson's nineteenth-century nuns exemplified Martha's commitment to action through tending to the sick, caring for the dying, assisting at surgery, and running apothecaries, missionary nurses at the NCM after 1923 took up Martha's emphasis on practical service. Margaret MacIntosh and Margaret Gay spent their energies on Bible teaching. Like the biblical Mary, they emphasized the eternal, the spiritual, and the state of the soul. Margaret Gay's decision to study nursing after ten years as an evangelistic worker underscores the shift from the spiritual to the corporeal, from eternal to temporal concerns. Missionary nurses who spent their energies on the task of establishing modern hospitals and nursing schools still considered the state of Chinese soul to be important; it simply was not their domain.

Ironically, although later nurses criticized MacIntosh's emphasis on evangelism, they also benefitted from it. That is, Chinese girls and boys, acculturated to a Christian worldview through education in mission schools and membership in the CCC comprised the main pool from which potential nursing students were drawn. Those who later became nursing leaders in their own right – such as Miss Li Shuying, Miss Liu Qing Yin, and Miss Chou – were children of active Chinese Christians, including biblewomen, pastors, and, notably, the first Christian convert in Henan. The family nature of religion experienced by the Canadians was replicated in China, not only because Chinese nurses had family ties to Christianity, but also because the Christian worldview encouraged nurses to re-image each other as part of the same spiritual family. Canadian nurses took seriously Paul's New Testament assertion to the Galatians that "ye are all the children of God by faith in Christ Jesus," regardless of ethnicity, nationality, class, or gender; they believed they were co-creating a nursing community where Canadian and Chinese nurses had similar values, beliefs, and assumptions. Being "brothers and sisters in Christ" with Chinese nurses offered another layer of protection for Canadian missionary nurses; indwelled by the same Holy Spirit of God, Chinese nurses could be expected to have the same spiritual inspiration, direction, and sustenance as Canadian nurses. This spiritual-familial relationship did not, however, always withstand the economic and political pressures of the day. While many of the Chinese nurses (and doctors) remained committed to the NCM during periods of national upheaval and armed conflict, some absconded. Sometimes Chinese staff saw loyalty to the Canadians as disloyalty to China – especially during the Nationalist movement of 1927. At other times, fleeing meant self-preservation – as when the Chinese nurses fled the Weihui compound during the Communist takeover in 1947, leaving Margaret Hossie and Clara Preston alone to care for seventy hospitalized patients. Although the Canadians themselves frequently chose to leave North Henan during periods of danger, they felt affronted and abandoned when Chinese exercised the same option. Leaving the mission amounted to forsaking their family of Christian believers.

Religion was a family affair. Protection was proffered by being part of a religious community or "family" of believers. More than that, God Himself promised protection to His followers. The missionaries depended on the Old Testament promise to Joshua that God would "never leave or forsake" them. Ever since the missionaries' dramatic escape from the Boxers in 1900, the mission placed much faith in divine protection from harm. Crises were retrospectively depicted as opportunities to experience God in new ways; God revealed Himself through suffering, pain, and struggle. The survival of missionaries during various rebellions, revolutions, and wars reinforced their belief that God was shielding them; God was intimately interested in and pleased with their work. As long as they were obedient to God's call, they did not have to fear. Yet while protection from harm was an example of divine favour, suffering was not considered divine punishment. Rather, suffering was a necessary part of the Christian experience. It provided opportunity to grow in faith and experience God in new ways. To the missionaries, God revealed Himself by blessing them as they "worked out their salvation" through individual and community prayer, scripture reading, and service to others. When tragedy did strike, God revealed Himself by giving them the strength to work through their own suffering.

Like nationality and religion, gender also played a protective role for Canadian missionary nurses at the NCM. All of the Canadian missionary nurses were female. Nursing was considered a suitable profession for young women because of the congruence between nursing and Christian values such as altruism and service to the poor and sick. Missionary nursing offered ambitious, bright, and adventurous single women unprecedented opportunities for world travel and challenging work. One might expect that family members would have resisted the idea of their daughters and sisters travelling halfway around the world, to a country characterized by turmoil, for three to six years at a time. Yet while there were hints of occasional family hesitancy or disapproval (for example, in the cases of Clara Preston and Margaret Gay), overall the material studied is conspicuously silent about any fears felt by those at home. Only one nurse – Miss Hargrave – decided against coming to China because of opposition from her family, in 1938. The lack of conflict between daughters and families might signify that such matters were too confidential to be documented, or that nurses benefited by writing about their experiences in a positive light. Or it might signify that parents did not think they were sending their daughters off unprotected. God would protect them – so would missionary men. As single women, missionary nurses (and female doctors) could count on the chivalry of the male-dominated mission organization. In this sense, gender and marital status could be used to the women's advantage.

Throughout the history of the NCM, otherwise fiercely independent and ambitious missionary women relied on the missionary men to support their cause. Male missionary physicians played pivotal roles in sponsoring and supporting the development of nursing in China: Harriet Sutherland, Jennie Graham, and Margaret MacIntosh would not have been in China if not for Dr. James Frazer Smith. Dr. Fred Auld, Dr. Bob Reeds, and Dr. Bob McClure were unequivocal in their support of nursing. By committing to nursing, missionary men also committed to the protection of all single missionary women. They ensured that separate residences were built for single female missionaries to protect their chaste reputations, and they went to great lengths to respond to calls for help. This was exemplified in 1900 when Rev.

W. Harvey Grant travelled nine hours to rescue Margaret MacIntosh and Martha MacKenzie at Chu-wang because of a message stating that they felt threatened. More dramatic still was Dr. James Menzies' response to calls for help by Sadie Lethbridge and Janet Brydon in 1920, and his subsequent murder. Through Menzies' death, single missionary women knew they could count on the protection of missionary men. When missionary nurses married, responsibility for their protection was shifted to husbands and their sponsoring missions.

To be a missionary nurse in North Henan also meant being part of an intimate household of single women. Gender brought together nurses with female physicians, teachers, and evangelistic workers who ate, slept, and played under a shared roof. Personal furnishings such as tables, chairs, photos, and gramophones helped to create a sense of home. With Chinese servants to care for domestic duties such as cooking, cleaning, and laundry, these women could return home after a day of work to an atmosphere of calm and a place of refreshment. An ebb and flow of work and refreshment was important to the missionaries, as evidenced by weekends of socializing, extended summer vacations at resort towns, and year-long furloughs back to Canada. Wherever they were, single female missionaries banded together into clusters of friendship and interdependence. The line between work and home blurred, especially between nurses and single female physicians such as Dr. Isabelle McTavish and Dr. Margaret Forster. Besides living together, Clara Preston and Isabelle McTavish were regular travel companions. The impact of their friendship on their work, and vice versa, is not clear from the record. Yet it appears that their intimate relationship helped to level power differences at work. Indeed, there is a surprising lack of evidence of power conflicts between missionary nurses and physicians. While it is possible that earlier missionary nurses kow-towed to physicians, the lack of conflict between later nurses and physicians might well be explained by the relatively high status given mishkids and senior missionaries. Having been reared together in North Henan, nurses and physicians such as Bob McClure and Jean Menzies had already established a relationship of equality that carried over into the hospital setting. Senior missionaries such as Margaret Gay, Janet Brydon, Jeanette Ratcliffe, and Clara Preston earned a level of respect through their decades-long commitment to the mission.

One of the most striking characteristics of the culture of nursing created at the NCM was the enduring presence of male Chinese nurses. Social mores in turn-of-the-century China demanded that illness care be provided by members of the same gender; males were attended to by males, females by females. Earlier Canadian missionary nurses adapted to these mores by providing nursing care to males in the presence of male physicians. Latter missionary nurses adapted by separating male and female patients into gender-segregated wards and hospitals. Such gender separation was also a feature of nursing in Chengdu, West China. Yet, where Chengdu had separate training schools for male and female nursing students, the NCM integrated male and female students into the same training program. When Chengdu tested the idea of co-education by opening up the men's hospital training school for nurses to female students in 1934, the school was integrated for only two years: by 1936, all the students entering the school were female. This was perceived as a sign of progress and professionalization; having an all-female staff was more in line with the values and beliefs in Western nursing practice. Yet at the NCM, males were integrated into hospital and public health nursing service, education, and administration throughout the history of the mission. Given the Canadians' acculturation to nursing as a female profession in Canada, it seems incredible that Canadian missionary nurses at the NCM consistently accepted and supported a role for Chinese men in nursing. Canadian nurses considered women to have a more compassionate and nurturing temperament, deemed essential for good nursing care. By creating a space for male Chinese nurses, they defied their own convictions that females made better nurses. Three possible explanations for this emerge from the data. First, in comparison with the progressive, university-affiliated West China Mission, the NCM was both conservative and less developed (having only a diploma program on-site). Because male attendants had always been part of ancient Chinese healing practices, and because gender separation was an important part of Chinese mores, the earliest caregivers for males naturally would have been men. The West China Mission associated the presence of male staff with a lack of development beyond the old Chinese traditions. Second, and in contrast, at the NCM it was not unusual for Canadian missionary nurses to privilege Chinese culture over Canadian culture if the needs of Chinese patients would be better served. For example, although schools such as the Peking Union Medical College taught nursing in English, the Canadians taught in Chinese. Keeping male nurses might have better served the needs of male Chinese patients. Third, the presence of male nurses offered some protection to the female nurses. Some female nurses, such as Margaret Gay and Clara Preston, had violent male patients. Others, such as Janet Brydon and Coral Brodie, had experience with brutal intruders and soldiers. Male students and graduate nurses may have added an element of safety to the culture of nursing.

Two questions resonated with me as I pored over the letters, photos, and memoirs. First, what brought – and kept – missionary nurses in such a violent setting? Second, what did missionary nurses actually accomplish in China? The first question can be most easily answered by summarizing the elements of the preceding discussion. Missionary nursing provided an unparalleled opportunity for personal and professional growth within a protected and privileged community. Within the cloistered boundaries of a national, religious, and gendered community, nursing flourished. Although they had opportunity to work elsewhere, the nurses in this study preferred work in China to mission work in Canada (home mission hospitals in northern settings), Korea, Japan, or India, or to mainstream nursing at places such as Vancouver General Hospital and Toronto General Hospital. Having invested in China, these nurses eschewed other settings because they did not seem to offer the same sense of challenge, privilege, and belonging. As a foreign mission field, China was unique. Not only was China exotic, with stunning ancient architecture and seaside resorts such as Bedaiho, but the newly emerging republic was also experiencing the effects of ongoing sociopolitical upheaval and natural disasters. During this period, disease, famine, trauma, and disenfranchisement were pervasive. The Canadian nurse's decision to become a missionary was partially based on her impulse to save and to heal Henan. The desire to return to China was more complex. Canadian missionary nurses developed enduring relationships with individual Chinese and with the community of Christians (Canadian and Chinese) in China. Their attachment to the unique features of the Henan mission cannot be overstated. They grieved each time doors to North Henan closed.

The answer to the second question can be understood only in relation to the first. The professional accomplishments of Canadian missionary nurses in China did not occur in a vacuum, but within the (solid) physical and (permeable) social walls of the mission. The most progressive decade of missionary nursing was the 1930s. This was a time of relative peace, when foundational relationships with the Chinese had been laid, and when the mission hierarchy wholeheartedly supported the development of modern nursing. Within a relatively short time frame, Canadian missionary nurses not only helped to establish and develop modern hospitals, training schools, and nursing services, but they also formed professional organizations that linked nursing in North Henan to other parts of China through membership in the National Association of China and the International Council of Nurses. As a group, the Canadian missionary nurses were accomplished and bright women who placed a high value on post-secondary education. While others portrayed missionary nurses as members of a noble and even beatific profession, nurses portrayed themselves as scientific, modern, and determined individuals who aimed to uphold the standards and traditions of the profession in Canada. For example, Margaret Gay endeavoured to transplant "a bit of the VGH [Vancouver General Hospital] in the Orient."[7] The missionary nurses incorporated Canadian nursing rituals, including the use of different nursing uniforms to indicate the level of training a nursing student held. They created a hierarchy of students, staff, educators, and administrators that reflected the organizational structure found in Canadian hospitals. They provided education, mentorship, and support to a growing cadre of both male and female Chinese nurses, and then moved aside as Chinese nurses stepped into leadership roles. Not only was missionary nursing a respectable vocation for these nurses, it was their identity. Single nurses hired through the Woman's Missionary Society contributed to an understanding of missionary nursing as skilled, paid work – a public role. Married nurses contributed to an understanding of missionary nursing as an extension of family duties – a private role. Even when they were no longer employed, remunerated, or acknowledged, married nurses could be counted on to provide nursing care in the homes of missionary families and, during crises, in the hospitals.

The hasty closure of the NCM in 1947 was fatal to missionary nursing there. At first glance, it appears that external forces were responsible for the closure; Communist soldiers literally forced their way into the sheltered space. On closer inspection, however, it is apparent that the world of missionary nursing at the NCM was crumbling long before Canadians were expelled from the mission compounds. The myriad of structures that had supported missionary nursing in the past had weakened over time. Missionary nursing in China had always been dependent on China's compliance, the United Church's financial solvency, and the Woman's Missionary Society's commitment to tend to administrative details. It was also dependent on a reliable pool of prospective missionary nurses. To be suitable for missionary nursing, one had to demonstrate a unique blend of characteristics. These included an ability to live under harsh and uncertain conditions, an interest and ability to learn the Chinese language, a willingness to leave family and friends for a period of years or even decades, a disinterest in material possessions, and a public commitment to religious ideals. One required mental tenacity, physical fortitude, and spiritual depth – an ability to recognize suffering, and to feel responsible for it. The pool of prospective missionaries had been dwindling since the 1920s; with the exception of the Henan mishkids, fewer nurses seemed interested in the life of a career missionary. And those nurses who were already part of the mission had been slowly losing their most precious resource: hope based on a sense of divine purpose. Even if China desired the continued presence of Canadians in North Henan, in reality, missionary nursing was unsustainable.

Before undertaking this project, I read through fourteen letters written by Canadian nurses and published in *Canadian Nurse* between 1935 and 1947. When I first read Clara Preston's 1947 letter – the last letter from China published by *Canadian Nurse* – it seemed to me that the story of Canadian missionary nursing in China had been left dangling mid-sentence. Indeed, it had been. After 1947, the voices of Canadian missionary nurses were silent, due to the women's fear of placing Chinese colleagues at risk in Communist China. Their stories were obscured by the political disagreement within the United Church over the meaning of Communist rule to missions in China.

And their modest accomplishments in North Henan were eclipsed by the dramatic expulsion of all foreigners from China in 1952. As successful as missionary nurses were at creating a culture of nursing within the boundaries of the NCM, external and internal pressures ultimately collapsed their cloistered world and eradicated their dreams. Those who participated in the last years of missionary nursing witnessed its slow and painful demise. The death of the NCM produced an overwhelming sense of loss – but also an ashamed sense of relief.

Epilogue
Return to Henan, 2003

As I stepped onto the train platform at Anyang in October 2003, it occurred to me I might be the only Canadian nurse to do so since the United Church North China Mission (NCM) was unceremoniously closed in 1947. Our train from Beijing through Shijiazhuang and Baoding to Henan had been crammed with young urban professionals toting cell-phones and snack bags. The high-tech twenty-first-century din that followed us from Beijing faded as my husband and I were escorted away from the train station and toward the heart of Anyang. Before leaving Canada, I had worked with a Toronto travel agency to arrange for a driver and interpreter in China to escort us through Anyang and Xinxiang (the larger centre of which Weihui is now a part) and to help us find sites of the former NCMs, I dubiously accepted reassurances that it would be no problem to locate the former mission stations, even though there was no way to confirm ahead of time whether or not any NCM buildings had survived the sixty-year interim. What if nothing was left? I reassured myself that, even if I found nothing tangible, it would be worth the trip to experience firsthand that which could not be divined from the data I had collected in Canada – that is, the feel of the Henan air, the smells and tastes of local cooking, the sounds of spoken Chinese, and the sense of geographic space. To be a foreigner in China, I reasoned, would help me to better understand the Canadian nurses' experience.

My expectations, then, were quite low. I realized that much had happened in the previous sixty years to obliterate the former connection between Canada and China: communication between the missionaries and their Chinese friends was severed after the Communist Revolution in 1949. I came to China with the belief that any sense of community that might have survived among the Henanese Christians themselves would have been severely tested, if not destroyed, during Mao Zedong's violent purge of all things foreign during the Great Proletarian Cultural Revolution (from 1966 until Mao's death in 1976). Although some Canadian missionaries were invited back to China during the 1980s as a way to acknowledge their humanitarian efforts in China, historic strands connecting Canadians with their Chinese friends and colleagues seemed tenuous at best. Neither country seemed anxious to re-establish missionary ties. From what I'd been told by Canadians, the Chinese who participated in the missionary era faced punishment and persecution by the Communist government. It would make sense for the Chinese not to admit past relationships with Canadians. In Canada, former missionaries and their children faced a different, subtle form of social pressure to hide their missionary past. Former China missionaries told me of making a conscious decision not to speak publicly of their experiences in China for fear that they might inadvertently place their Chinese friends in jeopardy. Never mind that China was half a world away: if "loose lips [could] sink ships," unintentional public identification of Chinese Christians could lead to persecution under the Communists. Severed communication ties between the countries left Canadian missionaries anxiously speculating about the fate of their Chinese peers for years.

By the time it was safe to voice their experiences in Canada, missionaries found that Canadians were no longer interested in what they had to say. Even the next generation of missionaries dismissed the "outdated" wisdom of their elders. The perceived "failure" of missionary efforts in China sparked debate among Canadian Christians on the topic of missionary methods and aims. As the Christian church grappled with questions of relevance and the role of foreign missions, the Canadian public began questioning the morality of mission work. Once portrayed as respected purveyors of the Christian faith, missionaries were now described as religious oppressors and cultural imperialists. Missions' historic ride on the coat-tails of British colonialism became a lightning rod for academic criticism. For Canadian mishkids, whose self-identity and self-worth was grounded in the belief that the efforts of their missionary parents and grandparents were noble and self-sacrificing, public and academic criticism of the missionary enterprise during the 1960s and 1970s triggered an identity crisis. In response, some mishkids chose to separate themselves from their family legacy, hiding their missionary past like a shameful secret. Ironically, by choosing not to openly challenge public and academic condemnation of missionary work, mishkids (like their missionary parents) inadvertently contributed to the silence surrounding missionary nursing in China. Yet the passion with which participants shared their memories with me belied the depth of their feelings for China, and the indelible mark that China had made on their lives. When it comes to China missions, disconnection with the past does not necessarily mean disinterest in it.

What happened to the Woman's Missionary Society (WMS) nurses after the NCM closed? By 1947, there were only five NCM nurses still under contract with the WMS. The three oldest nurses (Preston, Brydon, and Gay) soon retired. Louise Clara Preston was ill when she returned to Canada in October 1947. She took three months of sick leave and then was appointed to the WMS hospital at Burns Lake, British Columbia, where she served as a nursing superintendent until 1952. She died in 1959.[1] Janet Brydon retired in London, Ontario, in 1948, and died in 1982.[2] Margaret Gay retired in 1951, after an extended leave of absence. She died in 1973.[3] The two newest WMS recruits, Hossie and Turner, stayed in China for a few more years after the closure of the NCM. Helen Turner Nelson returned to Canada with her husband in 1951, and later settled in Scotland. She died from complications related to childbirth, in 1955.[4] Margaret Hossie married Mr. Bob Hart before returning with him to Canada.[5]

The richness of the archival data available in Canada for this project meant that I could probably have painted a fair portrait of Canadian missionary nursing at the NCM without ever visiting China. Yet to do so would be something akin to painting a portrait from a few postcards. To understand (and portray) nursing more fully, I had to experience Henan firsthand – however superficially. I hoped that by placing myself within the geographic context in which nurses lived and worked, I would be able to more clearly envision their world. Since I did not expect to pick up any threads of human connection between Canada and Henan (how *does* one build a relationship with brick buildings?), I could think of only one way to search for the NCM: by dragging my husband halfway around the world to the small and dusty cities of Anyang and Weihui to see it for myself. In the end, we found more than we bargained for.

It was not until our hired driver pulled into the Roman Catholic compound in Anyang that I began to doubt our young guide's competence, and my sanity for investing so much into the uncertain discovery of evidence linking China and Canada's past. Having been assured by the sister of one North China missionary that her brother found many or most of the brick buildings intact during his visit in the 1980s, I anticipated a cluster of buildings in both cities being used for retail or other businesses. The morning after our arrival at the Anyang train station, our interpreter met up with us for breakfast at the hotel. Armed with photocopies of NCM photos dating back to the 1920s, we climbed into our Chinese driver's battered sedan and headed through the dusty streets of Anyang. We passed by rows of Chinese taking their morning exercise on the cobblestone squares in front of office buildings – graceful, choreographed movements that looked similar to tai chi, except with swords and umbrellas. We drove by rows of modern storefronts interspersed with an occasional pagoda or temple. Then we turned into what looked like a gated parking lot.

As soon as I saw the crucifix above the compound gate, I knew we had the wrong place. The Chinese priest knew it too. After some discussion with our interpreter, the priest squeezed into the back seat with my husband and me and directed us to a second compound. Much like the first, this compound was located behind a six-foot wrought-iron gate and was enclosed on four sides by a whitewashed brick fence. Three elderly Chinese women and one man came to greet us. The spokeswoman was about seventy years old. After some discussion with our interpreter, they led the three of us past a crumbling, two-story brick building on our left, to a long, low building facing the centre courtyard from our right. In front of us was a large, new church building. After offering us tea and fruit, our Chinese hosts asked who we were and why we had come. I was feeling impatient by this time, certain that we had taken another wrong turn, and eager to keep moving. As our interpreter spoke with the elderly woman, she nodded. Suddenly I heard something vaguely familiar – she said *"Loa dai fu,"* which I recognized as the Chinese name for Dr. Robert McClure: *Loa Ming yuan,* the *dai fu* (doctor). I sat up straight: "Yes, yes, *Loa dai fu!"* I exclaimed. A feeling of relief washed over me as our hostess left the room to fetch a copy of the history of what is now called *dong yang fang* (East Overseas House).

This *was* the former site of the NCM in Anyang – the east compound that was used primarily for residences. Today the compound is much smaller than the original, comprising 4.7 *mu* (approximately four-fifths of an acre), compared with the original 85 *mu* (approximately fourteen acres). In 1952, the hospital (on the former west compound) was given to the government and renamed the "Anyang People's Hospital." The Anyang People's Hospital has occupied a new building since 1992. After the Communist takeover in 1949, the east compound was occupied by the hospital administration, and Chinese Christians were forced to meet elsewhere. They gathered at *Ma hao* Street until the Cultural Revolution, during which all religious activities were banned. Since 1978, religious freedom was slowly recovered, and in 1984, the Anyang City Christianity Association was established. In 1992, 4.7 *mu* of the original NCM property was returned to the association. In 1995, the group built a new church – a "roman style" building that can accommodate three thousand. Only two of the original NCM buildings remain in Anyang, both former missionary residences. The elderly spokeswoman lives in the one that is said to have belonged to Jonathan Goforth. The association hopes to restore both buildings as "historic relics."

As exciting as it was to wander through the four sparse bedrooms and rickety stairwell of the "Goforth's House," taking in the stark fixtures, views from the windows, and the bullet-ridden exterior ("from the war with Japan," we were told), the most moving part of the trip to Anyang occurred in the new church building. This church has the conventional structure of a Western Christian church – wooden pews facing a main platform with a pulpit, which is flanked by two pianos. Our hosts, somewhat wary of the reason for our visit, gave reserved answers to our initial questions. It was frustrating to be unable to communicate – even body language was indecipherable. Then my husband, a pianist, gestured toward the piano. "May I?" he asked. He started to play the old hymn *How Great Thou Art*. Then the elderly spokeswoman started to sing, in Chinese. I joined her, in English. The others looked on and smiled as the two of us stumbled our way through *Lead Me; Guide Me* and *Amazing Grace*. By the end of the song, we were arm in arm, eyes glistening. Time, nationality, language, and distance melted away, and for a moment I understood what it meant for a Canadian nurse to connect with someone halfway around the world in China.

Having discovered that the Canadian missionaries left a tangible legacy at Anyang, I was less anxious about what we would or would not find at Weihui. The trip from Anyang to Weihui was a mere ninety minutes by car along a paved highway – a far cry from the sedan chairs and mule carts of a century earlier. As we wound through the narrow, dirt streets of Weihui asking for directions, I had more confidence in our driver and interpreter's ability to sniff out the former NCM site. They stopped at virtually every street corner, asking the oldest person sitting there for help. Weihui struck me as having more in common with rural towns in Kenya or Uganda than other parts of China I had visited: dusty, one-story buildings were crowded together, many selling wares or fresh food. People were crouched in front of buildings, washing dishes, visiting, and playing games. Once again, we came upon a Catholic compound. And once again someone there gave directions to the Protestant compound – apparently alongside a highway. Finding a gate with a small iron cross above it, we pulled over. The gate was locked, and there was no one inside. Helpful neighbours suggested we go to the fields to locate the resident minister – apparently he was helping with the wheat and cotton harvest. After two fruitless hours of driving along the edge of Weihui, we decided to return to the Protestant compound, to at least take photos from the outside. To our delight, the gate was open.

Awaiting us were six young men and women, to whom I showed old photos of the NCM, including the hospital. One woman began to nod and point. She scrambled into the car with us to direct us. Apparently we were at the new location for Chinese Christians, not at the actual NCM site. We drove for twenty minutes back through the narrow streets of town, and then turned a corner through a gate, into what looked like a large hospital compound. The cluster of buildings inside was not unlike a hospital complex in Canada, with multi-storeyed, modern buildings facing a small central park, complete with a gazebo. What caught my attention was the smaller building directly ahead of us. I recognized it from the old photos: the original Weihui (Huimin) hospital.

The hospital was essentially boarded up. As I peeked through the windows of the front door, I noticed a clutter of furniture and boxes – how I would have loved to wander through! Its exterior had recently been painted – gray-blue with white lines to set off the outline of the original bricks. It was being preserved, we were told. The city was hoping to restore the building as a tourist site – not to depict mission history, but as an example of older Chinese hospitals. It is now on the grounds of the First Affiliated Hospital of the Xinxiang Medical University. By bringing to light the story of Canadian missionary nurses, I hope that *Healing Henan* will help to close the circle that signifies the Chinese-Canadian relationship that began in Henan in 1888.

Appendices

Missionary nurses at the North China Mission (NCM)

	Chinese name	Date of birth	Birthplace	Father's occupation	Dates in China under WMS	Total years as WMS nurse
Woman's Missionary Society (WMS) nurses						
Harriet Sutherland (Corbett)[a]	?	?	?	?	1888-89	1
Jennie Graham	?	?	Simcoe County, ON	? (Sister to Dr. Lucinda Graham)	1889-91	2
Margaret MacIntosh	Ma Chiao Shih	6 Jan. 1857	Guelph, ON	?	1889-1927	38
Margaret Gay	Gai Magu	12 Aug. 1886	Toronto, ON	?	1910-41	31 (10 in Canada)
M.E. (Maisie) McNeeley (Forbes)[a]	?	?	?	?	1914-16	2
Mrs. Jeanette (McCalla) Ratcliffe[b]	Yao Xiuzhen	5 Oct. 1876	St. Catharines, ON	? (Sister to Dr. Susan [McCalla] Grant)	1916-40	24
Janet L. Brydon	?	30 Sept. 1886	Eramosa Township, ON	Farmer	1917-39	22
Margaret Mitchell	?	?	Scotland	?	1916-35	19

▶

◄   *Appendix 1*

WMS nurses	Chinese name	Date of birth	Birthplace	Father's occupation	Dates in China under WMS	Total years as WMS nurse
Isabel Leslie *(Fleming)*[a]	Lei Runtian	?	?	?	1920-37	17
Eleanor Galbraith *(Bridgman)*[a]	?	11 April 1896	St. John County, NB	?	1920	1
Margaret M. Straith *(Fuller)*[a]	?	3 July 1890	Holstein, ON	?	1921	1
L. Clara Preston	Peng Hu Shih	23 March 1891	Boissevain, MB	Businessman (industrialist)	1922-47	25
Jean Menzies *(Stockley)*[a]	?	9 March 1898	Anyang, Henan, China	NCM missionary (James R. and Davina Robb Menzies)	1923-27	4
Coral Brodie	?	3 May 1897	Bethesda, ON	Farmer	1923-40	17
Georgina Menzies *(Lewis)*[a]	?	27 Sept. 1906	Huaiqing, Henan, China	NCM missionary (James R. and Davina Robb Menzies)	1931-39	8
Allegra Doyle *(Smith)*	?	12 Nov. 1905	Sperling, MN	?	1931-35	4
Mary Boyd *(Stanley)*[a]	?	10 April 1916	Huaiqing, Henan, China	NCM missionary (Rev. H.A. and Mrs. Boyd)	1939-40	1
Dorothy Boyd *(Johnston)*	?	21 Sept. 1913	Huaiqing, Henan, China	NCM missionary (Rev. H.A. and Mrs. Boyd)	1939-41	2
Elizabeth Thomson *(Gale)*[a]	?	22 June 1911	Anyang, Henan, China	NCM missionary (Andrew and Margaret McKay Thomson)	1939-40	1

►

◄ *Appendix 1*

WMS nurses	Chinese name	Date of birth	Birthplace	Father's occupation	Dates in China under WMS	Total years as WMS nurse
Helen Turner (*Nelson*)[a]	?	1 Aug. 1918	Carlingford, ON	?	1947-50	3
Margaret Hossie	?	?	?	?	1947-49	2

Married nurses at the NCM (under auspices of husband's mission board)

Missionary wives	Date of birth	Birthplace	Father's occupation	Dates in China	Total years in China as missionary
Christina *Malcolm*	?	?	?	1892-96 (died)	4
W.C. *Netterfield*	?	?	?	1921-23?	2
M. *Roulston*	?	?	?	1926-40	14
Anna Marion Fisher *Faris*	?	?	?	1925-37	12
Mrs. *MacKinley*[c]	?	?	?	1931-33	2
Florence MacKenzie *Liddell*[d]	?	North Henan	NCM missionary (Hugh and Agnes MacKenzie)	1934-39	5
Dorothy Lochead *MacKenzie*	?	North Henan	NCM missionary (Arthur and Jessie Lochead)	1945-50?	5
Harriet Brown *Alexander*[e]	?	?	?	1946	0.5

Other

Church of England (Anglican) nurse	Date of birth	Birthplace	Father's occupation	Dates in China	Total years in China
Susie Kelsey	?	?	?	1924-49	27

a Married China missionary after arrival; stayed in China, but no longer under the WMS.
b Widowed before coming to China.
c Volunteered with husband.
d Returned to China after nurses' training, but not under the NCM.
e At NCM for 6 months with FAU.
Note: Miss M.L. Hargrave was hired by the WMS in 1937. She resigned in 1938 before coming to China because of opposition from her family.

Appendix 2

WMS nurses who resigned to be married

Name	Date of arrival in China	Date of resignation	Husband	Husband's mission (China)	Date of departure from China	Total years in China
Harriet Sutherland	1888	1889	Rev. Dr. Hunter Corbett	American Presbyterian	unknown, died in China	?
Maisie McNeeley	1914	1916	Rev. H. Stewart Forbes	North China Mission	1940	26
Isabel Leslie	1920	1937	J.T. Fleming	North China Mission	1939	19
Eleanor Galbraith	1920	1920	Rev. H.T. Bridgman	South Presbyterian Mission (United States)	?	?
Margaret Straith	1921	1921	Glen Fuller	?	?	?
Jean Menzies	1923	1927	Dr. Handley Stockley	English Baptist Mission	1945?	22?
Georgina Menzies	1931	1939	Dr. John Lewis	Baptist Missionary Society	1945?	14?
Allegra Doyle	1931	1935	Douglas Smith	N/A	1935	4
Mary Boyd	1939	1940	Charles Johnson Stanley	Foreign student at Peiping [Beijing]	1945?	6?
Dorothy Boyd	1939	1941	Phillip Johnston	N/A	1941	2
Elizabeth Thomson	1939	1940	Dr. Godfrey Gale	London Missionary Society (England)	1945	6
Helen Turner	1947	1950	Peter Nelson	English Baptist Missionary Society	1951	4

Appendix 3

Three types of missionary nurses

Unmarried Woman's Missionary Society nurses	Woman's Missionary Society nurses who resigned to be married	Foreign Mission Board missionary wives who were also nurses
Jennie Graham*	Harriet Sutherland	Christina Malcolm
Margaret MacIntosh	Maisie McNeeley	M. Roulston
Margaret Gay	Isabel Leslie	W.C. Netterfield
Jeanette Ratcliffe (previously widowed)	Eleanor Galbraith	Anna Marion Fisher Faris
Janet Brydon	Margaret Straith	Mrs. MacKinley
Margaret Mitchell	Jean Menzies**	Harriet Alexander
Clara Preston	Georgina Menzies**	Dorothy Lochead MacKenzie**
Coral Brodie	Allegra Doyle	
Margaret Hossie*	Mary Boyd**	
	Dorothy Boyd**	
	Elizabeth Thomson**	
	Helen Turner	

* It is not clear whether these nurses married after returning to Canada.

** These nurses were also mishkids.

Note: Anglican nurse Susie Kelsey was also included in this study for her role with the North China Mission nurses, and Florence MacKenzie Liddell was a Henan mishkid who returned to China as a missionary wife after graduating from the Toronto General Hospital training school for nurses.

Appendix 4

Missionary nurse education

	Basic nurse's training (RN)	Graduation date	Date of arrival in China	Post-graduate nursing education	Other education	Language study
Woman's Missionary Society (WMS) nurses						
Harriet R. Sutherland	TGH	?	1888	?	–	?
Jennie Graham	TGH	?	1889	?	–	Yes
Margaret MacIntosh	TGH	1889	1889	?	–	Yes
Margaret Gay	VGH	1926	1910	–	Missionary training (Toronto, 1910)	Yes
M.E. (Maisie) McNeeley	?	?	1914	–	–	Yes
Mrs. Jeanette *Ratcliffe*	?	?	1916	U of T (1917) Qilu (1918)	–	Yes
Janet L. Brydon	Victoria Hospital (London, ON)	1910	1917	–	Teacher's certificate (Kingston, 1916?)	Yes
Margaret Mitchell	? (Scotland)	?	1916	–	–	?
Isabel Leslie	?	?	1920	–	–	?
Eleanor Galbraith	Rhode Island Hospital	?	1920	–	Missionary training (Toronto, 1919)	Yes
Margaret M. Straith	WGH	1919	1921	–	–	Yes
L. Clara Preston	Royal Victoria Hospital (Montreal, QC)	1922	1922		McGill (Education, 1928); UWO (Hosp. Admin., 1931); UWO (Public Health, 1938)	Yes

▶

◀ *Appendix 4*

WMS nurses	Basic nurse's training (RN)	Graduation date	Date of arrival in China	Post-graduate nursing education	Other education	Language study
Jean Menzies	TGH	1922	1923	–	–	Yes
Coral Brodie	TGH	1921	1923	Cleveland Clinic (1927); U of T (Public Health, 1936)	Missionary training (Toronto, 1922)	Yes
Georgina Menzies	TGH	1929	1931	–	–	Yes
Allegra Doyle	TGH	1929	1931	–	–	Yes
Mary Boyd	TGH	193?	1939	U of T (BA, 19??)	–	Yes
Dorothy Boyd	TGH	193?	1939	U of T (Public Health, 193?)	–	?
[M.L. Hargrave][a]	?	?	–	BA	–	–
Elizabeth Thomson	TGH	1935	1939	U of T (Hosp. Admin., 1938)	–	Yes
Helen Turner	TGH	1941	1947	U of T (Public Health, 1944)	–	Yes
Margaret Hossie	Woman's College Hospital	?	1947	–	–	?
Married nurses: Missionary wives with nurses' training						
Christina *Malcolm*	? (Guelph)	?	1892	?	?	?
Mrs. *Netterfield*	?	?	1922	?	?	?
M. *Roulston*	?	?	1926	?	?	?
Anna Marion Fisher *Faris*	UBC	1923	1925	BScN (UBC, 1925)	?	?

▶

◄ *Appendix 4*

	Basic nurse's training (RN)	Graduation date	Date of arrival in China	Post-graduate nursing education	Other education	Language study
Amy *McClure* [b]	TGH	Not complete	1925	–	–	?
Florence *Liddell*	TGH	?	1934	?	?	?
Harriet *Alexander*	?	?	1946	?	?	?
Dorothy *MacKenzie*	?	?	1945	?	?	?
Mrs. *MacKinley* [c]	?	?	1931	?	?	?

a Resigned before coming to China.

b Married to Dr. Robert McClure. Amy McClure completed two of three years of nurses' training at TGH.

c Volunteered with her husband for two years.

Abbreviations:

TGH = Toronto General Hospital, Toronto, ON
U of T = University of Toronto, Toronto, ON
UWO = University of Western Ontario, London, ON
VGH = Vancouver General Hospital, Vancouver, BC
UBC = University of British Columbia, Vancouver, BC
WGH = Winnipeg General Hospital, Winnipeg, MB
McGill = McGill University, Montreal, QC
Qilu = Shandong Christian University, Jinan, Shandong, China

Appendix 5

Summary of 1947 Confidential Report

1 Pastor Niu, an elderly classical scholar, evangelist, and pastor, died in prison.
2 Pastor Peter Wang was accused of not being a productive worker, and was dragged behind a rope by a crowd around his village until "the flesh of his body was torn and lacerated." Pastor Wang's sister was coerced into confessing that Pastor Wang forced her to become a Nationalist spy – a charge that would bring a death sentence. Wang's sister escaped without knowing her brother's fate.
3 Elder Chiao was charged in a mob trial with having a son in the Nationalist army. He was barely alive after being dragged [by a mule?] three times; his grandson crushed his skull with a large stone to "bring his sufferings to a speedy end."
4 The wife of Pastor Liu of Anyang was dragged [?] for being the wife of a church treasurer, then placed under house arrest for two months. She later escaped to Anyang city.
5 Evangelist Lei of Huaiqing was arrested without trial and shot.
6 Evangelist Li Hung Chung accompanied "two missionary doctors" (McClure and Allen) on visits to see three churches. Shortly afterward, the Communists arrested more than one hundred men, including twenty-six who had been in contact with the doctors. Some who escaped reported that Li and sixteen others were "liquidated."
7 Pastor Chang Hsin Shu of Hwahsien was reportedly killed by "cruel torture," but a footnote in pencil reads, "Later, Pastor Chang is well at Sinhsiang."
8 A pregnant woman was killed, and then her unborn child was "taken from her" and "dashed to pieces on the hard ground."
9 Deacon Liu Hsing Yung escaped with his son to Anyang from a nearby village (and was joined later by his daughter). His wife was robbed of her family possessions and forced to live on the property of a wrecked temple property and beg.
10 Elder Chung Hsueh En was put on trial, but nine men openly supported him. These nine were later arrested, tied, hanged from a tree, and beaten with a bamboo stick. Chung was then arrested and fined 300,000 lbs. of grain, which bankrupted him. Later, his son was arrested but escaped; both fled to Anyang as refugees. Chung's daughter was later strangled and his wife was dragged to her death.
11 Che'eng Tao Shen of T'ai Pao (outside of Anyang) was a Nationalist military official. He was captured by the Communists, placed in a cauldron of boiling water, and drowned — a "white boil." In a "red boil," arms and legs are taken off, and then the body is placed in a boiling cauldron.

Authors of the report wrote, "These are but a selection from the many gruesome stories that are current. Those here recorded have come from original sources and we have been careful to restrain from overstatement. They are not given for propaganda purposes but to indicate the general conditions of life under Communist rule."[1]

---

1 Summarized from "Conditions in North Honan," Kaifeng, 1 June 1947. UCCVUA 83.045C, box 12, file 213. Only three copies of this report were made. They were neither circulated nor published.

Notes

Spellings

1 Developed by Victorian linguists Sir Thomas Wade and Professor Herbert Giles, the Wade-Giles system was replaced by Pinyin in the 1960s. Peter Stursberg, *No Foreign Bones in China: Memoirs of Imperialism and Its Ending* (Edmonton: University of Alberta Press, 2001), xv.

Introduction

1 From http://www.bloorstreetunited.org/history_hist.htm.
2 Also among this group was Dr. Victoria Cheung, a physician born in Victoria to parents of Chinese descent, who was headed to the Presbyterian mission in South China.
3 Dr. George Leslie MacKay established a mission in Taiwan under the Presbyterian Church in Canada in 1870. George Leslie MacKay, *From Far Formosa: The Island, Its People and Missions*, 4th ed. (New York: Fleming H. Revell Company, 1895).
4 According to the United Church website, Menzies went to China in 1902.
5 Dr. Robert McClure, interview by Peter Stursberg, transcripts, 14 July 1976. Library and Archives Canada, MG 31 Series D78 vol. 44, file 44-29.
6 Our Outgoing Missionaries, 1923. United Church of Canada/Victoria University Archives [hereafter UCCVUA] Bio Files Jean Menzies, Coral Brodie.
7 Liu Chung-tung, "From San Gu Liu Po to 'Caring Scholar': The Chinese Nurse in Perspective," *International Journal of Nursing Studies* 28, 4 (1991): 315-24.
8 Sioban Nelson, *Say Little, Do Much: Nursing, Nuns, and Hospitals in the Nineteenth Century* (Philadelphia: University of Pennsylvania Press, 2001). For recent comprehensive reviews of Florence Nightingale, see Lynn McDonald, ed., *Florence Nightingale: An Introduction to Her Life and Family. Volume One of the Collected Works of Florence Nightingale* (Waterloo, ON: Wilfred Laurier Press, 2001); Barbara Montgomery Dossey, *Florence Nightingale, Mystic, Visionary, Healer* (Springhouse, PA: Springhouse, 2000).
9 Christina Bates, Dianne Dodd, and Nicole Rousseau, eds., *On All Frontiers: Four Centuries of Canadian Nursing* (Ottawa: University of Ottawa Press and Canadian Museum of Civilization, 2005).
10 Kathryn McPherson, *Bedside Matters: The Transformation of Canadian Nursing, 1900-1990* (Toronto: Oxford University Press, 1996).
11 *Vancouver General Hospital Training School Annual, 1926*. Vancouver General Hospital Alumnae Association.
12 Chung-tung, "Caring Scholar"; Nelson, *Say Little, Do Much;* Pauline Paul, "The History of the Relationship between Nursing and Faith Traditions," in Margaret B. Clark and Joanne K. Olson, eds., *Nursing within a Faith Community* (Thousand Oaks, CA: Sage, 2000), 59-75; Kaiyi Chen, "Missionaries and the Early Development of Nursing in China," *Nursing History Review* 4 (1996): 129-49; Mary Ellen Doona, "Linda Richards and Nursing in Japan," *Nursing History Review* 4 (1996): 99-128. Stephen Endicott, *James G. Endicott: Rebel out of China* (Toronto: University of Toronto Press, 1980); Rosalind Goforth, *Goforth of China*

(Toronto: McClelland and Stewart, 1937); Sydney Gordon and Ted Allen, *The Scalpel, the Sword: The Story of Doctor Norman Bethune*, 3rd ed. (New York: Monthly Review Press, 1973); Munroe Scott, *The China Years of Dr. Bob McClure* (Toronto: Canec, 1977); Ruth Compton Brouwer, *New Women for God: Canadian Presbyterian Women and India Missions, 1876-1914* (Toronto: University of Toronto Press, 1990); Rosemary Gagan, *A Sensitive Independence: Canadian Methodist Women Missionaries in Canada and the Orient, 1881-1925* (Montreal and Kingston: McGill-Queen's University Press, 1992); Rosemary Gagan, "The Methodist Background of Canadian WMS Missionaries," in Neil Semple, ed., *Canadian Methodist Historical Society Papers* 7 (1992): 115-36; Peter Kong-Ming New and Yuet-wah Cheung, "Early Years of Medical Missionary Work in the Canadian Presbyterian Mission in North Honan, China, 1887-1900," *Asian Profile* 12, 5 (1984): 409-23; Yuet-wah Cheung, *Missionary Medicine in China: A Study of Two Canadian Protestant Missions in China before 1937* (Lanhan, MD: University Press of America, 1988).

13 Erleen J. Christensen, *In War and Famine: Missionaries in China's Honan Province in the 1940s* (Montreal and Kingston: McGill-Queen's University Press, 2005). Although Christensen states that the Anglican Church began mission work in Henan in 1907, it appears that it did not formalize the mission until 1910.

14 Ibid., 77.

15 Cora E. Simpson, *A Joy Ride through China for the NAC* (Shanghai: Kwang Hsueh House, 1926).

16 Cheung, *Missionary Medicine;* Alvyn Austin, *Saving China: Canadian Missionaries in the Middle Kingdom, 1888-1959* (Toronto: University of Toronto Press, 1987); Grant Maxwell, *Assignment in Chekiang: Seventy-one Canadians in China, 1902-1954* (Scarborough, ON: Scarboro Foreign Mission Society, 1984).

17 Austin, *Saving China*, 32-35. See also MacKay, *From Far Formosa*.

18 Kenneth Beaton, *Serving with the Sons of Shuh: Fifty Fateful Years in West China, 1891-1941* (Toronto: United Church of Canada, 1941), 233-35. According to a list of West China missionaries between 1891 and 1939, there were fourteen female physicians and thirty-two married registered nurses (RN). Added to Beaton's count of twenty-four single RNs between 1894 and 1952, the ratio of female RNs to medical doctors (MD) was 56:14 at West China. Also Janet Beaton, "Canadian Missionary Nurses in China: 1894-1951," paper presented at the fourteenth Annual Conference of the Canadian Association for the History of Nursing (9 June 2001). It appears that the Grey Sisters who went as nurses were Sisters St. Oswald, Mary Anthony, Mary Genevieve Anderchuk, St. Angela Lynch, and Mary Daniel O'Connor. The record, however, is not clear regarding their training. Mary Catherine Doyle was apparently trained as a pharmacist. Nine Grey Sisters went to China altogether between 1929 and 1952. Sister Rita McGuire, *Grey Sisters in China, 1929-1943; 1946-1952*. Unpublished history of the Grey Sisters of Immaculate Conception, Pembroke Archives.

19 This estimate includes married nurses; the West China Mission, for example, had thirty-two married nurses in addition to the twenty-four Woman's Missionary Society (WMS) nurses.

20 McGuire, "Grey Sisters," 126-42.

21 "Woman's Search for Nirvana," *North China Herald*, 12 January 1932: 45. In this newspaper article, French Canadian nurse "Sister Alice," who was moving to Chengdu, West China, after ten years of working in Tachienlu, where she had been in charge of the "French Hospital at the South Gate" in Shanghai. For further study on the missionary work of nurses in Catholic religious orders, see Pauline Paul, "The Contribution of the Grey Nuns to the Development of Nursing in Canada: Historiographic Issues," *Canadian Bulletin of Medical History* 11, 1 (1994): 207-17; and Sioban Nelson, *Say Little, Do Much*.

22 Jean Ewen, *China Nurse, 1932-1939: A Young Canadian Witnesses History* (Toronto: McClelland and Stewart, 1981); Scott, *McClure*. Coral Brodie, Jean Menzies, and Bob McClure, among others, were "designated" to mission work in China on 17 June 1923 at Bloor Street Church in Toronto. Bob McClure married Amy Hislop, who took partial nurses' training at Toronto General Hospital starting in 1923; Jonathan Goforth and Rosalind Goforth, *Miracle Lives of China* (Grand Rapids: Zondervan, 1931); and Rosalind Goforth, *Goforth of China*. While nurse Margaret Gay is credited in these early versions for taking dictation from the blind

Jonathan for *Miracle Lives of China,* later versions omit references to Gay – for example, Rosalind Goforth, *Jonathan Goforth* [based on *Goforth of China*] (Minneapolis: Bethany, 1986); Ellen Caughey, *Heroes of the Faith – Eric Liddell: Olympian and Missionary* (Uhrichsville, OH: Barbour, 2000); "Toronto General Hospital Alumnae Association," *Canadian Nurse* 27, 10 (1926): 547.

23 Austin, *Saving China,* 172. Canadian female physicians in China are also, as a group, under-studied. One exception is Margaret Negodaeff-Tomsik's *Honour Due: The Story of Dr. Leonora Howard King* (Ottawa: Canadian Medical Association, 1999). See also Ruth Compton Brouwer's *Modern Women Modernizing Men: The Changing Missions of Three Professional Women in Asia and Africa, 1902-69* (Vancouver: UBC Press, 2002) for in-depth analyses of the professional lives of missionary physicians Dr. Chone Oliver (India) and Dr. Florence Murray (Korea).

24 Austin also names Miss Amelia Brown as a registered nurse; Austin, *Saving China,* 52. According to West China Mission historian Dr. Janet Beaton, however, Amelia Brown was not a nurse; Jennie Ford was the first West China Mission nurse.

25 Many of the early contributors to Sino-Canadian mission scholarship had personal ties to China. For example, Peter Kong-Ming New's grandfather was among the first group of Chinese boys sent to study in the United States in 1872, and his father – one of the first Chinese to receive the MD degree from Harvard Medical School – became a prominent figure in early Western medicine in China. Yuet-wah Cheung was New's doctoral student. Historians Stephen Endicott, Peter Stursberg, and Alvyn Austin spent their childhood as Canadians in China: Endicott's grandfather arrived in China as a Methodist missionary in 1895, and his father became a United Church missionary in 1925; Stursberg's grandfather was a marine captain working in China in the mid-1800s, and his father was a China postal commissioner; and Austin, the son of missionaries, lived in China until age six. The intercultural experiences of these authors may account for their collective insight into Sino-Canadian relations before 1950. See Austin, *Saving China;* Cheung, *Missionary Medicine;* Endicott, *Rebel;* New and Cheung, *North Honan;* Scott, *McClure;* Peter Stursberg, *The Golden Hope: Christians in China* (Toronto: United Church Publishing House, 1987). Yong Wang, "Mission Unfinished: The United Church of Canada and China, 1925-1970" (PhD diss., Department of History, University of Waterloo, 1999).

26 Stursberg, *Golden Hope.*

27 Murdoch MacKenzie, *Twenty-five Years in Honan* (Toronto: Board of Foreign Missions, 1913), 181-89. There was reason to feel that this was a successful method: the first convert in North Honan was a formerly blind man, "Mr. Chou," who was able to see after cataract surgery.

28 Stursberg, *Golden Hope,* 61.

29 Cheung, *Missionary Medicine.*

30 New and Cheung, *Early Years.*

31 John Watt, "The Development of Nursing in Modern China, 1870-1949," *Nursing History Review* 12 (2004): 67-96.

32 A. Donald MacLeod, "Our Mission to China," *Channels* 17, 1 (2001), http://renewalfellowship. presbyterian.ca/channels/r01171-2.html.

33 The Huaiqing hospital was irreparably damaged during the Sino-Japanese War. Information on the Anyang church, the Anyang People's Hospital, and Xinxiang Hospital comes from personal communication with church elders, the hospital director, and the president during my visit to Anyang and Weihui in October 2005.

34 The change from "Women's" to "Woman's" came after the church union in 1925. According to Bob Burrows, this change was made to reflect the belief that each person was unique and had a contribution to make. Bob Burrows, *Healing in the Wilderness: A History of United Church Mission Hospitals* (Madeira Park, BC: Harbour Publishing, 2004).

35 Janet Beaton and Marion McKay, "Carolyn Wellwood: Pragmatic Visionary," *Canadian Journal of Nursing Leadership* 12, 4 (1999): 30-33; Sonya Grypma, "Neither Angels of Mercy nor Foreign Devils: Re-Visioning Canadian Missionary Nurses in China, 1935-1947," *Nursing History Review* 12 (2004): 97-119. Jean Ewen has written an important memoir of her work with Dr. Norman Bethune, but it is not a scholarly work, and is not representative of Canadian missionary nurse experience in China. See Jean Ewen, *China Nurse.*

36 Myra Rutherdale, *Women and the White Man's God: Gender and Race in the Canadian Mission Field* (Vancouver: UBC Press, 2002). Here Rutherdale cites from Mary Louise Pratt's *Imperial Eyes: Travel Writing and Transculturation*.

37 Jane Hunter, *The Gospel of Gentility: American Women Missionaries in Turn of the Century China* (Westford, MA: Yale University Press, 1984).

38 Brouwer, *New Women for God.*

39 Gagan, *Sensitive Independence;* Gagan, "Methodist Background."

40 Gagan, "Methodist Background," 118.

41 Ibid., 129.

42 Gagan, *Sensitive Independence,* 116. Gagan does not identify Brown as a nurse, but Austin does. See Austin, *Saving China.*

43 By 1913, nineteen missionary children had died of illness.

44 Gagan, *Sensitive Independence,* 211.

45 Margaret Brown, *History of the Honan (North China) Mission of the United Church of Canada, Originally a Mission of the Presbyterian Church in Canada,* UCCVUA, 6: 8; Mary Ellen Kelm, *Colonizing Bodies: Aboriginal Health and Healing in British Columbia, 1900-1950* (Vancouver: UBC Press, 1999), xviii.

46 Kelm, *Colonizing Bodies,* xix; Rutherdale, *White Man's God,* xx.

47 Kelm, *Colonizing Bodies,* xix.

48 Cited in ibid., 147.

49 Ibid., 149.

50 Rutherdale, *White Man's God,* xx.

51 Burrows, *Healing in the Wilderness.*

52 Rev. Doug Brydon, interview with S. Dunlop, 31 May 1993. Brydon (Eramosa Township) Family File. Wellington County Museum and Archives, A1994.129.

53 Chung-tung, "Caring Scholar"; Chen, "Early Development."

54 Citation of E. Brown in Chung-tung, "Caring Scholar," 323.

55 Chen, "Early Development," 143.

56 Ibid.; Chung-tung, "Caring Scholar." Although Chen makes mention of the study by Peter Kong-Ming New and Yuet-wah Cheung on the North China Mission before 1900, his supposition is that Canadian missionary work ended with the Boxer Uprising.

57 Beaton, "Missionary Nurses," 6.

58 Grypma, "Angels of Mercy."

59 For further examples of the powerful influence of missionary women, see Ruth Compton Brouwer's *Modern Women, Modernizing Men.*

60 Beaton, *Serving with the Sons of Shuh,* 233-35. According to a list of West China missionaries, between 1891 and 1939 there were fourteen female physicians and thirty-two married RNs. See also Beaton, "Missionary Nurses."

61 The Toronto General Hospital training school was initially a two-year program; other early nursing programs in Canada may have been the same length. All but one of the North China Mission nurses graduated in Canada: Margaret Mitchell likely graduated in Scotland.

62 Geertje Boschma, *Faculty of Nursing on the Move: Nursing at the University of Calgary, 1969-2004* (Calgary: University of Calgary Press, 2005), 15. These programs were the result of the influential leadership of Toronto General Hospital nurse superintendent Jean Gunn.

63 Harold Balme and Milton T. Shauffer, "An Enquiry into the Scientific Efficiency of Mission Hospitals in China," 1-39, paper presented at the annual conference of the China Medical Missionary Association, 21-27 February 1920, Beijing. J.W. Scott Library, University of Alberta, RT 02 004 ANO483 Microfiche.

64 The Church of Christ in China was formed in 1927. In 1938, the membership was more than 100,000, with sixteen synods. It was a united church, largely composed of Presbyterian, but also Methodist, Baptist, Congregational, Dutch Reformed, and Lutheran groups. *T'ien Kuo (Kingdom of Heaven): Jubilee of North Honan Mission souvenir booklet,* 1938.

65 Chung-tung, "Caring Scholar," 316.

66 Christopher Maggs, "A History of Nursing: A History of Caring?" *Journal of Advanced Nursing* 23, 3 (1996): 630-35.

67 Sioban Nelson, "The Fork in the Road: Nursing History versus the History of Nursing?" *Nursing History Review* 10 (2002): 175-88.

68 Patricia D'Antonio, "Revisiting and Rethinking the Rewriting of Nursing History," *Bulletin of the History of Medicine* 73, 2 (1999), 268-90; Sonya Grypma, "Critical Issues in the Use of Biographic Methods in Nursing History, *Nursing History Review* 13 (2005): 171-87.

69 Maggs, "History of Caring," 632; Nelson, "Fork in the Road," 178.

70 Kathleen Cruikshank, "Education History and the Art of Biography," *American Journal of Education* 107, 3 (1999): 231-39.

71 Bruce Lawrie, "Summary of North China Mission," UCCVUA FA 186.

72 M. Louise Fitzpatrick, "Historical Research: The Method," in Patricia Munhall and Carolyn Oiler Boyd, eds., *Nursing Research: A Qualitative Perspective,* 2nd ed. (New York: National League for Nursing Press, 1993).

73 Cheung, *Missionary Medicine,* 121.

74 Ibid., 122.

75 Margo S. Gewurtz, "'Their Names May Not Shine': Narrating Chinese Christian Converts," in Alvyn Austin and Jamie S. Scott, eds., *Canadian Missionaries, Indigenous Peoples: Representing Religion at Home and Abroad* (Toronto: University of Toronto Press, 2005), 134-51.

76 Ibid., 148.

77 Evelyn Richer, Overview of WMS History in Honan. United Church of Canada Woman's Missionary Society Overseas Missions: Honan, UCCUVA 83.05C, series 3.

Chapter 1: The Gospel of Soap and Water, 1888-1900

1 Bruce Lawrie, "Summary of North China Mission," United Church of Canada / Victoria University Archives [hereafter UCCVUA] FA 186.

2 Letter from Jonathan Goforth to the Foreign Mission Board in 1888, in Margaret Brown, *History of the Honan (North China) Mission of the United Church of Canada, Originally a Mission of the Presbyterian Church in Canada,* UCCVUA, 4: 8.

3 James Frazer Smith, *Life's Waking Part: Being the Autobiography of Reverend James Frazer Smith* (Toronto: Thomas Nelson and Sons, 1937), 75.

4 Celebrating Our History, Toronto General Hospital School for Nurses, www.uhn.ca/teahing/historical_archives/tghexhibit/panel2.html. See also Christina Bates, Dianne Dodd, and Nicole Rousseau, eds., *On All Frontiers: Four Centuries of Canadian Nursing* (Ottawa: University of Ottawa Press and Canadian Museum of Civilization, 2005).

5 Cora E. Simpson, *A Joy Ride through China for the NAC* (Shanghai: Kwang Hsueh House, 1926).

6 Isabel A. Hampton, "The Aims of the Johns Hopkins Hospital Training School for Nurses," *Johns Hopkins Hospital Bulletin* 1 (December 1889): 2. University of British Columbia Woodward Library Archives, Ethel Johns Collection.

7 Ibid., 3.

8 Henry Hurd, "The Relation of the Training School for Nurses to the Johns Hopkins Hospital," *Johns Hopkins Hospital Bulletin* 1 (December 1889): 7. University of British Columbia Woodward Library Archives, Ethel Johns Collection [emphasis in original].

9 Hampton, "Johns Hopkins," 3.

10 Hurd, "Johns Hopkins," 7.

11 Brown, *History of NCM,* 3: 8.

12 Frazer Smith, *Waking Part,* 74. It is interesting that later missionaries would point to the first seven *men* as the Henan pioneers: Smith, Goforth, McClure, MacGillivray, MacKenzie, MacVicar, and MacDougall. See Dr. Alfred Gandier, "Happy Fellowship in Troubled Times," *Honan Messenger* 13, 6, UCCVUA 83.058C, box 57, file 16, series 3.

13 Arriving in other provinces of China soon afterward were Canadian missionaries with the China Inland Mission (1888) and the Methodist Church of Canada (1891).

14 Lawrie, "Summary."

15 Ernest B. Struthers, *A Doctor Remembers: Days in China and Korea* (publication by author, 1976).

16 Lawrie, "Summary."

17 Brown, *History of NCM,* 4: 11. She was married the following September.

18 It is not clear whether typical terms were five, six, or seven years. It is most likely that they were six years, with a seventh year of furlough.

19 Frazer Smith, *Waking Part,* 134.
20 There is no record of the date of Harriet Sutherland's death in the United Church records. She is listed on a 1925 document as still living, but was deceased before Frazer Smith published his book in 1937.
21 Brown, *History of NCM,* 7: 4.
22 Ibid., 7: 1, 2.
23 Ibid., 7: 1; Murdoch MacKenzie, *Twenty-five Years in Honan* (Toronto: Board of Foreign Missions, 1913).
24 According to Alvyn Austin, one wag suggested the North Mission change its name to "McAll Mission" because of the predominance of Scottish names. Alvyn Austin, *Saving China: Canadian Missionaries in the Middle Kingdom, 1888-1959* (Toronto: University of Toronto Press, 1987), 40.
25 UCCVUA Bio Files Margaret MacIntosh and Jennie Graham.
26 B.F. Austin, *Woman, Her Character, Culture and Calling: A Full Discussion of Woman's Work in the Home, the School, the Church, and the Social Circle* (Brantford, ON: Book and Bible House, 1890), 180.
27 Brown, *History of NCM,* 7: 5; UCCVUA Bio File MacIntosh.
28 Mrs. J.C. Griffith, "Pioneer WMS Worker," *Honan Messenger* 13, 5 (May 1927): 17-18. UCCVUA BV 3420.H6hmps.
29 Brown, *History of NCM,* 7: 5.
30 Ibid., 14: 6.
31 Ibid., 14: 5.
32 Frazer Smith, *Waking Part,* 275.
33 Margaret MacIntosh, "Encouraging Incidents" letter from Sincheng, 25 January 1893, UCCVUA 83.045C, box 7, file 113.
34 Brown, *History of NCM,* 16: 8.
35 Frazer Smith, *Waking Part,* 196. They were still awaiting entrance to Anyang.
36 Brown, *History of NCM,* 16: 5; 18: 10.
37 Frazer Smith, *Waking Part,* 196-97.
38 Brown reported that Mrs. Malcolm died of peritonitis. Brown, *History of NCM,* 18: 10.
39 Ibid.
40 He later married Eliza Pringle and returned with her to China in 1897. List of missionaries who served in the Henan (North China Mission) before 1925. UCCVUA 83.045C, box 1, file 1.
41 Brown, *History of NCM,* 58: 13.
42 Ibid., 22: 3; 34: 4. In 1894, MacIntosh had managed to get a number of boys and girls together for elementary Christian instruction, teaching them to read and sing some hymns. This work lasted for approximately one year, until she left Sincheng.
43 Louise Clara Preston, *Flowers amongst the Debris: A Canadian Nurse in War Torn China* (Brockville, ON: Preston Robb, *n.d.*).
44 Of thirty-six missions established in 1888 or earlier, thirty reported that they had hospitals or dispensaries by 1904. See Harlan P. Beach, "Statistics of Missions in China for 1904," in *Dawn on the Hills of T'ang: Missions in China* (New York: Student Volunteer Movement for Foreign Missions, 1905, originally published in 1898), Appendix E.
45 Erleen J. Christensen, *In War and Famine: Missionaries in China's Honan Province in the 1940s* (Montreal and Kingston: McGill-Queen's University Press, 2005); Harold Balme and Milton T. Shauffer, "An Enquiry into the Scientific Efficiency of Mission Hospitals in China," paper presented at the annual conference of the China Medical Missionary Association, 21-27 February 1920, Beijing. J.W. Scott Library, University of Alberta, RT 02 004 ANO483 Microfiche.
46 MacKenzie, *Twenty-five Years,* 139.
47 R. Goforth, *Goforth of China* (Toronto: McClelland and Stewart, 1937), 346 [emphasis in original].
48 Geo J. Bond, *Our Share in China and What We Are Doing with It* (Toronto: Missionary Society of the Methodist Church, 1909), 57; Henry Beets, "China as a Mission Field," in *Toiling and Trusting: Fifty Years of Christian Reformed Missions* (Grand Rapids, MI: Grand Rapids Printing, 1940), 220; Beach, *T'ang,* 11.

49 F.L. Hawks Pott, *The Emergency in China* (New York: Missionary Education Movement of the United States and Canada, 1913), 221.
50 MacKenzie, *Twenty-five Years,* 143.
51 Brown, *History of NCM,* 17: 12. A chapel was usually built adjacent to the dispensary and was typically used as a patient waiting room.
52 Frazer Smith, *Waking Part,* 102.
53 Ibid., 104-8.
54 Ibid.
55 Ibid., 246.
56 Beach, *T'ang,* 110.
57 Cited in Mrs. Howard Taylor, *Guinness of Honan* (Toronto: China Inland Mission, 1930), 242-43. Dr. Gibson was of the China Inland Mission at Kaifeng, Henan – south of the Yellow River from the Canadian Presbyterian North Henan Mission. Quotes are from "an article" written by Dr. Gibson.
58 Dr. Robert McClure, interview by Peter Stursberg, transcripts, 14 July 1976. Library and Archives Canada, MG 31 Series D78 vol. 44, file 44-29.
59 MacKenzie, *Twenty-five Years,* 231. See Sonya Grypma, "James R. Menzies: Healing and Preaching in Early 20th Century China," *Canadian Medical Association Journal* 170, 1 (2004): 84-85.
60 Jonathan and Rosalind Goforth, "Earliest Trophies of Grace: The Blind Chief," in *Miracle Lives of China* (Grand Rapids, MI: Zondervan, 1931), 1-9; MacKenzie, *Twenty-five Years,* 183-98; *The Honan Messenger* 6, 4 (20 April 1920), UCCVUA Bio File James R. Menzies.
61 Margo S. Gewurtz, "'Their Names May Not Shine': Narrating Chinese Christian Converts," in Alvyn Austin and Jamie S. Scott, eds., *Canadian Missionaries, Indigenous Peoples: Representing Religion at Home and Abroad* (Toronto: University of Toronto Press, 2005), 134-51.
62 Brown, *History of NCM,* 66: 7.
63 Austin, *Woman,* 177-81.
64 MacKenzie, *Twenty-five Years,* 154.
65 Austin, *Woman,* 180.
66 Ibid. [emphasis in original].
67 Ibid., 163-64.
68 Ibid., 164.
69 Ibid.
70 MacKenzie, *Twenty-five Years,* 153.
71 Brown, *History of NCM,* 16: 1.
72 Austin, *Woman,* 181.
73 Frazer Smith, *Waking Part,* 105.
74 Ibid., 103-4.
75 MacKenzie, *Twenty-five Years,* 140.
76 Taylor, *Guinness,* viii.
77 Frazer Smith, *Waking Part,* 103; Hawks Pott, *Emergency,* 220.
78 Hawks Pott, *Emergency,* 220.
79 Frazer Smith, *Waking Part,* 103.
80 Hawks Pott, *Emergency,* 221.
81 MacKenzie, *Twenty-five Years,* 42.
82 Goforth, *Goforth of China,* 98.
83 Ibid., 100.
84 Frazer Smith, *Waking Part,* 155.
85 Goforth, *Goforth of China,* 80.
86 Frances Wood, *No Dogs and Not Many Chinese: Treaty Port Life in China, 1843-1943* (London, UK: John Murray, 1998), 6-65; Peter Stursberg, *The Golden Hope: Christians in China* (Toronto: United Church Publishing House, 1987), 49-59.
87 Goforth, *Goforth of China,* 138. The phrase "our thousand miles of miracle" may have been a reference to a book published in 1904 by Archibald E. Glover entitled *A Thousand Miles of*

Miracle. According to Frances Wood, this was one among many books written to commemorate the massacre of Protestants – and a particularly angry and defiant one.

88 Honan Mission Chronological Record [hereafter HMCR], p. 21, dated 16 July 1937, UCCVUA 83.058C, series 3.
89 Goforth, *Goforth of China*, 127-28.
90 Brown, *History of NCM*, 27: 11, 12.
91 HMCR, 21.
92 They presumably travelled on to Japan, since they were there on 27 July. Brown, *History of NCM*, 28: 2.
93 Ibid., 27: 8, 9.
94 HMCR, 21.
95 Brown, *History of NCM*, 27: 8
96 MacKenzie, *Twenty-five Years*, 94; Goforth, *Goforth of China*, 130.
97 Brown, *History of NCM*, 27: 7.
98 MacKenzie, *Twenty-five Years*, 94.
99 HMCR, 21.
100 Rev. Murdoch and Martha MacKenzie and son Douglas; Miss Margaret MacIntosh; Dr. Jean Dow; Miss Minnie Pyke; Dr. Percy and Mrs. Isabella Leslie; Rev. Jonathan and Rosalind Goforth and children Paul, Helen, Ruth, and one other; Rev. John Griffith; Rev. James and Elizabeth Slimmon and infant; Rev. T. Craigie Hood; Rev. R.A and Jennie Mitchell. Also among them was Cheng Pi-Yueh, who later was the first Chinese in North Henan to be ordained a minister. Brown, *History of NCM*, 27: 19. It is possible that the other Chinese Christian, Goforth's *amah* Mrs. Cheng, was Cheng Pi-Yueh's wife.
101 John Griffith, "Escape from Honan in 1900," memoirs written in 1937, UCCVUA 83.058C, series 3, pp. 46-47.
102 Ibid., 47.
103 Ibid.
104 Goforth, *Goforth of China*, 137.
105 MacKenzie, *Twenty-five Years*, 48.
106 Isabella O. Leslie, "Flight to Safety," 5, UCCVUA 83.045C, box 13, file 244. This record was written in pencil on a Chinese houseboat during the latter part of this journey. The notes were found in Mrs. Leslie's personal effects after her death in 1949. They had been intended for her family in 1900 should she have died during the events.
107 Brown, *History of NCM*, 28: 1-2. The British government had appealed for interpreters and nurses. Brown is not clear regarding what initiated the appeal.
108 Ibid., 29: 4.
109 Ibid., 28: 10.
110 Ibid., 28: 9.
111 Goforth, *Goforth of China*, 128, 130. Brown, *History of NCM*, 27: 9, 23.
112 Percy C. Leslie, "A Survivor of the Boxer Outbreak," pamphlet written in the spring of 1961. UCCVUA 83.045C, box 13, file 244.

Chapter 2: Visions Interrupted, 1901-20
1 Margaret Brown, *History of the Honan (North China) Mission of the United Church of Canada, Originally a Mission of the Presbyterian Church in Canada,* United Church of Canada/Victoria University Archives [hereafter UCCVUA] 30: 2-5.
2 The amount was for $50,000. This included a claim for a new Bible for Mrs. Chang of Chuwang. It is not clear what currency Brown refers to here. It may be Chinese currency, Mexican silver, or Canadian dollars – most likely the amount given is in Chinese currency. After some criticism of the mission, this amount was later reduced.
3 Brown, *History of NCM*, 31: 8.
4 UCCVUA Bio File Margaret MacIntosh.
5 Brown, *History of NCM*, 32: 1.
6 Ibid.
7 UCCVUA Bio File Margaret MacIntosh.

8 Brown, *History of NCM*, 32: 2.

9 Ibid., 32: 3.

10 Ibid., 32: 9.

11 Dr. Robert McClure, interview by Peter Stursberg, transcripts, 14 July 1976. Library and Archives Canada, MG 31 Series D78 Vol. 44, File 44-29.

12 Brown, *History of NCM*, 31: 9.

13 Creighton Lacy, "The Missionary Exodus from China," *Pacific Affairs* 28, 4 (1955): 301-14. Lacy questioned the value of some typical mission practices, such as walled compounds, refrigerators, and mountain holidays. He suggested that, for an effective ministry, missionary standards should be "as simple and close to the community level as possible." Although the missionaries perceived themselves as self-sacrificial, they did enjoy economic and class advantages over most Chinese citizens.

14 Brown, *History of NCM*, 32: 8.

15 Ibid., 32: 9.

16 Ibid., 21: 2.

17 Murdoch MacKenzie, *Twenty-five Years in Honan* (Toronto: Presbyterian Board of Foreign Missions, 1913), 143.

18 Brown, *History of NCM*, 21: 2.

19 James Frazer Smith, *Life's Waking Part: Being the Autobiography of Reverend James Frazer Smith* (Toronto: Thomas Nelson and Sons, 1937), 180.

20 The Henan missionary doctors and nurses moved around the various mission stations as the need arose. It is a daunting, if not impossible, task, to keep track of who was where, when. That the McClure family was in Weihui in 1901 comes from Munroe Scott, *The China Years of Dr. Bob McClure* (Toronto: Canec, 1977), 7.

21 McClure, interview by Stursberg.

22 Brown, *History of NCM*, 33: 17-19.

23 Ibid.

24 Harlan P. Beach, "Statistics of Missions in China for 1904," *Dawn on the Hills of T'ang: Missions in China* (New York: Student Volunteer Movement for Foreign Missions, 1905, originally published in 1898): Appendix E. In that year, medical missionaries in China reportedly cared for 880,304 patients, including 3,946 from Henan. This number does not reconcile with Henan Mission figures reported by Brown (including more than 34,000 patients treated at Anyang and Huaiqing alone). It is possible that Beach's number represents in-patients rather than outpatients, or patients rather than treatments (if patients received more than one treatment).

25 Erleen J. Christensen, *In War and Famine: Missionaries in China's Honan Province in the 1940s* (Montreal and Kingston: McGill-Queen's University Press, 2005), 77.

26 F.L. Hawks Pott, *The Emergency in China* (New York: Missionary Education Movement of the United States and Canada, 1913). Statistics of the Work of Protestant Missions in China for 1910 (includes 1911 and 1912).

27 Brown, *History of NCM*, 33: 20.

28 Ibid., 33: 21.

29 See Margaret Negodaeff-Tomsik, *Honour Due: The Story of Dr. Leonora Howard King* (Ottawa: Canadian Medical Association, 1999). Dr. King, a female Canadian physician, worked in the treaty port of Tianjin from 1877 to 1925. Chinese gentry supported her work after she successfully treated the (secluded) wife of viceroy Li Hung-chang in 1879. Although it was customary practice for missionaries to operate separate facilities for men and women in Tianjin, Dr. King and her colleagues treated men and women on the same premises.

30 Brown, *History of NCM*, 57: 10.

31 Ibid., 57: 11.

32 Peter Stursberg, *The Golden Hope: Christians in China* (Toronto: United Church Publishing House, 1987), 61-62. Stursberg's description is based on his interview with Dr. Scott's son.

33 Ibid.

34 McClure, interview by Stursberg.

35 Murray McCheyne Thomson, *A Daring Confidence: The Life and Times of Andrew Thomson in China, 1906-1942* (Ottawa: publication by author, 1992), 106.

36 Brown, *History of NCM,* 57: 12.
37 Ibid., 46: 2. With no nurses forthcoming, the Foreign Mission Board sent out an appeal for two female doctors instead.
38 Frances Wood, *No Dogs and Not Many Chinese: Treaty Port Life in China, 1843-1943* (London, UK: John Murray, 1998), 169-74.
39 Brown, *History of NCM,* 46: 4.
40 Yuet-wah Cheung, *Missionary Medicine in China: A Study of Two Canadian Protestant Missions in China before 1937* (Lanhan, MD: University Press of America, 1988).
41 McClure, interview by Stursberg.
42 Brown, *History of NCM,* 46: 11.
43 Ibid., 57: 12.
44 Cora E. Simpson, *A Joy Ride through China for the NAC* (Shanghai: Kwang Hsueh House, 1926), 11.
45 Kaiyi Chen, "Missionaries and the Early Development of Nursing in China," *Nursing History Review* 4 (1996): 129-49; Kaiyi Chen, "Quality Versus Quantity: The Rockefeller Foundation and Nurses Training in China," *Journal of American East Asian Relations* 5, 1 (1996): 77-104.
46 Liu Chung-tung, "From San Gu Liu Po to 'Caring Scholar': The Chinese Nurse in Perspective." *International Journal of Nursing Studies* 28, 4 (1991): 315-24; Brown, *History of NCM,* 57: 12; Simpson, *Joy Ride.*
47 Simpson, *Joy Ride,* 14.
48 Brown, *History of NCM,* 57: 1-10.
49 Ibid., 57: 2.
50 "List of missionaries of the Henan (North China) mission before 1925 under the Presbyterian Church in Canada," UCCVUA 83.045C, box 1, file 1.
51 It is not clear if the Christian Medical Association of China was a separate group from the China Medical Missionary Association. It seems that these names were used interchangeably for the same organization, although it is possible that the latter was a larger organization that included missionaries and Chinese Christians.
52 Ernest B. Struthers, *A Doctor Remembers: Days in China and Korea* (publication by author, 1976). Dr. Ernest Struthers' brother, Dr. R. Gordon Struthers, was appointed to Weihui one year after Ernest, in 1915.
53 Brown, *History of NCM,* 57: 13.
54 Margaret Gay, "Above All that Ye Ask or Think: How I got my RN in 1926," unpublished memoir. Private collection of Muriel Gay.
55 Ibid.
56 Brown, *History of NCM,* 57: 13-14.
57 McClure, interview by Stursberg.
58 Brown, *History of NCM,* 57: 13-14.
59 Thomson, *Daring Confidence,* 85.
60 UCCVUA Bio File Jeanette Ratcliffe.
61 A footnote in the memoirs of L. Clara Preston states that Mrs. Ratcliffe was a widow and that she was the sister of Mrs. Harvey Grant. See Louise Clara Preston, *Flowers amongst the Debris: A Canadian Nurse in War Torn China* (Brockville, ON: Preston Robb, n.d.), 18.
62 Ruth Compton Brouwer, *New Women for God: Canadian Presbyterian Women and India Missions, 1876-1914* (Toronto: University of Toronto Press, 1990).
63 Ibid., 79.
64 Brown, *History of NCM,* 32: 1. The Grants worked in Henan until 1937.
65 UCCVUA Bio File Jeanette Ratcliffe.
66 Brown, *History of NCM,* 57: 14-16.
67 UCCVUA Bio File Jeanette Ratcliffe.
68 Struthers, *Doctor Remembers,* 20; Thomson, *Daring Confidence,* 66-67. According to Thomson, for twelve months beginning March 1917, about eighty thousand Chinese men were transported across the Pacific and then across Canada in guarded train cars. They were loaded onto ships for the trans-Atlantic voyage. In France, they did heavy labour, including moving ammunition, digging communication trenches, and moving food supplies.
69 Thomson, *Daring Confidence,* 67.

70 Brown, *History of NCM,* 57: 16. It is interesting that Margaret Brown does not call Janet Brydon the "third nurse," since Margaret MacIntosh was still at the Henan Mission. Apparently MacIntosh was peripheral to the subsequent nursing developments in China.

71 The physicians at Henan during that year were Jean Dow, Isabelle McTavish, E.B. Struthers, R. Gordon Struthers, Fred Auld, Percy Leslie, James Menzies, William McClure, F.F. Carr Harris and W.R. Reeds. Since Margaret Brown states that five doctors went to France, and lists "Dr. Menzies and Dr. Isabelle McTavish" as the only doctors left in Henan, it is possible that the others were on furlough in Canada.

72 Howard Parkinson, nephew of Janet Brydon. Letter to author, 27 February 2003.

73 Brydon (Eramosa township) Family File, WCMA, A1994.129.

74 "Going to Mission Field," *Fergus News Record,* 19 July 1917: 1, WCMA.

75 Brown, *History of NCM,* 57: 16.

76 Rev. Doug Brydon, interview with S. Dunlop, 31 May 1993. Brydon (Eramosa Township) Family File, WCMA, A1994.129.

77 McClure, interview with Stursberg. When asked why he did not include events of the Second World War in his biography, McClure responded that he had not written much about the war at all – it was, he said, "too complicated."

78 Brown, *History of NCM,* 59: 1-2.

79 Later, Janet Brydon's uncle, Rev. Doug Brydon, recalled Janet telling him that Menzies had shouted at the nurses to "run and hide in the __, a code word for a safe hiding place." Brydon and Lethbridge accordingly "ran to the garret and hid under an eave." It seems unlikely that this is the order of events since Brown's account was based on her own correspondence with Lethbridge immediately after the incident, whereas Doug Brydon's account was second-hand and more than seventy years later. See Brydon, interview with S. Dunlop.

80 Brown, *History of NCM,* 59: 3; "An Heroic End," *The Honan Messenger* 6, 4 (April 1920): 3, UCCVUA Bio File James R. Menzies. The next morning, the body of one of the robbers was found; apparently one of the shots that hit Menzies also hit him. It was important to the missionaries to clarify that Menzies was unarmed and did not attack the man.

81 Brown, *History of NCM,* 59: 4-6.

82 Ibid.

83 "Period of 1920-1930: Death of Dr. J.R. Menzies," 64, UCCVUA 83.058C, box 17, file 57, series 3.

84 *The Honan [Henan] Messenger* 6, 4 (April 1920): 1-4, UCCVUA Bio File James R. Menzies.

85 Brydon, interview with S. Dunlop.

86 List of missionaries of the Honan (North China) Mission, UCCVUA 83.045C, box 1, file 1.

87 Brown, *History of NCM,* 59: 12.

88 Ibid., 59: 12-14, 60: 1-2.

89 Ibid., 60: 3-5.

90 "Our Outgoing Missionaries," *The Presbyterian Witness,* 6 December 1923: 5, UCCVUA, box 9001.A40PS, Microfilm #25, 6 July 1923-16 October 1924.

91 Brown, *History of NCM,* 59: 11-12.

92 Ibid., 59: 12-14. Jimmy Ainsworth was from Chiastso and the son of a non-Henan missionary.

93 Ibid.

94 Ibid., 59: 4.

95 There is no bio file on Isabel Leslie at the UCCVUA. She is listed on the UCCVUA "List of Missionaries who served in the Honan (North China) Mission before 1925" as having arrived in China in 1920, and on the "Honan Nurses 1888-1938" list as arriving in 1921. It is most likely that she sailed from Canada in late 1920, arriving in Henan in early 1921. UCCVUA 83.058C, box 57, file 17, series 3; UCCVUA 83.145C, box 1, file 1.

96 UCCVUA Bio File Eleanor May Galbraith.

Chapter 3: Modern Nursing at Last, 1921-27

1 Cora E. Simpson, *A Joy Ride through China for the NAC* (Shanghai: Kwang Hsueh House, 1926), 26.

2 Margaret Brown, *History of the Honan (North China) Mission of the United Church of Canada, Originally a Mission of the Presbyterian Church in Canada,* United Church of Canada/Victoria University Archives [hereafter UCCVUA] 66: 4.

3 Ibid., 1-14.
4 R.G. Struthers, "The New Hospital at Weihwei," UCCVUA 83.014C, box 3, file 13.
5 The currency is not specified, but is most likely in Canadian dollars since Dr. R.G. Struthers wrote to the supporters in Canada that the cost was $50,000. See Struthers, "New Hospital."
6 Lillian Bertha Craigie, "Woman's Missionary Society Notes," 1926, Glenbow Museum and Archives [hereafter GMA], M 285, box 3, file 25. By 1926, Canadian Presbyterian, Methodist, and Congregationalist churches had combined into the United Church of Canada.
7 Craigie, "WMS Notes," file 26.
8 Ibid., file 24.
9 Central United Church. GMA M1365, box 19, file 164; box 18, file 153. Author of *Serving with the Sons of Shuh* is Rev. J.K. Beaton; authors of *China Rediscovers Her West* are Yi-Fang Wu and Frank W. Price. *"Fourth Daughter of China"* may refer to *Lady Fourth Daughter of China: Sharer of Life*, written by Mary Brewster Hollister in 1932. The Presbyterian Church of Canada had become part of the United Church of Canada by this time.
10 Craigie, "WMS Notes," file 24.
11 See Louise Clara Preston, *Flowers amongst the Debris: A Canadian Nurse in War Torn China* (Brockville, ON: Preston Robb, *n.d.*), 45-51.
12 Struthers, "New Hospital."
13 "Dr. Jean Isabel Dow," *Honan Messenger* 13, 4, UCCVUA 83.058C, box 17, file 16, series 3.
14 Harold Balme and Milton T. Shauffer, "An Enquiry into the Scientific Efficiency of Mission Hospitals in China," 1-39, paper presented at the annual conference of the China Medical Missionary Association, 21-27 February 1920, Beijing. J.W. Scott Library, University of Alberta, RT 02 004 ANO483 Microfiche. Since only "78%" of the Henan missions replied to the survey, it is unclear whether it was the Canadian Presbyterians who responded. Since anecdotes by nurse Clara Preston are consistent with the findings of the CMMA study, however, it seems likely that the Presbyterians were included. In addition, in his role as president of the Shandong Christian University (Qilu), Dr. Harold Balme would have worked closely at Qilu with North China missionaries such as Dr. William McClure, who worked at Weihui until 1916.
15 Erleen J. Christensen, *In War and Famine: Missionaries in China's Honan Province in the 1940s* (Montreal and Kingston: McGill-Queen's University Press, 2005), index under "hospitals."
16 Anna C. Jamme, "Nursing Education in China," *American Journal of Nursing* 23 (1923): 667.
17 Liu Chung-tung, "From San Gu Liu Po to 'Caring Scholar': The Chinese Nurse in Perspective," *International Journal of Nursing Studies* 28, 4 (1991): 321.
18 Balme and Shauffer, "Scientific Efficiency," 31.
19 Ibid., 1.
20 L. Clara Preston, "Nursing in China," *Canadian Nurse* 43, 3 (1947): 217-18.
21 Chung-tung, "Caring Scholar," 321. Although the admission of Chinese members to the Nurses Association of Canada (NAC) was made possible only after 1922, by 1930, all the officers of the NAC were Chinese. According to Brown, the school of nursing opened a year before the main hospital at Weihui. *History of NCM,* 66: 7.
22 Margaret Straith was at language school in Beijing in 1921 with fellow Winnipeg alumna Mabel Naisbett. Other Winnipeg alumnae working in China were Irene Harris and Grace Bedford and, later, Susie Kelsey. Letter from Mabel Naisbett to Miss Polyxphen, 22 January 1922, Winnipeg General Hospital/Health Sciences Centre Archives [hereafter WGH/HSCA].
23 Preston, *Flowers,* 21.
24 Ibid., 2.
25 Ibid., 3-5.
26 Ibid., 4.
27 Ibid.
28 Ibid., 20.
29 Ibid., 3.
30 Ibid., 11.
31 Dr. Percy Leslie had already retired, but returned to Henan after hearing about the death of Dr. Menzies. Brown, *History of NCM,* 66: 2.
32 Preston, "Nursing in China."

33 Preston, *Flowers,* 45.
34 Ibid., 49. This section is based on memoirs written by Clara Preston in 1938. It seems surprising that intravenous injections would have been given during the time period described by Preston (1920s), but Margaret Brown's record of the use of "injections of brandy" as a treatment for Rev. Harold M. Clark in 1903 corroborates the early use of injections, although perhaps not intravenously (see below).
35 Ibid., 46.
36 Ibid., 49.
37 Struthers, "New Hospital."
38 Ibid. Struthers is quoting "a writer" but does not say whom.
39 Brown, *History of NCM,* 66: 13.
40 Struthers, "New Hospital."
41 Brown, *History of NCM,* 66: 1-14.
42 Ibid., 66: 5; Struthers, "New Hospital."
43 Preston, *Flowers,* 49.
44 From "The planting of the faith," Women's Missionary Society 1921, quoted by Brown, *History of NCM,* 66: 8.
45 Ibid.
46 Ibid., 66: 7.
47 Ratcliffe, "Weihwei Hospital," *Honan Messenger* 13, 4: 14-15, UCCVUA 83.058C, box 57, file 16, series 3.
48 Ibid.
49 Brown, *History of NCM,* 66: 7.
50 Preston, "Nursing in China," 217.
51 Quoted in Isabel M. Stewart, "Report on Nursing Education in Countries Affiliated with the International Council of Nurses," *Canadian Nurse* 27, 1 (1926): 27, 43.
52 Ratcliffe, "Weihwei Hospital," 14-15.
53 For some reason, twelve reportedly finished the year's work: four from Weihui and three each from Huaiqing and Wuan, and one each from Hsiuwu and Daokou. Brown, History of NCM, 66: 9.
54 Ibid., 66: 7. Also spelled "Chow."
55 Lillian [Janet] Brydon, "The Nurses' Association," *Honan Messenger* 8, 4: 4, UCCVUA BV 3420.H6hmps. Brydon reports the attendance of six Chinese nurses from Guangdong "whose passage money to the amount of three hundred dollars had been provided by ..." (the rest of the sentence is indecipherable). Their reliance on external funding might explain why Chinese nurses had not been present at NAC meetings in previous years.
56 Ibid. [emphasis in original].
57 Preston, "Nursing in China," 218.
58 Jamme, "Nursing Education," 666-74.
59 Brown, *History of NCM,* 66: 9.
60 Ibid., 66: 13.
61 Ibid., 66: 14.
62 Preston, *Flowers,* 48.
63 Preston, "Nursing in China," 217.
64 Brown, *History of NCM,* 66: 11-12.
65 I have made liberal use of the term "mishkid," based on a memoir by Marion F. Menzies Hummel entitled *Memoirs of a Mishkid.* However, according to Dr. Mary (Struthers) McKim MacKenzie, also born in China to missionary parents, the term "mishkid" was never used by missionaries or their families. She first heard the term used by American expatriates in India in the 1960s. Dr. Mary McKim MacKenzie, personal communication with author, 28 February 2005.
66 Dr. Robert McClure, interview by Peter Stursberg, transcripts, 14 July 1976, Library and Archives Canada, MG 31 Series D78 vol. 44, file 44-29.
67 UCCVUA Bio File Jean McClure Menzies.
68 Later there would be a residence for missionary kids at the Weihui school, but in the early days mishkids boarded with Weihui families.
69 McClure, interview with Stursberg.

70 Brown, *History of NCM,* 65: 1.
71 Others were Georgina Menzies, Mary Boyd, Dorothy Boyd, Elizabeth Thomson, and Florence MacKenzie.
72 UCCVUA Bio File Coral May Brodie.
73 Munroe Scott, *The China Years of Dr. Bob McClure* (Toronto: Canec, 1977), 81.
74 Ibid., 82-83.
75 Assembly Minutes, 1924, "List of Missionaries – VII – North China," UCCVUA, FA 138. Here Jean is listed at Huaiqing in 1924; her UCCVUA Bio File lists her at Weihui the same year.
76 McClure, interview with Stursberg.
77 Assembly Minutes, 1924. Although only Anyang, Weihui, and Huaqing developed modern hospital facilities, in 1924, there was still some question of constructing a new hospital at Wuan, since one Canadian family had donated money expressly for this purpose.
78 Brown, *History of NCM,* 71: 1.
79 Ranbir Vohra, *China's Path to Modernization: A Historical View from 1800 to the Present* (Upper Saddle River, NJ: Prentice Hall, 2000), 97, 115.
80 See ibid., 124-25.
81 Scott, *McClure,* 115-20.
82 Preston, *Flowers,* 34.
83 Ibid.
84 Brown, *History of NCM,* 73: 14-15.
85 Ratcliffe, "Weihwei Hospital."
86 Brown, *History of NCM,* 73: 15.
87 Ibid., 73: 16.
88 Ibid., 95: 13-14.
89 Elizabeth Thomson Gale, personal diary written 1941-45. Personal collection of Margaret (Gale) Wightman.
90 Brown, *History of NCM,* 108: 4.
91 Ibid., 88: 2; 111: 7. Mr. and Mrs. Alexander were from the Friends Ambulance Unit, and helped with postwar hospital rehabilitation.
92 See Glennis Zilm and Ethel Warbinek, *Legacy: History of Nursing Education at the University of British Columbia, 1919-1994* (Vancouver: University of British Columbia School of Nursing, 1994).
93 Mrs. D.K. Faris, "Pollyanna," *Henan Messenger* 13, 6, UCCVUA 83.058C, box 57, file 16, series 3.
94 Letters from Dorothy Lochead MacKenzie to her mother, 14 January 1948 to 14 February 1949, Norman MacKenzie Papers, UCCVUA 89.155.
95 Louise MacKenzie McLean, telephone interview with author, 8 April 2003.
96 Ibid. See also David McCasland, *Eric Liddell: Pure Gold* (Grand Rapids, MI: Discovery House, 2001).
97 Margaret Gay spent ten years away from Henan, from 1922 to 1931, during which she took nurses' training (from 1923 to 1926).
98 "Evangelistic Committee Report," *Honan Messenger* 8, 3, UCCVUA BV 3420.H6hmps.
99 Dr. W.R. Reeds, "The Crisis in China," *Honan Messenger* 13, 5, UCCVUA BV 3420 H6hmps.
100 M. Shipley, "Dr. Jean Isabel Dow," *Honan Messenger* 13, 4, UCCVUA 83.058C, box 57, file 16, series 3.
101 Preston, *Flowers,* 35.
102 Brown, *History of NCM,* 75: 7.
103 Preston, *Flowers,* 36-37.
104 Ibid.
105 Ibid., 37; Brown, *History of NCM,* 75: 8. Brown recalled four cottages.
106 Alvyn Austin, *Saving China: Canadian Missionaries in the Middle Kingdom, 1888-1959* (Toronto: University of Toronto Press, 1987), 219-20.

Chapter 4: Golden Years, 1928-37

1 Margaret Brown, *History of the Honan (North China) Mission of the United Church of Canada, Originally a Mission of the Presbyterian Church in Canada,* United Church of Canada/Victoria University Archives [hereafter UCCVUA] 77: 1-10.

2 Ibid., 79: 7; Letter to Mrs. Inksater (no sender listed), 28 January 1930, UCCVUA 83.058C, box 56, file 2, series 3. Because Jinan was a relatively expensive treaty port city, Brodie received additional salary allowances.

3 Ernest B. Struthers, *A Doctor Remembers: Days in China and Korea* (publication by author, 1976), 47-49; Brown, *History of NCM*, 80: 1.

4 Struthers, *Doctor Remembers*, 48.

5 Letter from W.B. Djang to "a list of friends," 29 May 1928, UCCVUA83.045C, box 3, file 42.

6 Letter from Djang, 29 May 1928.

7 Arthur Kennedy Sr., telephone conversation with author, 19 March 2004. Brodie related this incident to Kennedy on an occasion when the latter was helping to prepare her will.

8 Brown, *History of NCM*, 81: 2; See also "Report of Conditions on North Honan Field, 1928," UCCVUA 83.045C, box 3, file 42.

9 Brown, *History of NCM*, 81: 3-5.

10 Ibid., 81: 6. It is not clear what "balopticon" refers to.

11 It is difficult to decipher the currency rates of exchange. Between the different types of currency used by the Canadians in China (i.e., Mexican silver, Mexican dollars, Canadian dollars, gold, and Chinese currency), the fluctuating exchange rates, and the fact that the type of currency is often not specified, it is difficult to understand the relative value of the dollar amounts given in the NCM reports. In 1928, the rate was given as Cdn$1 gold = $2.15 Mexican. By 1932, this was Cdn$1 gold = $4.00 Mexican.

12 Letter from W. Harvey Grant to Helen R. Inksater, 23 September 1930, UCCVUA 83.058C, box 56, file 2, series 3.

13 Brown, *History of NCM*, 83: 7-9.

14 Ibid., 83: 12-13.

15 Letter from W. Harvey Grant to Mrs. Anson Spotton, 30 October 1933, UCCVUA 83.058C, box 56, file 5, series 3.

16 Ibid.

17 Letter from W. Harvey Grant to Dr. A.E. Armstrong, 21 July 1933, UCCVUA 83.058C, box 56, file 6, series 3.

18 Brown, *History of NCM*, 88: 1.

19 Ibid., 88: 2. Dr. Pierson Struthers took care of MacKinlay's medical practice in Sarnia while the latter worked in China. Dr. Struthers, born in 1900, was the third Struthers brother to study medicine in order to become a China missionary. His goal was thwarted after an "elective" appendectomy he underwent was followed by a pulmonary embolus. Dr. Mary McKim MacKenzie, personal communication with author, 12 December 2005.

20 Letter to Helen Inksater, 28 January 1930, UCCVUA 83.058C, box 56, file 2, series 3.

21 UCCVUA Bio Files Georgina Menzies and Allegra Doyle.

22 Letter from Mission Secretary (Weihui) to Mrs. Inksater, 15 October 1931, UCCVUA 83.058C, box 56, file 3, series 3. The mission secretary expressed both surprise and delight at the arrival of Margaret Gay, having received "no word of her appointment or sailing," but also asked, "but now, what about some new full time evangelists?"

23 Margaret Gay, "How I got my RN in 1926," unpublished letter. Private collection of Muriel Gay.

24 While the nature of her "nervous breakdown" is not clear, Gay was sent to Shanghai "for health reasons" in 1920 and stayed there, helping the MacGillivrays to distribute Christian literature, until her return to Canada in 1922. UCCVUA Bio File Margaret Gay.

25 Gay, "RN." She tied Elizabeth Smith for the top spot in her graduating class.

26 Muriel Gay, telephone interview with author, 12 December 2003.

27 *Vancouver General Hospital Training School Annual*, Vancouver General Hospital [hereafter VGH] Alumnae Association, 1926, courtesy of Muriel Gay. Copies were also obtained from the VGH Archives, courtesy of Ethel Warbenik and Glennis Zilm of the BC History of Nursing Group.

28 Cora E. Simpson, *A Joy Ride through China for the NAC* (Shanghai: Kwang Hsueh House, 1926), 7-8.

29 Ibid., 9.

30 VGH, 1926 *Annual*.

31 Gay, "RN."

32 Clara Preston, "Unknown Ships that Pass in the Night," memoir written on 3 March 1947. Private collection of Skinner Family.

33 Gay, "RN."

34 Letter from Mission Secretary (Weihui) to Mrs. Inksater, 24 October 1931, UCCVUA 83.058C, box 56, file 3, series 3.

35 Ibid.

36 The mission used coded messages for the public cables. For example, "IPKES, OARYT, AOKAK" when decoded read, "What has been decided about furlough. Miss M.H. Brown. Require a definite answer at once. Telegraph immediately." Hugh MacKenzie, the author of this particular cablegram, sent a follow-up letter apologizing for the abrupt sentence: "The codebook does not seem to lend itself to more polite language." Letter from Hugh MacKenzie to Mrs. Anson Spotton, 6 July 1934, UCCVUA 83.058C, box 56, file 6, series 3.

37 Extract from letter from Dr. Grant to Mrs. Ratcliffe, 24 August 1931, UCCVUA 83.058C, box 56, file 3, series 3. This "Dr. Grant" is most likely Ratcliffe's sister Susan (McCalla) Grant, although it might have been Susan's husband, W. Harvey (a minister), or daughter Mary (a physician). This letter was noted in the North China Mission notes on 24 August 1931, but was originally written on 20 July.

38 Ibid. [emphasis in original].

39 Menzies and Doyle took language study on site, rather than in Beijing. They successfully completed their exams in 1934. Letter from W.H. Grant to Mrs. Spotton, 20 February 1934. Item 36, UCCVUA 83.058C, box 56, file 6, series 3; UCCVUA Bio Files Georgina Menzies and Allegra Doyle.

40 Louise Clara Preston, *Flowers amongst the Debris: A Canadian Nurse in War Torn China* (Brockville, ON: Preston Robb, *n.d.*), 72-73.

41 Ibid., 73.

42 Ibid.

43 This nurse was the "wife of the Chinese doctor" at Anyang. This was probably either Mrs. Li or Mrs. Duan ("Tuan" in Wade-Giles). Since Dr. Li was Director of Rural Medicine, Preston was probably referring to Dr. Duan, who was at the Anyang hospital before 1935. Brown, *History of NCM*, 88: 14.

44 Preston, *Flowers*, 74.

45 Ibid., 73-74.

46 Ibid., 73.

47 Brown, *History of NCM*, 88: 5, 11.

48 Letter from Norman and Violet Knight to "Friends," 23 November 1932.

49 Brown, *History of NCM*, 88: 8.

50 For further study, see Munroe Scott, *The China Years of Dr. Bob McClure* (Toronto: Canec, 1977).

51 Preston, *Flowers*, 74.

52 Brown, *History of NCM*, 89: 1-3.

53 Ibid., 89: 8.

54 Ibid., 89: 6, 9. By 1936, the North China Mission Medical Committee reported 91,000 in-patients at the mission hospitals.

55 Margaret Gay, "Nursing in China," *Canadian Nurse* 29, 8 (1933): 414-16.

56 Preston, *Flowers*, 47.

57 Struthers, *Doctor Remembers*, 79-81.

58 Preston, *Flowers*, 47.

59 Struthers, *Doctor Remembers*, 81. After the Sino-Japanese War, Struthers returned to Qilu to find that 1,200 case histories of kala azar, bound in a series of volumes and including photographs of one hundred patients, had been sold to the Japanese as waste paper. Regrettably, he was therefore unable to prepare a monograph on his work at Qilu. See also Brown, *History of NCM*, 80: 6-10.

60 Gay, "Nursing," 414.

61 Ibid., 415.

62 Brown, *History of NCM*, 89: 6, 9.

63 Ibid., 89: 7-11; Preston, *Flowers*, 73.

64 Isabel Leslie, "A Good Word from China," *Canadian Nurse* 30, 5 (1934): 210.

65 Gay, "Nursing," 415.
66 Leslie, "A Good Word," 210.
67 Letter to W.H. Grant from Executive Mission Secretary, 2 October 1933; Letter from W. Harvey Grant to Mrs. Anson Spotton, 23 November 1934, UCCVUA 83.058C, box 56, file 6, series 3.
68 "Report of the Menzies Memorial Hospital for 1936 (Hwaiking Medical System)," 13 January 1937, UCCVUA 83.045C, box 8, file 119.
69 Ibid., 1; see also Brown, *History of NCM,* 89: 7-11.
70 "Menzies Memorial Hospital 1936," 3.
71 One of the reasons that the "Honan Mission" was renamed the "North China Mission" was that many of the "Honan missionaries" were actually working outside of Henan province – at Tianjin, Jinan, and Shanghai. The Honan Council did not actually approve of the name change until 1939.
72 Coral'Brodie, "Cheeloo University Hospital," UCCVUA 83.045C, box 8, file 119.
73 Preston, *Flowers,* 50. See also p. 73.
74 L. Clara Preston, "In a Chinese Setting," *Canadian Nurse* 32, 10 (1936): 480.
75 L. Clara Preston, "Report of L.C. Preston," 1936, UCCVUA 83.058C, box 58, file 29, series 3; W. Robert Reeds, "Changte [Anyang] Hospital Report 1936," UCCVUA 83.045C, box 8, file 119, series 3.
76 Jeanette Ratcliffe, "Report 1936," UCCVUA 83.058C, box 58, file 31, series 3.
77 Ibid.
78 Ibid.; Jeannette Radcliffe [sic], "War in Weihwei," *Canadian Nurse* 34, 7 (1938): 356-58.
79 Georgina Menzies, "Ward Rounds," 1936/37 [emphasis added], UCCVUA 83.058C, box 58, file 26, series 3.
80 Margaret Gay, "Annual Report," 1936/37, UCCVUA 83.058C, box 58, file 16, series 3.
81 Menzies, "Rounds."
82 Ibid.
83 Preston, "Report of L.C. Preston."
84 Preston, "Chinese Setting."
85 Preston, *Flowers,* 43.
86 Ibid.
87 Commission on the work of the Rural Church, "Health," General Assembly of The Church of Christ in China for the Fourth Quadrennial Assembly, Qingdao, July 1937. Private collection of Skinner Family.
88 Commission on the Rural Church, "Health."
89 "Reply to Questionnaire of Policy Committees of the Foreign Missionary Board and of Woman's Missionary Society to the Men and Women of the Field," 1936, section 9, "Production and Use of Christian Literature," UCCVUA 83.045C, box 8, file 121.
90 Liu Ze's Nurses Association of China 1935 certificate is on public display at the newly opened Huimin Hospital Museum at Weihui (opened October 2006). Liu's grandson Liujing is currently on staff at the First Affiliated Hospital of the Xinxiang Medical University at Weihui.
91 Brown, *History of NCM,* 88: 12-13; 89: 4; Ratcliffe, "Report 1936."
92 Radcliffe [sic], "War in Weihwei," 356. Dr. Bob McClure later commented on the dignity with which Ratcliffe turned over her position to those who had been her subordinates. McClure, interview with Stursberg.
93 Radcliffe [sic], "War in Weihwei," 356.
94 John Watt, "The Development of Nursing in Modern China, 1870-1949," *Nursing History Review* 12 (2004): 67-96.
95 Muriel MacIntosh, "Nursing in China," *Canadian Nurse* 37, 1 (1941): 17-20.

Chapter 5: Scattered Dreams, 1937-40

1 "Heavy Fighting in North China," *North China Herald,* 14 July 1937.
2 Margaret Brown, *History of the Honan (North China) Mission of the United Church of Canada, Originally a Mission of the Presbyterian Church in Canada,* United Church of Canada/Victoria University Archives [hereafter UCCVUA] 94: 4. The Nationalists changed the name of Beijing

(then called Peking) to "Peiping" after Nanjing became the capital of China, in order to denote the lesser status of the former capital.

3 Louise Clara Preston, *Flowers amongst the Debris: A Canadian Nurse in War Torn China* (Brockville, ON: Preston Robb, *n.d.*), 38.

4 Jeannette Radcliffe [sic], "War in Weihwei," *Canadian Nurse* 34, 7 (1938): 356-58 at 356.

5 Brown, *History of NCM*, 94: 8.

6 Jeanette Ratcliffe, "Foreword," 31 December 1939, UCCVUA 83.058C, box 58, file 31, series 3.

7 Radcliffe [sic], "War in Weihwei," 356.

8 Ibid.

9 Brown, *History of NCM*, 95: 1. Canadians were subjects of Great Britain.

10 Gay had planned to take the scenic route home, and together the women circumnavigated the world, travelling through Singapore, Ceylon, India, the Suez Canal, Malta, Marseilles, England, and then across the Atlantic to Canada. Preston, *Flowers*, 77-84; Margaret Gay, "Betty and Alice." Private collection of Muriel Gay.

11 Radcliffe [sic], "War in Weihwei," 357.

12 Jeanette Ratcliffe, "Foreword."

13 Radcliffe [sic], "War in Weihwei," 357-58.

14 Brown, *History of NCM*, 95: 9-10.

15 Ibid., 95: 12.

16 "Extracts of a letter from Bob McClure to Dr. McCulloch," 20 April 1938. Private collection of Skinner Family.

17 Brown, *History of NCM*, 96: 7.

18 Ibid., 95: 18.

19 Quoted in ibid., 95: 18.

20 Mrs. Ethel (Craig) Fleming married Rev. Fleming shortly after they both came to China, in 1921. She died in 1935. "List of Missionaries of the Honan Mission," UCCVUA 83.045C, box 1, file 1; Brown, *History of NCM*, 98: 1.

21 Letter from unnamed author to Mrs. Taylor, 10 March 1938, UCCVUA 83.058C, box 56, file 10, series 3; Brown, *History of NCM*, 94: 8.

22 Letter from Mrs. Taylor, 3 May 1938, UCCVUA 83.058C, box 56, file 10, series 3.

23 Brown, *History of NCM*, 98: 1. It is not clear when five-year terms replaced the original six- or seven-year terms.

24 At the time of the current study, the Toronto General Hospital [hereafter TGH] archives were in temporary storage while TGH alumnae sought a permanent storage site. They were therefore inaccessible to the researcher.

25 "Missionary Nurses at Home and Abroad," *Nurses Alumnae Annual* 1928, Alumnae Association of the Winnipeg General Hospital. These included Susie Kelsey, Mable Naisbitt, Emily Neill, Edith Howland, Irene Harris, and Kathryn Ross. The others worked with the Canadian Methodists in Sichuan and the Anglican mission in Henan.

26 Munroe Scott, *The China Years of Dr. Bob McClure* (Toronto: Canec, 1977), 247.

27 Muriel (Thomson) Valentien, telephone interview with author, 3 November 2003.

28 UCCVUA Bio File Elizabeth (Betty) Thomson Gale.

29 Valentien, interview.

30 Margaret (Gale) Wightman, interview with author, 15 October 2003.

31 Janet L. Brydon, "Opportunities in China," *Canadian Nurse* 33, 6 (1937): 272.

32 Valentien, interview.

33 Preston, *Flowers*, 88; Brown, *History of NCM*, 100: 6. Jen visited Preston and McTavish when they were under house arrest in July and "threw her arms around the doctor's neck and wept."

34 Ratcliffe, "Foreword."

35 Letter from Brydon to "House Folks," 1938.

36 Dr. Mary McKim MacKenzie, personal communication with author, 10 March 2005. Ernest B. Struthers, *A Doctor Remembers: Days in China and Korea* (publication by author, 1976), 78-87. Dr. Struthers joined other Qilu staff at the West China Union University in September 1939.

37   C.H. Corbett quoted in Brown, *History of NCM,* 99: 2.

38   Ibid., 100: 4-19.

39   Preston, *Flowers,* 88-89.

40   Clara Preston, "Unknown Ships that Pass in the Night," memoir written on 3 March 1947. Private collection of Skinner Family.

41   Preston, *Flowers,* 90.

42   Clara Preston, "Difficult Times in China," *Canadian Nurse* 35, 12 (1939): 689-90.

43   Brown, *History of NCM,* 100: 10.

44   Preston, *Flowers,* 92.

45   Margaret Gay, "Events in the Autumn of 1939 in Henan," undated letter. Private collection of Muriel Gay.

46   Dr. Duan was also known as Tuan Chia Pin.

47   Gay, "Autumn of 1939."

48   Confidential letter from G.K. King to Dr. Armstrong, 26 August 1939, UCCVUA 83.058C, box 56, file 11, series 3. Mr. Fleming's illness is not identified.

49   Ratcliffe, "Foreword."

50   "The general situation in the newly established period (1896-1948) of the first affiliated hospital of Xinxiang medical college." Unpublished history of Huimin Hospital provided courtesy of Ren Jijuan and Dr. Zhang Xinzhong of Weihui.

51   Ibid.

52   Brown, *History of NCM,* 100: 16.

53   Letter from H.A. Boyd and H.S. Forbes to the Officer Commanding, Military Police Headquarters, Imperial Japanese Army, Huaiqing, 29 October 1939, UCCVUA 83.045C, box 9, file 156.

54   Letter from Boyd and Forbes, 29 October 1939, 7.

55   Gay, "Autumn of 1939."

56   Letter from G.K. King to Dr. Armstrong, 14 December 1939, UCCVUA 83.058C, box 56, file 11, series 3; Margaret Gay reported meeting Dr. Chang a few months later, in West China. Gay, "Autumn of 1939."

57   Gay, "Autumn of 1939."

58   Jonathan Goforth and Rosalind Goforth, "The Idol Maker," in *Miracle Lives of China* (Grand Rapids, MI: Zondervan, 1931), 32-39.

59   Gay, "Autumn of 1939."

60   Although it is not clear what happened to this particular group during the Sino-Japanese War, Catholic missionaries as a whole were among the last foreigners to leave China after the Communist takeover in 1949. See Creighton Lacy, "The Missionary Exodus from China." *Pacific Affairs* 28, 4 (1955): 301-14.

61   G.K. King, "Events Which Led Missionaries of the United Church of Canada to Withdraw from Weihui, Henan, October 12, 1939," UCCVUA 83.045C, box 9, file 56.

62   Andrew Thomson, dressed in Chinese clothing, managed to remain at the small mission centre of Daokou for another seven months. He left Henan in May for Qilu, where he officiated at the wedding ceremony of his daughter Elizabeth in September 1940. Andrew Thomson, "Report, July-December 1940," UCCVUA 83.045C, box 10, file 163.

63   Gay, "Autumn of 1939."

64   G.K. King, "NCM Who's Who and Where," 14 February 1940, UCCVUA 83.058C, box 56, file 12, series 3.

65   King, "Who's Who"; Letter from Ruth Taylor (Foreign Mission Executive Secretary) to G.K. King, 2 April 1940, UCCVUA 83.05C, box 56, file 12, series 3. Thomson was originally asked to refund three-quarters of her outfit allowance to the Women's Missionary Society ($288.80), but this request was later waived.

66   Letter from Helen MacDougall to Mrs. Ruth Taylor, 14 December 1939, UCCVUA 83.058C, box 56, file 11, series 3.

67   Ibid.

68   Letter from G.K. King to Dr. Armstrong, 14 December 1939.

69   King, "Who's Who"; Brown, *History of NCM,* 102: 7.

70   Gay, "Autumn of 1939."

71 Margaret Gay, untitled, undated letter. Private collection of Muriel Gay.
72 Gay, "Autumn of 1939."
73 Ibid.
74 Letter from Helen MacDougall to Mrs. Taylor, 11 September 1939, UCCVUA 83.058C, box 56, file 11, series 3.
75 Letter from MacDougall to Taylor, 14 December 1939.
76 Letter from King to Armstrong, 14 December 1939.
77 King, "Who's Who."
78 Letter from G.K. King to Mrs. Taylor, 29 January 1940. Dr. E.B. Struthers considered Coral's stroke to be a complication of malaria. Dr. Mary McKim MacKenzie, personal communication with author, 12 December 2005.
79 Letter from G.K. King to Mrs. Taylor, 22 April 1941.
80 Dave Shepperd, Arthur Kennedy, and Frances Kennedy Fraser, telephone and email correspondence with author, April 2004 and January 2005.
81 "Our Outgoing Missionaries," *Presbyterian Witness*, 6 December 1926: 5-6, UCCVUA, BX 9001.A40, PS Microfilm #25.
82 Brown, *History of NCM*, 102: 11.
83 Letter from Coral Brodie to Mrs. Taylor, 10 September 1940; Letter from Coral Brodie, no recipient, no date, UCCVUA 83.058C, box 58 file 8, series 3. Mexican silver was a common currency circulated in China at that time.
84 Dr. Mary McKim MacKenzie, correspondence with author.
85 Letter from R. Taylor to G.K. King, 30 April 1940, UCCVUA 83.058C box 56, file 12, series 3.
86 Arthur Kennedy Sr., telephone interview with author, 19 March 2004.
87 Letter Brodie to Taylor, 10 September 1940.
88 Letter to G.K. King from Mrs. Taylor, 30 September 1940, UCCVUA 83.058C, box 56, file 12, series 3.
89 UCCVUA Bio File Coral May Brodie.
90 Letter from G.K. King to Mrs. H. Taylor, 18 April 1940, UCCVUA 83.058C, box 56, file 12, series 3.
91 Letter from King to Taylor, 23 April 1940.
92 Ibid.
93 Ibid.
94 Letter from G.K. King to Mrs. Taylor, 30 May 1940.
95 Rev. Doug Brydon, interview with S. Dunlop, 31 May 1993. Brydon (Eramosa Township) Family File. Wellington County Museum and Archives, A1994.129.
96 Brown, *History of NCM*, 104: 7; Letter from Mrs. Taylor to G.K. King, 26 October 1940, UCCVUA 83.058C, box 56, file 13, series 3.
97 Brown, *History of NCM*, 104: 11, 102: 12; Letter from Taylor to King, 26 October 1940.
98 Letter from Mrs. Taylor to G.K. King, 29 November 1940, UCCVUA 83.058C, box 56, file 13, series 3.
99 David McCasland, *Eric Liddell: Pure Gold* (Grand Rapids, MI: Discovery House, 2001).
100 "Biographical Sketch of Norman Hall MacKenzie." Norman MacKenzie Papers, UCCVUA 86.004C, FA 316. While Norman MacKenzie reportedly worked in China from 1943 to 1950, it is not clear whether his wife Dorothy remained with him during this entire time. Correspondence between Dorothy and her mother indicates that she was in Sichuan between January 1948 and February 1949, however. UCCVUA 89.155C, FA 316.

Chapter 6: War Years, 1941-45

1 Dr. C.T. Tuan (Duan Mei-Qing), "Weihwei General Hospital Report of 1940," UCCVUA 83.045C, box 10, file 163.
2 Stephen Endicott, *James G. Endicott: Rebel out of China* (Toronto: University of Toronto Press, 1980), 106-9. Dr. James Endicott, moderator of the United Church of Canada and father of West China missionary James G. Endicott, led a small delegation to China in 1927, where he met with exiled West China missionaries in Shanghai, and North China missionaries in Tianjin. At the height of Chinese Nationalism, the Chinese Church sought to transfer administrative power from the missionaries to local Chinese Church representatives.

According to Stephen Endicott, the Canadian "colonizers" frustrated any Chinese attempts to achieve genuine independence over the next two decades by insisting on keeping their basic structures, and the "colonized" were doomed to perpetuate their own dependence by accepting the colonizers' gifts for development within their structures.

3 "North China (Honan) 1940," UCCVUA 83.045C, box 10, file 163.
4 Margaret Gay, "Dr. Oliver." Private collections of Muriel Gay and Irene Pooley; Letter from Clara Preston to "Friends," 16 April 1947. Private collection of Skinner Family.
5 "Church of England Missionary Home," undated newspaper clipping in Alumnae Scrap Book, Winnipeg General Hospital/Health Sciences Centre Archives [hereafter WGH/HSCA]. Apparently there was another Canadian on the premises in October 1941. Miss F. May Watts was the mission treasurer. It is not clear when or how Miss Watts left. Letter from G.K. King to Mrs. Taylor, 3 October 1941, UCCVUA 83.058C, box 56, file 14, series 3.
6 Letter from King to Taylor, 3 October 1941.
7 Louise Clara Preston, *Flowers amongst the Debris: A Canadian Nurse in War Torn China*. Letters compiled by Dr. Preston Robb (Brockville, ON: Preston Robb, *n.d.*), 101.
8 Letter from Rev. G.A. Andrew to the UCC General Secretary, 19 May 1940, UCCVUA 83.058C, box 56, file 12, series 3.
9 Letter from Mary Boyd to Mrs. Taylor, 16 January 1941, UCCVUA 83.058C, box 58, file 6, series 3.
10 "The Girls," in WGH yearbook *Blue and White*, Class of 1923: 22, WGH/HSCA.
11 Letter from G.K. King to Mrs. Taylor, 30 May 1940, UCCVUA 83.058C, box 56, file 12, series 3.
12 Letter from G.K. King to Dr. I. McTavish, 29 October 1940, UCCVUA 83.058C, box 56, file 13, series 3.
13 Stanley was a former librarian at the College of Chinese Studies at Qilu.
14 Letter from Mrs. Taylor to G.K. King, 18 November 1940; Letter from G.K. King to Mrs. Taylor, 28 November 1940, UCCVUA 83.058C, box 56, file 13, series 3.
15 Susie Kelsey, "In a Concentration Camp in China," *Canadian Nurse* 40, 7 (1944): 480-82.
16 Preston, *Flowers*, 101.
17 Letter [from Adelaide Harrison?] to Mrs. Taylor, 6 April 1940, UCCVUA 83.058C, box 61, file 12, series 5.
18 Yuet-wah Cheung, *Missionary Medicine in China: A Study of Two Canadian Protestant Missions in China before 1937* (Lanhan, MD: University Press of America, 1988).
19 "West China Nurses," UCCVUA 83.058C, box 61, file 15, series 5; Janet Beaton, "Canadian Missionary Nurses in China: 1894-1951," paper presented at the 14th Annual Conference of the Canadian Association for the History of Nursing (9 June 2001).
20 Beaton, "Missionary Nurses."
21 Preston, *Flowers*, 101 [emphasis added].
22 Janet Sutherland MacDonald MacHattie, "MacHattie Chronicles." Memoir of life in China, 1913 to 1949. Private collection of Dr. Mary McKim MacKenzie.
23 Preston, *Flowers*, 102.
24 Letter from Clara Preston to Mrs. Taylor, no date, received in Toronto 21 April 1941, UCCVUA 83.058C, box 58, file 29, series 3.
25 Preston, *Flowers*.
26 Letter from Preston to Taylor, 21 April 1941.
27 Clara Preston, "Nursing in Chungking," *Canadian Nurse* 39, 2 (1943): 144-45.
28 Preston, *Flowers*, 103.
29 Ibid., 104.
30 "Missionary Tells about War in China," *Whig-Standard*, 16 March [no year]. Private collection of Skinner Family.
31 Margaret Gay, "Events of 1939 and 1940." Private collections of Muriel Gay and Irene Pooley.
32 Preston, *Flowers*, 104.
33 Ibid.
34 Ibid.
35 Gay, "1939 and 1940."

36 Ibid.
37 Ibid.
38 Letter from Winifred Harris to Mrs. Taylor, 25 November 1940, UCCVUA 83.058C, box 61, file 12, series 5.
39 Gay, "1939 and 1940."
40 Letter from Harrison to Knight, 18 February 1941, UCCVUA 83.058C, box 62, file 20, series 5. Cited in Beaton, "Missionary Nurses."
41 Letter from G.K. King to Mrs. H. Taylor, 18 April 1940, UCCVUA 83.058C, box 56, file 12, series 3.
42 Letter from Adelaide Harrison to Mrs. Taylor, 7 May 1941, UCCVUA 83.058C, box 61, file 13, series 5.
43 Brown, *History of NCM,* 104: 6.
44 Letter from Mrs. Taylor to G.K. King, 30 September 1941, UCCVUA 83.058C, box 56, file 14, series 3.
45 Letter from Adelaide Harrison to Mrs. Taylor, 7 May 1941, UCCVUA 83.058C, box 61, file 13, series 5.
46 Gay, "1939 and 1940."
47 Letter from Mrs. Ruth Taylor to G.K. King, 5 May 1941.
48 Gay, "1939 and 1940."
49 Letter from Taylor to King, 5 May 1941; Letter from G.K. King to Margaret Gay, 19 May 1941, UCCVUA 83.058C, box 56, file 14, series 3.
50 Irene Pooley, telephone conversation with author, 20 January 2003. Irene Pooley, who is Gay's niece, recalls Margaret's return home in 1941. It was a "dreadful trip" from Hong Kong to San Francisco, and on to Vancouver. At that time, Margaret's brother and father were living in Vancouver.
51 Letter from Mrs. Taylor to G.K. King, 30 September 1941, UCCVUA 83.058C, box 56, file 14, series 3.
52 Margaret Gay was later nurse to the Lieutenant Governor's wife in Victoria. Muriel Gay, telephone conversation with author, 12 December 2003.
53 UCCVUA Bio File Margaret R. Gay.
54 Dorothy Boyd sailed for China in March 1939 with Mary Boyd and Elizabeth Thomson.
55 Letter from Mrs. Taylor to G.K. King, 14 May 1941, UCCVUA 83.058C, box 56, file 14, series 3.
56 Brydon, interview with S. Dunlop.
57 Letter from Mrs. Taylor to G.K. King, 25 June 1941, UCCVUA 83.058C, box 56, file 14, series 3.
58 Letter from G.K. King to Mrs. Taylor, 18 June 1941, UCCVUA 83.058C, box 56, file 14, series 3.
59 Letter from Mrs. Taylor to G.K. King, 30 September 1941, UCCVUA 83.058C, box 56, file 14, series 3.
60 Letter from Taylor to King, 30 September 1941.
61 Letter from G.K. King to Mrs. Taylor, 3 December 1941, UCCVUA 83.058C, box 56, file 14, series 3.
62 Grace W. Gibberd, "A Call to Service," *Canadian Nurse* 36 (1940): 210.
63 Letter from G.K. King to Mrs. Taylor, 3 October 1941, UCCVUA 83.058C, box 56, file 14, series 3.
64 Letter from G.K. King to Mrs. Taylor, 3 December 1941.
65 Letter from G.K. King to Mrs. Taylor, 2 November 1943, UCCVUA 83.058C, box 56, file 16, series 3.
66 See "Had to Guard Writing While in Hands of Japs, Missionary Says Here," *Globe and Mail,* 28 August 1942; Letter from King to Taylor, 3 December 1942, UCCVUA 83.058C, box 56, files 14-16, series 3; Letter from King to Taylor, 2 November 1942, UCCVUA 83.058C, box 56, files 14-16, series 3. Also Brown, *History of NCM,* 108: 4.
67 Margaret Gale was cared for by a Chinese *amah* named C.T. Sao. Journal of Betty Gale, 1941-45. Private collection of Margaret Gale Wightman.
68 Brown, *History of NCM,* 104: 11.

69 Ibid., 104: 8.
70 Ibid., 104: 9.
71 "Guard Writing," *Globe and Mail.*
72 Peter Nelson, correspondence with author, 10 April 2004.
73 Brown, *History of NCM,* 106-8.
74 G.K. King, 19 May 1942, cited in ibid., 104: 10.
75 Brown, *History of NCM,* 104: 10. It is not clear what a "bloodless knife" is.
76 Letter from Mary Boyd Stanley to Mrs. Taylor, 14 July 1941, UCCVUA 83.058C, box 58, file 6, series 3.
77 According to E.B. Struthers' daughter, Mary McKim MacKenzie, her uncle Dr. R.G. Struthers spent time at the Weixian camp before being repatriated on the first *Gripsholm.* Mary McKim MacKenzie, personal communication with author, 12 December 2005.
78 Sonya Grypma, *Canadian Nurses Interned under the Japanese in China, 1941-1945* (a study in progress).
79 Betty Gale journal.
80 "Guard Writing," *Globe and Mail.*
81 Betty Gale journal. Dr. Gale smuggled supplies when a Japanese commandant was ill and requested care, allowing Dr. Gale temporary access to the hospital.
82 Brown, *History of NCM,* 104: 9; Mrs. Faris returned to Canada with her children in December 1940.
83 Copy of letter from Isabelle McTavish to Clara Preston, 2 February 1942, UCCVUA 83.058C, box 58, file 29, series 3.
84 Copy of letter from Clara Preston to Annie Waddell, 26 February 1942, UCCVUA 83.058C, box 58, file 29, series 3.
85 This is probably the London Missionary Society hospital. Letter from Clara Preston to Florence MacKenzie Liddell, 1 March 1942, with copy of letter from Eric A. Liddell to Clara Preston, 23 January 1942, UCCVUA 83.058C, box 58, file 29, series 3.
86 Letter from Eric A. Liddell to Clara Preston, 1 February 1942, UCCVUA 83.058C, box 58, file 29, series 3.
87 Betty Gale journal.
88 Ibid.
89 Ibid.
90 One American doctor also stayed: Arabella Gault.
91 Margaret Wightman, interview with author, 15 October 2005.
92 Godfrey Gale, introduction to Betty Gale journal, added years later.
93 Betty Gale journal. Barb Putnam, personal communication with author, 6 October 2003.
94 Barb Putnam, personal communication with author.
95 Brown, *History of NCM,* 104: 9; Murray McCheyne Thomson, *A Daring Confidence: The Life and Times of Andrew Thomson in China, 1906-1942* (Ottawa: publication by author, 1922), 174.
96 "Guard Writing," *Globe and Mail;* Brown, *History of NCM,* 104: 10.
97 Betty Gale journal.
98 David McCasland, *Eric Liddell: Pure Gold* (Grand Rapids, MI: Discovery House, 2001).
99 United Church North China Mission missionary Winifred Warren was interned at Loonghwa Camp at Shanghai, where she remained until the end of the war.
100 Muriel Valentien, Margaret Gale Wightman, interviews with author, June 2005. According to Muriel and Margaret, Mary Boyd Stanley was also an internee. A letter handwritten by G.K. King to Mrs. Taylor on 2 November 1943 (while aboard the *MS Gripsholm*) corroborates this, suggesting that Betty Thomson Gale, Georgina Menzies Lewis, and Mary Boyd Stanley remained in China, interned with their families. UCCVUA 83.058C, box 56, file 16, series 3.
101 McCasland, *Pure Gold.*
102 Kelsey, "Concentration Camp."
103 McCasland, *Pure Gold.*
104 Kelsey, "Concentration Camp."
105 Ibid.
106 Letter from King to Taylor, 2 November 1943.

107 Letter from L.A. Dixon to Mrs. Taylor, 2 February 1945; Letter from Foreign Mission Executive Secretary to Canon L.A. Dixon, 9 February 1945, UCCVUA 83.058C, box 56, file 17, series 3.
108 "China – 1948," Alumnae Scrap Book, WGH/HSCA.
109 Peters spent twenty-one years at St. Paul's before the war. "Interesting People," *Canadian Nurse* 42, 12 (1946): 1038.
110 "China – 1948."
111 Letter from King to Taylor, 2 November 1943.
112 McCasland, *Pure Gold.*
113 Cited in ibid., 280.
114 Clara Preston heard about Eric Liddell's death in November 1945, after Winifred Warren had safely returned from Weixian. Letter from Clara Preston to Mrs. Taylor, 1 November 1945, UCCVIA 83.058C, box 56, file 13, series 3.
115 Circular letter from Clara Preston to Friends, 24 July 1942, UCCVUA 83.058C, box 58, file 29, series 3.
116 Letter from Preston to Taylor, 21 April 1941; Preston, "Chungking."
117 Preston, "Chungking."
118 Letter from Preston to Taylor, 21 April 1941 [emphasis in original].
119 Ibid.
120 Letter from Preston to Friends, 24 July 1942. Unfortunately, Preston does not provide his name.
121 Ibid.
122 Ibid.
123 Ibid. There is a discrepancy regarding the numbers of graduate nurses: Preston gives the number of graduate nurses on staff when she arrived as twenty-one, twenty, and twenty-four in various sources.
124 Preston, *Flowers,* 106.
125 Letter from Preston to Friends, 24 July 1942.
126 It is not clear who these patients were – they may have been British refugees from Hong Kong, for example. It is unlikely that they would have been American, Canadian, or British soldiers, since the armies had their own hospital bases.
127 Letter from Preston to Friends, 24 July 1942.
128 Letter from Adelaide Harrison to Mrs. Taylor, 18 January 1943, UCCVUA 83.058C, box 61, file 15, series 5.
129 Preston, *Flowers;* "Interesting People," *Canadian Nurse* 42, 10 (1946): 886.
130 Preston, *Flowers.*
131 Letter from Adelaide Harrison to Miss Buck, 6 April 1943, UCCVUA 83.058C, box 63, file 1, series 5.
132 Preston, *Flowers.* Also convalescing with Preston was missionary Lottie McRae.
133 Letter from Clara Preston, 1 November 1945, UCCVUA 83.058C, box 56, file 13, series 3.
134 UCCVUA Bio File L. Clara Preston.

Chapter 7: The Last Days, 1946-47

1 Oswald Chambers, *My Utmost for His Highest: Special Updated Edition* (Grand Rapids, MI: Discovery House, 1995). Chambers was a YMCA chaplain in Egypt when he died, in 1917. This devotional book comprises a collection of sermons compiled by his wife and originally published in 1935. It was a favourite among some Canadian missionaries to China.
2 The others were Mr. King, Mr. Boyd, Mr. Knight, Mr. Copland, Dr. E.B. Struthers, and the newly appointed Ervin Newcombe, as well as Miss Stewart, Miss Sommerville, Miss MacDougall, Miss Durrant, and the recently appointed Anne Davison. Margaret Brown, *History of the Honan (North China) Mission of the United Church of Canada, Originally a Mission of the Presbyterian Church in Canada,* United Church of Canada/Victoria University Archives [hereafter UCCVUA] 109: 3.
3 Ibid., 109: 4.
4 Munroe Scott, *The China Years of Dr. Bob McClure* (Toronto: Canec, 1977), 383. The ditty was penned by Doug Crawford, a "dour Scots hospital mechanic of Tengchung" (at 383).

5 Scott, *McClure*, 291-307.
6 Brown, *History of NCM*, 109: 6-7.
7 Ibid., 110: 3. Brown notes that Ch.$2 million was the rough equivalent of Cdn$2 thousand, representing an exchange rate of approximately 1000:1.
8 Ibid., 109: 7.
9 The two mission boards were the Overseas Mission Board and the Woman's Missionary Society.
10 Brown, *History of NCM*, 109: 8 ($5000 from each board).
11 Scott, *McClure*, 382-94.
12 Janet Sutherland MacDonald MacHattie, "MacHattie Chronicles." Memoir of life in China, 1913 to 1949. Private collection of Dr. Mary McKim MacKenzie.
13 Brown, *History of NCM*, 110: 3.
14 For example, in a letter written in February 1947, Preston stated: "the money has gone up from 6,000 to one American dollar to 20,000 and we are just getting $3,300." One month later she wrote: "We hear that money is to [be] exchanged at $1,200 which will make a big difference to us as we were only getting $3,300 for our money before." Since the rate of exchange between Chinese and Canadian dollars was reportedly 1000:1 the previous year, a rate of 20,000:1 represents a twenty-fold increase in just one year (assuming the Canadian dollar and the American dollar were relatively equal). Apparently this was only the beginning. In a family memoir entitled *Wild Swans*, Jung Chang wrote that by the end of 1947, inflation in China had risen to the unimaginable figure of 100,000 percent – and it was to go to 2,870,000 percent by the end of 1948 (p. 106). Letter from Clara Preston to Janie, 18 February 1947, and letter from Clara Preston to Janie, 16 March 1947. Private collection of Skinner Family; Jung Chung, *Wild Swans: Three Daughters of China* (New York: Random House, 1991).
15 "Memo of Conference with Dr. Stewart Allen, Weihwei, Honan, April 30-May 1, 1946," UCCVUA 93.045C, box 12, file 200.
16 Or, 5 million Chinese "dollars" to completely renovate the hospital and completely re-equip the wards and operating theatre. "Hwei Min [Huimin] Hospital Report for July 1946," UCCVUA 83.045C, box 12, file 200.
17 Brown, *History of NCM*, 110: 3. This was for Ch.$2 million. It is not clear whether this was a separate grant, or if Brown was referring to the original "International Relief Committee" grant.
18 "Hwei Min Hospital Statement of Receipts and Payments for the Month of July 1946," UCCVUA 83.045C, box 12, file 200.
19 "Sundry items" adding up to $2.87 accounted for the difference ($2,289,585 = $1,505,312.13 + $784,270 + $2.87).
20 Brown, *History of NCM*, 110: 9.
21 Ibid., 111: 10.
22 Scott, *McClure*, 393.
23 "North China (Honan) 1940," UCCVUA 83.045C, box 10, file 163.
24 Dr. C.T. Tuan (Duan Mei Qing), "Weihwei General Hospital Report of 1940," UCCVUA 83.045C, box 10, file 163.
25 Brown, *History of NCM*, 111: 5.
26 G.K. King, mission correspondence, 21 February 1946. Cited in ibid.
27 Letter from Jean Sommerville to Miss Courtice [WMS?], 22 July 1946, Weihui, UCCVUA 83.058C, box 56, file 18, series 3.
28 Scott, *McClure*, 392.
29 "Hwei Min Hospital Report for July 1946," UCCVUA 83.045C, box 12, file 200. According to Brown, Alexander was a "United Church Toronto man." Brown, *History of NCM*, 111: 7.
30 "Hwei Min Hospital Report for July 1946."
31 Scott, *McClure*, 392.
32 Walter Alexander, "Hwei Min Hospital Monthly Report for July 1946."
33 The Friends Ambulance Unit [hereafter FAU] paid out Ch.$1,570,527.00 in severance salaries.
34 "Hwei Min Hospital Report for July 1946."

35 Ibid.
36 "The general situation in the newly established period (1896-1948) of the first affiliated hospital of Xinxiang medical college," unpublished historical record housed at Xinxiang, courtesy of Ren Jijuan and Dr. Zhang Xinzhong, current president of the First Affiliated Hospital of Xinxiang Medical University (December 2006) [emphasis added].
37 Brown, *History of NCM*, 111: 6.
38 "Hwei Min Hospital Report for July 1946."
39 "Hwei Min Hospital FAU Report for August 1946," UCCVUA 83.045C, box 12, file 200.
40 Ch.$60,000 at Weihui compared to Ch.$150,000 by United Nations Relief and Rehabilitation Administration. Brown, *History of NCM*, 111: 9.
41 Ibid., 111: 10. Nurse Margaret Hossie was due to arrive in December but did not actually arrive until the following March.
42 Ibid., 111: 9. Li had anticipated the arrival of ten or more new students. It is not clear how many actually came.
43 Clara Preston identifies Miss Li as the first graduate of the Anyang program (1936), whereas Margaret Brown identifies her as one the first Weihui graduates. Louise Clara Preston, *Flowers amongst the Debris: A Canadian Nurse in War Torn China* (Brockville, ON: Preston Robb, n.d.), 135-36; Brown, *History of NCM*, 111: 9.
44 That is, two photos on display at the newly opened Huimin Hospital Museum in Weihui show graduating classes in 1941 and 1942. Personal visit to Huimin Hospital Museum, Weihui, October 2006. Translations graciously provided by the museum curator and Ren Jijuan of the First Affiliated Hospital of the Xinxiang Medical University in Weihui.
45 Brown, *History of NCM*, 111: 13; Lillian Taylor, interview with author, 18 December 2003. Lillian Taylor was a missionary nurse at the West China Mission. She travelled to China in 1947 with Margaret Hossie and Helen Turner.
46 "Hospital Report for December 1946," UCCVUA 83.045C, box 12, file 200.
47 Brown, *History of NCM*, 110: 1.
48 Ibid., 110: 4.
49 "Memo of Conference with Dr. Stewart Allen, Weihwei, Honan, April 30-May 1, 1946," UCCVUA 93.045C, box 12, file 200. Originally called the Canadian Relief Committee, it was also referred to as the China War Emergency Relief Committee.
50 Scott, *McClure*, 397; "Dr. Stewart Allen," UCCVUA 93.045C, box 12, file 200.
51 According to the account of events recorded by North China Mission missionary Margaret Brown (then in Shanghai), based on her own notes of a visit with Dr. Allen when he passed through Shanghai after his tour, and a confidential report written by Rev. G.K. King on 1 June 1947. Brown, *History of NCM*, 110: 12.
52 "Conditions in North Honan," Report to United Church Foreign Mission Board, 1 July 1947, UCCVUA 83.045C, box 12, file 213; Brown, *History of NCM*, 110: 12.
53 In addition to visiting Huaiqing and other Canadian hospitals, Allen had also visited some of the Peace Hospitals in Communist areas, based on an invitation by Madame Sun Yat-sen. The Peace Hospitals were memorials to Dr. Norman Bethune, a classmate of Dr. Allen's who died in China in 1938 after working with Mao Zedong's Eighth Route Army.
54 Dr. Robert McClure, interview by Peter Stursberg, transcripts, 14 July 1976. Library and Archives Canada, MG 31 series D78 vol. 44, file 44-29. According to McClure, Allen was put under house arrest for nearly two years. McClure was also blacklisted, but escaped arrest; Brown, *History of NCM*, 110: 10.
55 Brown, *History of NCM*, 110: 4.
56 Ibid., 110: 7. The record does not clarify who or which organization sponsored the Canadian Aid to China Committee. It may have been a subsidiary of the Canadian Red Cross. It is also not clear why Weihui did not secure similar funds (if, indeed, it did not).
57 Park Woodrow, "Kwang Sheng Hospital August 1946 Report, Changte, Honan," UCCVUA 83.045C, box 12, file 200.
58 Brown, *History of NCM*, 111: 12.
59 Ibid., 111: 13. The FAU was a wartime organization whose purpose had been served. The North China Mission was reluctant to see the FAU go. The home board offered the FAU personnel a three-year contract under the United Church if they would stay on at Henan,

but this was declined, for vague reasons. In response to a cable from Mrs. Taylor, G.K. King cabled back that the FAU was unavailable. Apparently, it had another hospital project to complete – most likely in Zhengzhou.

60 Letter from Jean Somerville to Mrs. Taylor, 12 October 1946, UCCVUA 83.058C, box 56, file 18, series 3.
61 Brown, *History of NCM,* 112: 1.
62 Preston, *Flowers,* 131; Letter from Clara Preston to Louise and Leslie, 11 February [year unclear; probably 1947]. Private collection of Skinner Family.
63 Letter from Clara Preston to Friends, 13 December 1946. Private collection of Skinner Family.
64 Ibid.
65 L. Clara Preston, "Nursing in China," *Canadian Nurse* 43, 3 (1947): 217-18.
66 Ibid.
67 Ibid.
68 Letter from Preston to Friends, 13 December 1946; Preston, *Flowers,* 135.
69 Brown, *History of NCM,* 111: 10.
70 Letter from Clara Preston to Jeff and Grace, 12 January 1947. Private collection of Skinner Family.
71 Letter from Jean Sommerville to Mrs. Taylor, 12 October 1946. UCCVUA 83.058C, box 56, file 18, series 3.
72 Letter from Preston to Louise and Leslie, 11 February [year unclear; probably 1947]. Private collection of Skinner Family.
73 Letter from Clara Preston to Elizabeth, 12 January 1947. Private collection of Skinner Family.
74 Letter from Clara Preston to Janie, 18 February 1947. Private collection of Skinner Family.
75 Probably the same Li Shuying who was in charge of the Weihui nursing school. Letter from Clara Preston to Louise and Leslie, 11 February [year unclear; probably 1947]. Private collection of Skinner Family.
76 Letter from Preston to Jeff and Grace, 12 January 1947.
77 Ibid.
78 Lillian Taylor, telephone interview with author, 18 December 2003; Peter Nelson, correspondence with author, 10 April 2004. According to Lillian Taylor, who was Helen Turner's classmate at the University of Toronto and fellow missionary nurse in China, Turner did travel to Henan – although Turner's United Church of Canada Bio File notes that she was first appointed to West China and then transferred to Henan in September 1947. While Turner did not go to West China, the "transfer to Henan" might have been to Qilu, rather than to Weihui or Anyang, since Qilu is where she met her husband, pharmacist Peter Nelson.
79 Letter from Clara Preston to Janie, 16 March 1947. Private collection of Skinner Family.
80 "Information re: Fighting in North Henan." Private collection of Skinner Family.
81 Letter from Clara Preston to Friends, 16 April 1947. Private collection of Skinner Family.
82 G.K. King, "Honan Mission, United Church of Canada Withdrawal of Staff from Weihui; Confidential Report – not for publication," 25 April 1947, UCCVUA 83.045C, box 12, file 213. King criticized Hsiung for deserting his hospital staff and the seventy patients under his care.
83 Ibid.
84 "Confidential – Not for Publication: Communist Attack on Weihwei, 11 April 1947," UCCVUA 83.045C, box 12, file 213. The author is not identified, but was likely G.K. King.
85 Ibid.
86 Brown, *History of NCM,* 113: 2; "Confidential," 11 April 1947.
87 United Church of Canada 1948 Yearbook, cited by Brown, *History of NCM,* 113: 3.
88 Letter from Preston to Friends, 16 April 1947.
89 United Church of Canada 1948 Yearbook, cited by Brown, *History of NCM,* 113: 3.
90 "Confidential," 11 April 1947.
91 Letter from Preston to Friends, 16 April 1947.
92 "Information re: Fighting in North Honan." Private collection of Skinner Family.
93 Letter from Preston to Friends, 16 April 1947.

94 "Confidential," 11 April 1947.
95 Ibid.
96 Letter from Preston to Friends, 16 April 1947.
97 Because the "First Affiliated Hospital of the Xinxiang Medical University" is in Weihui, the names Xinxiang and Weihui are sometimes used to refer to the same place. Xinxiang is actually south of Weihui, however. According to Preston, Xinxiang was a three-hour drive away from Weihui at that time. Today, the same drive takes approximately thirty minutes by freeway.
98 King, "Withdrawal from Weihwei."
99 Ibid.
100 Mr. King, Pastor Chi, and Miss Sykes returned to Weihui sometime in late April or early May to make further plans to evacuate the hospital. The mission compound had been turned into a military stronghold. Nationalist troops were deeply entrenched in the compound. Some buildings and walls had been torn down, brick fortresses had been constructed in front of each gate, and "loop holes" had been punched in the walls. Mr. Chi – now the hospital superintendent – consulted with the remaining hospital staff in Weihui city. They unanimously decided to move hospital personnel and as much equipment and medicines as they could to Zhengzhou. Letter from Rev. D.K. Faris to Mr. Mitchell, 25 April 1947 (excerpt), UCCVUA 83.045C, box 12, file 213.
101 Letter from Faris to Mitchell, 25 April 1947.
102 Ibid. [emphasis in original].
103 King, "Withdrawal from Weihwei."
104 Miss Tsoa was to be the first young woman from Henan to study in Canada. It is not clear whether she made it to Canada.
105 "Confidential Statement of Changte Station Evacuation," 13 May 1947, UCCVUA 83.058C, box 56, file 19, series 3.
106 Ibid. Surplus funds of Ch.$1,126,900 were passed over to the Henan Church Synod Chairman, and an additional "CN half million" from relief funds was given to assist poor patients. According to Louise McLean, her brother Norman MacKenzie returned to China in 1987. The same elders who were left in charge of the church when he had departed welcomed him. They were now in their eighties. Louise McLean, interview with author, 8 April 2003.
107 G.K. King, 12 July 1947, cited in Brown, *History of NCM,* 114: 2.
108 Letter from Clara Preston to Friends, 8 June 1947, Kaifeng; Letter from Clara Preston to Irene, 12 June 1947, from Kaifeng; Letter from Clara Preston to Friends, 22 August 1947, from Chi Kung Shan. Private collection of Skinner Family.
109 Others present were Mr. and Mrs. Boyd, Mr. N. Knight, Miss Stewart, Miss Sommerville, Mrs. N. MacKenzie, Mr. and Mrs. Newcombe, and Mr. and Mrs. King. G.K. King, "Memorandum of Meeting with Dr. Stewart Allen," UCCVUA 83.058C, box 56, file 19, series 3.
110 "Confidential Extracts from letter of May 15 from Rev G.K. King to Dr. Armstrong," UCCVUA 83.058C, box 56, file 19, series 3 [emphasis added].
111 Rev. G.K. King, Honan correspondence 8 April 1948, cited in Brown, *History of NCM,* 113: 13.
112 Brown, *History of NCM,* 113: 12.
113 Doris Weller, interview with author, June 2002. According to China Inland Mission missionary nurse Doris Weller – who was in China from 1947 to 1952 – returning missionaries kept silent because of the fear of repercussions to Chinese colleagues and friends. In later years, when it was deemed safe to talk about China, people were no longer interested.
114 "Conditions in North Honan," report to United Church Foreign Mission Board, 1 July 1947, UCCVUA 83.045C, box 12, file 213 [emphasis in original]. This is the extremely sensitive report noted by Margaret Brown.
115 Nym Wales [Helen Foster Snow], *Inside Red China* (New York: Doubleday, Doran and Company, 1939); Edgar Snow, *Red Star over China* (London: V. Gollancz, 1937); Edgar Snow, *Random Notes on China, 1936-1945,* 4th ed. (Cambridge, MA: Harvard University Press, 1974); Agnes Smedley, *Battle Hymn of China* (New York: A.A. Knopf, 1943).
116 "Conditions in North Honan."

117 Honan Mission Council Minutes 18 August 1947, cited in Brown, *History of NCM*, 114: 4.
118 Peter Nelson, correspondence with author. Helen (Turner) Nelson and her husband Peter Nelson were among the last missionaries to leave Jinan, in June 1951.
119 Preston, *Flowers*, 140.
120 Brown, *History of NCM*, 115: 1.
121 Ibid., 115: 2.
122 H.A. Boyd and G.K. King, "Report on Visit to Weihwei, to Board of Overseas Missions and Woman's Missionary Society, United Church of Canada," 10-12 September 1947, UCCVUA 83.045C, box 12, file 213.
123 Nelson, correspondence with author.
124 Jesse H. Arnup, "China and Missions," circulated to various missionaries in February and March 1951, UCCVUA 83.058C, box 56, file 19, series 3.
125 Arnup, "China and Missions."

Conclusion: Creating a Cloistered Space

1 Among the first missionary nurses to Canada were Catholic sisters belonging to the religious order Hospitalières de la Miséricorde de Jésus in Dieppe. These nurses moved from France to staff the Hôtel-Dieu at Quebec in 1639. Two centuries later, the Sisters of Charity of Montreal (Grey Nuns) were sent from Quebec to distant regions of Canada and the United States. The Grey Nuns' establishment of a mission in St. Boniface, Manitoba, in the 1840s marked the beginning of Canadian missionary nursing activities. Pauline Paul, "The Contribution of the Grey Nuns to the Development of Nursing in Canada: Historiographic Issues," *Canadian Bulletin of Medical History* 11, 1 (1994): 207-17; Sioban Nelson, *Say Little, Do Much: Nursing, Nuns, and Hospitals in the Nineteenth Century* (Philadelphia: University of Pennsylvania Press, 2001).
2 To use Rosemary Gagan's term. Rosemary Gagan, *A Sensitive Independence: Canadian Methodist Women Missionaries in Canada and the Orient, 1881-1925* (Montreal and Kingston: McGill-Queen's University Press, 1992).
3 Jan Wong, *Jan Wong's China: Reports from a Not-So-Foreign Correspondent* (Toronto: Doubleday, 1999).
4 Kathryn McPherson, *Bedside Matters: The Transformation of Canadian Nursing, 1900-1990* (Toronto: Oxford University Press, 1996).
5 Alvyn Austin, *Saving China: Canadian Missionaries in the Middle Kingdom, 1888-1959* (Toronto: University of Toronto Press, 1987).
6 Nelson, *Say Little, Do Much*.
7 Vancouver General Hospital, *1926 Annual:* 17.

Epilogue: Return to Henan, 2003

1 United Church of Canada/Victoria University Archives [hereafter UCCVUA] Bio File Clara Preston.
2 UCCVUA Bio File Janet Brydon.
3 UCCVUA Bio File Margaret Gay.
4 Peter Nelson, telephone conversation with author, 10 April 2004.
5 Ibid. Mr. Nelson had corresponded with Margaret (Hossie) Hart as recently as 2003. I sent a letter of inquiry to a home address he provided, but it was returned by the post office.

Bibliography

Archive Collections

Alumnae Association of the Winnipeg General Hospital
Winnipeg General Hospital Yearbook *Blue and White,* class of 1923
Alumnae Scrapbook
Alumnae Journal, 1914-42

Emory University Robert W. Woodruff Library
Philip Jaffe Fonds

Glenbow Museum
Craigie, Lillian Bertha. Women's Missionary Society Minutes and Reports, 1926-49
Central United Church. Women's Missionary Society Papers, 1933-49
Photo Collection
Red Cross Files, 1941-45

Grey Sisters of Immaculate Conception of Pembroke Archives
Grey Sisters in China 1929-52

Library and Archives Canada
Peter Stursberg Fonds (interview of Dr. Robert McClure)
Ted Allen Fonds

United Church of Canada/Victoria University Archives
Presbyterian Church in Canada Woman's Missionary Society, 1876-1927
    Accession no. 79.205 C.
    Fonds 127, FA 226.
    Boxes 12, 19.
United Church of Canada Board of Overseas Missions
    Accession no. 83.045C.
    Fonds 502, FA 186.
    Series 4/3: China (Henan) Mission 1912-52.
    Boxes 1-3, 5-10, 12, 13, 16-18, 40, 41.
United Church of Canada Board of World Missions
    Accession no. 83.041.
    Fonds 503, FA 321.
    Series 5: China 1888-1969.
    Box 3.

United Church of Canada Woman's Missionary Society
  Accession no. 83.058C.
  Fonds 505, FA 90.
  Series 3: China (Henan) 1925-55.
  Boxes 56-58.
United Church of Canada Woman's Missionary Society
  Accession no. 83.058C.
  Fonds 505, FA 90.
  Series 5: China (West) 1935-52.
  Boxes 61-63.
United Church of Canada Biographical Files (Bio Files)
United Church of Canada Photograph Collection (Graphic Files)
United Church of Canada Microfilm Collection
  BX 9001. A40 PS Microfilm 25.
Honan Messenger. Accession no. BV 3420.H6hmps
Brown, Margaret (n.d.). *History of the Honan (North China) Mission of the United Church of Canada, Originally a Mission of the Presbyterian Church in Canada.* Volumes 1-4 (1,500 pages)
Norman MacKenzie Papers. Accession no. 89.155C FA 316

University of Alberta JW Scott Library
Balme, Harold, and Milton T. Shauffer, "An Enquiry into the Scientific Efficiency of Mission Hospitals in China," 1-39. Presented at the *Annual Conference of the China Medical Missionary Association,* 21-27 February 1920, Beijing (microfiche).

Wellington County Museum and Archives
Brydon (Eramosa township) Family File.
"Going to Mission Field," *Fergus News Record,* 19 July 1917

Vancouver General Hospital Alumnae Association
Vancouver General Hospital Training School Annual, 1926

Xinxiang Medical College (First Affiliated Hospital), Weihui, Henan, People's Republic of China
"The general situation in the newly established period (1896-1948) of the first affiliated hospital of Xinxiang medical college." Unpublished history of Huimin Hospital.

Other Sources
Austin, Alvyn. *Saving China: Canadian Missionaries in the Middle Kingdom, 1888-1959.* Toronto: University of Toronto Press, 1987.
Austin, Alvyn, and Jamie S. Scott. *Canadian Missionaries, Indigenous Peoples: Representing Religion at Home and Abroad.* Toronto: University of Toronto Press, 2005.
Austin, B.F. *Woman, Her Character, Culture and Calling: A Full Discussion of Woman's Work in the Home, the School, the Church, and the Social Circle.* Brantford, ON: Book and Bible House, 1890.
Bates, Christina, Dianne Dodd, and Nicole Rousseau, eds. *On All Frontiers: Four Centuries of Canadian Nursing.* Ottawa: University of Ottawa Press, 2005.
Beach, Harlan P. "Statistics of Missions in China for 1904." In *Dawn on the Hills of T'ang: Missions in China.* New York: Student Volunteer Movement for Foreign Missions, 1905 [1898].
Beaton, Janet. "Canadian Missionary Nurses in China: 1894-1951." Paper presented at the fourteenth Annual Conference of the *Canadian Association for the History of Nursing,* 9 June 2001.
Beaton, Janet, and Marion McKay. "Carolyn Wellwood: Pragmatic Visionary." *Canadian Journal of Nursing Leadership* 12, 4 (1999): 30-33.
Beaton, Kenneth. *Serving with the Sons of Shuh: Fifty Fateful Years in West China, 1891-1941.* Toronto: United Church of Canada, 1941.

Beets, Henry. "China as a Mission Field." In *Toiling and Trusting: Fifty Years of Christian Reformed Missions*. Grand Rapids, MI: Grand Rapids Printing, 1940.

Bloor Street United Church, Toronto. http://www.bloorstreetunited.org/history_hist.htm.

Bond, Geo J. *Our Share in China and What We Are Doing with It*. Toronto: Missionary Society of the Methodist Church, 1909.

Boschma, Geertje. *Faculty of Nursing on the Move: Nursing at the University of Calgary, 1969-2004*. Calgary: University of Calgary Press, 2005.

Brouwer, Ruth Compton. *Modern Women Modernizing Men: The Changing Missions of Three Professional Women in Asia and Africa, 1902-69*. Vancouver: UBC Press, 2002.

–. *New Women for God: Canadian Presbyterian Women and India Missions, 1876-1914*. Toronto: University of Toronto Press, 1990.

Brydon, Janet L. "Opportunities in China." *Canadian Nurse* 33, 6 (1937): 272.

Burrows, Bob. *Healing in the Wilderness: A History of United Church Mission Hospitals*. Madeira Park, BC: Harbour Publishing, 2004.

Cameron, Elspeth. "Truth in Biography." In R.B. Fleming, ed., *Boswell's Children: The Art of the Biographer*, 27-32. Toronto: Dundurn Press, 1992.

Caughey, Ellen. *Heroes of the Faith: Eric Liddell – Olympian and Missionary*. Uhrichsville, OH: Barbour, 2000.

Chambers, Oswald. *My Utmost for His Highest: Special Updated Edition*. Grand Rapids, MI: Discovery House, 1995 [1930].

Chapleau, J.A. "The Chinaman in China." In *Report on the Royal Commission on Chinese Immigration: Report and Evidence*. Ottawa: Royal Commission, 1885.

Chen, Kaiyi. "Missionaries and the Early Development of Nursing in China." *Nursing History Review* 4 (1996): 129-49.

–. "Quality versus Quantity: The Rockefeller Foundation and Nurses Training in China." *Journal of American East Asian Relations* 5, 1 (1996): 77-104.

Cheung, Yuet-wah. *Missionary Medicine in China: A Study of Two Canadian Protestant Missions in China before 1937*. Lanhan, MD: University Press of America, 1988.

Chong, Thelma. "Adventure in Canton." *Canadian Nurse* 39, 2 (1943): 131-34.

Christensen, Erleen J. *In War and Famine: Missionaries in China's Honan Province in the 1940s*. Montreal and Kingston: McGill-Queen's University Press, 2005.

Chung, Jung. *Wild Swans: Three Daughters of China*. New York: Random House, 1991.

Chung-tung, Liu. "From San Gu Liu Po to 'Caring Scholar': The Chinese Nurse in Perspective." *International Journal of Nursing Studies* 28, 4 (1991): 315-24.

Copland, Marnie. *Moon Cakes and Maple Sugar*. Burlington, ON: G.R. Welch, 1980.

Cruikshank, Kathleen. "Education History and the Art of Biography." *American Journal of Education* 107, 3 (1999): 231-39.

D'Antonio, Patricia. "Revisiting and Rethinking the Rewriting of Nursing History." *Bulletin of the History of Medicine* 73, 2 (1999): 268-90.

Doona, Mary Ellen. "Linda Richards and Nursing in Japan." *Nursing History Review* 4 (1996): 99-128.

Dossey, Barbara Montgomery. *Florence Nightingale: Mystic, Visionary, Healer*. Springhouse, PA: Springhouse, 2000.

Endicott, Stephen. *James G. Endicott: Rebel out of China*. Toronto: University of Toronto Press, 1980.

Ewen, Jean. *China Nurse, 1932-1939: A Young Canadian Witnesses History*. Toronto: McClelland and Stewart, 1981.

Fitzpatrick, M. Louise. "Historical Research: The Method." In Patricia Munhall and Carolyn Oiler Boyd, eds., *Nursing Research: A Qualitative Perspective*, 2nd ed. New York: National League for Nursing Press, 1993.

Frazer Smith, James. *Life's Waking Part: Being the Autobiography of Reverend James Frazer Smith*. Toronto: Thomas Nelson and Sons, 1937.

Gagan, Rosemary. "The Methodist Background of Canadian WMS Missionaries." In Neil Semple, ed., *Canadian Methodist Historical Society Papers* 7 (1992): 115-36.

–. *A Sensitive Independence: Canadian Methodist Women Missionaries in Canada and the Orient, 1881-1925*. Montreal and Kingston: McGill-Queen's University Press, 1992.

Gay, Margaret. "Nursing in China." *Canadian Nurse* 29, 8 (1933): 414-16.

Genevieve, Sister M. "From China." *Canadian Nurse* 21, 12 (1935): 542.

Gewurtz, Margo S. "'Their Names May Not Shine': Narrating Chinese Christian Converts." In Alvyn Austin and Jamie S. Scott, eds., *Canadian Missionaries, Indigenous Peoples: Representing Religion at Home and Abroad,* 134-51. Toronto: University of Toronto Press, 2005.

Gibberd, Grace W. "A Call to Service." *Canadian Nurse* 36 (1940): 210.

Goforth, Jonathan, and Rosalind Goforth. *Miracle Lives of China.* Grand Rapids: Zondervan, 1931.

Goforth, Rosalind. *Goforth of China.* Toronto: McClelland and Stewart, 1937.

–. *Jonathan Goforth.* Minneapolis: Bethany, 1986; originally published as *Goforth of China.* Toronto: McClelland and Stewart, 1937.

Gordon, Sydney, and Ted Allen. *The Scalpel, the Sword: The Story of Doctor Norman Bethune,* 3rd ed. New York: Monthly Review Press, 1973.

Grypma, Sonya. "Critical Issues in the Use of the Biographic Method." *Nursing History Review* 13 (2005): 171-87.

–. "James R. Menzies: Healing and Preaching in Early 20th Century China." *Canadian Medical Association Journal* 170, 1 (2004): 84-85.

–. "Neither Angels of Mercy nor Foreign Devils: Re-Visioning Canadian Missionary Nurses in China, 1935-1947." *Nursing History Review* 12 (2004): 97-119.

Hampton, Isabel A. "The Aims of the Johns Hopkins Hospital Training School for Nurses." *Johns Hopkins Hospital Bulletin* 1, December 1889: 2. University of British Columbia Woodward Library Archives, Ethel Johns Collection.

Harrold, Trudy A. *On Highest Mission Sent: The Story of Health Care in Lamont, Alberta.* Lamont, AB: Lamont Health Care Centre, 1999.

Hawks Pott, F.L. *The Emergency in China.* New York: Missionary Education Movement of the United States and Canada, 1913.

"Heavy Fighting in North China." *North China Herald* (14 July 1937): 52-53.

Hermanson, Hilda. "Letters from Near and Far." *Canadian Nurse* 42, 11 (1946): 978-79.

Huizenga, Lee S. *Unclean! Unclean.* Grand Rapids, MI: Smitter Book, 1927.

Hummel, Marion F. Menzies. *Memoirs of a Mishkid.* Compiled and edited by Elizabeth Mittler. Editor, 2001.

Hunter, Jane. *The Gospel of Gentility: American Women Missionaries in Turn of the Century China.* Westford, MA: Yale University Press, 1984.

Hurd, Henry. "The Relation of the Training School for Nurses to the Johns Hopkins Hospital." *Johns Hopkins Hospital Bulletin* 1, December 1889: 7. University of British Columbia Woodward Library Archives, Ethel Johns Collection.

"Interesting People." *Canadian Nurse* 42, 10 (1946): 886.

"Interesting People." *Canadian Nurse* 42, 12 (1946): 1038-39.

James, Peter D. "Book Review: Saving China – The History behind the Mission." *Quill and Quire* 52 (1986): 47.

Jamme, Anna C. "Nursing Education in China." *American Journal of Nursing* 23 (1923): 666-74.

Johns, Martin W. *Bamboo Sprouts and Maple Buds.* Publication by author, 1992.

Kelm, Mary Ellen. *Colonizing Bodies: Aboriginal Health and Healing in British Columbia, 1900-1950.* Vancouver: UBC Press, 1999.

Kelsey, Susie. "In a Concentration Camp in China." *Canadian Nurse* 40, 7 (1944): 480-82.

Kipling, Rudyard. "The White Man's Burden, 1899." www.fordham.edu/halsall/mod/Kipling.html.

Lacy, Creighton. "The Missionary Exodus from China." *Pacific Affairs* 28, 4 (1955): 301-14.

Leslie, Isabel. "A Good Word from China." *Canadian Nurse* 30, 5 (1934): 210.

Lum, Noreen. "From a Chinese School." *Canadian Nurse* 31, 12 (1935): 542.

Lynaugh, Joan. "The Importance of Writing History as Narrative: Bringing Nurses and Nursing Events Alive." *Nursing History Review* 8 (2000): 1.

MacIntosh, Muriel. "Nursing in China." *Canadian Nurse* 37, 1 (1941): 17-20.

MacKay, George Leslie. *From Far Formosa: The Island, Its People and Missions,* 4th ed. New York: Fleming H. Revell Company, 1895.

MacKenzie, Murdoch. *Twenty-Five Years in Honan.* Toronto: Presbyterian Board of Foreign Missions, 1913.

MacLeod, A. Donald. "Our Mission to China." *Channels* 17, 1 (2001). http://renewal fellowship.presbyterian.ca/channels/r01171-2.html.

Maggs, Christopher. "A History of Nursing: A History of Caring?" *Journal of Advanced Nursing* 23, 3 (1996): 630-35.

Martin, Ged. "Foreword: Biography and History." In R.B. Fleming, ed., *Boswell's Children: The Art of the Biographer,* ix-xv. Toronto: Dundurn Press, 1992.

Maxwell, Grant. "Partners in Mission: The Grey Sisters." In *Assignment in Chekiang: Seventy-one Canadians in China, 1902-1954,* 126-42. Scarborough, ON: Scarboro Foreign Mission Society, 1984.

McCasland, David. *Eric Liddell: Pure Gold.* Grand Rapids, MI: Discovery House, 2001.

McDonald, Lynn, ed. *Florence Nightingale: An Introduction to Her Life and Family. Volume One of the Collected Works of Florence Nightingale.* Waterloo, ON: Wilfred Laurier University Press, 2001.

McPherson, Kathryn. *Bedside Matters: The Transformation of Canadian Nursing, 1900-1990.* Toronto: Oxford University Press, 1996.

Morley, Patricia. "Book Review: Holier than Mao." *Books in Canada* 16 (1987): 29.

Murray, Constance. "A Repatriate from Hong Kong." *Canadian Nurse* 42, 3 (1946): 242-43.

Negodaeff-Tomsik, Margaret. *Honour Due: The Story of Dr. Leonora Howard King.* Ottawa: Canadian Medical Association, 1999.

Nelson, Sioban. "The Fork in the Road: Nursing History vs. the History of Nursing?" *Nursing History Review* 10 (2002): 175-88.

–. *Say Little, Do Much: Nursing, Nuns, and Hospitals in the Nineteenth Century.* Philadelphia: University of Pennsylvania Press, 2001.

New, Peter Kong-Ming, and Yuet-wah Cheung. "Early Years of Medical Missionary Work in the Canadian Presbyterian Mission in North Honan, China, 1887-1900." *Asian Profile* 12, 5 (1984): 409-23.

Nurse Who Knows. "The Mission Field." *Canadian Nurse* 31, 4 (1935): 163.

Paul, Pauline. "The Contribution of the Grey Nuns to the Development of Nursing in Canada: Historiographic Issues." *Canadian Bulletin of Medical History* 11, 1 (1994): 207-17.

–. "The History of the Relationship between Nursing and Faith Traditions." In Margaret B. Clark and Joanne K. Olson, eds., *Nursing within a Faith Community,* 59-75. Thousand Oaks, CA: Sage, 2000.

Preston, L. Clara. "Difficult Times in China." *Canadian Nurse* 35, 12 (1939): 689-90.

–. *Flowers amongst the Debris: A Canadian Nurse in War Torn China.* Letters compiled by Dr. Preston Robb. Brockville, ON: Preston Robb, *n.d.*

–. "In a Chinese Setting." *Canadian Nurse* 32, 10 (1936): 480.

–. "Nursing in China." *Canadian Nurse* 43, 3 (1947): 217-18.

–. "Nursing in Chungking." *Canadian Nurse* 39, 2 (1943): 144-46.

Radcliffe [Ratcliffe], Jeannette. "War in Weihwei." *Canadian Nurse* 34, 7 (1938): 356-58.

"Refugees at Hankow: Good Work by Gallant Doctors and Nurses." *North China Herald* (26 January 1932): 119.

Reimer, Helena. "Letters from Near and Far." *Canadian Nurse* 42, 10 (1946): 899-900.

Rutherdale, Myra. *Women and the White Man's God: Gender and Race in the Canadian Mission Field.* Vancouver: UBC Press, 2002.

Scott, Munroe. *The China Years of Dr. Bob McClure.* Toronto: Canec, 1977.

Simpson, Cora E. *A Joy Ride through China for the NAC.* Shanghai: Kwang Hsueh House, 1926.

Sinclair, Donna. *Crossing Worlds: The Story of the Woman's Missionary Society of the United Church of Canada.* Toronto: United Church Publishing House, 1992.

Smedley, Agnes. *Battle Hymn of China.* New York: A.A. Knopf, 1943.

Smith, William Edward. *A Canadian Doctor in West China: Forty Years under Three Flags.* Toronto: Ryerson Press, 1939.

Snow, Edward. *Random Notes on China, 1936-1945,* 4th ed. Cambridge, MA: Harvard University Press, 1974.

–. *Red Star over China*. London: V. Gollancz, 1937.

Stewart, Isabel M. "Report on Nursing Education in Countries Affiliated with the International Council of Nurses." *Canadian Nurse* 27, 1 (1926): 43.

The Story of Eric Liddell: An Olympic Gold Medalist's Lifelong Race to Spread the Gospel. A Day of Discovery Television Production. Produced by RBC Ministries. 90 min. videocassette.

Struthers, Ernest B. *A Doctor Remembers: Days in China and Korea*. Publication by author, 1976.

Stursberg, Peter. *The Golden Hope: Christians in China*. Toronto: United Church Publishing House, 1987.

–. *No Foreign Bones in China: Memoirs of Imperialism and Its Ending*. Edmonton: University of Alberta Press, 2002.

Thomson, Murray McCheyne. *A Daring Confidence: The Life and Times of Andrew Thomson in China, 1906-1942*. Ottawa: Publication by author, 1992.

T'ien Kuo (Kingdom of Heaven): Jubilee of North Honan Mission souvenir booklet. North China Mission, 1938.

Taylor, Mrs. Howard. *Guinness of Honan*. Toronto: China Inland Mission, 1930.

"Toronto General Hospital Alumnae Association." *Canadian Nurse* 27, 10 (1926): 547.

Vohra, Ranbir. *China's Path to Modernization: A Historical View from 1800 to the Present*. Upper Saddle River, NJ: Prentice Hall, 2000.

Wales, Nym [Helen Foster Snow]. *Inside Red China*. New York: Doubleday, Doran and Company, 1939.

Wang, Yong. "Mission Unfinished: The United Church of Canada and China, 1925-1970." PhD diss., University of Waterloo, 1999.

Watt, John. "The Development of Nursing in Modern China, 1870-1949." *Nursing History Review* 12 (2004): 67-96.

"Woman's Search for Nirvana." *North China Herald* (12 January 1932): 45.

Wong, Jan. *Jan Wong's China: Reports from a Not-So-Foreign Correspondent*. Toronto: Doubleday, 1999.

Wood, Frances. *No Dogs and Not Many Chinese: Treaty Port Life in China, 1843-1943*. London: John Murray, 1998.

Zilm, Glennis, and Ethel Warbinek. *Legacy: History of Nursing Education at the University of British Columbia, 1919-1994*. Vancouver, BC: UBC School of Nursing, 1994.

Index